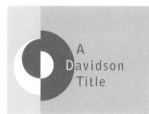

A Davidson Title

Davidson's
100 Clinical Cases

Commissioning Editor: Laurence Hunter
Development Editor: Carole McMurray
Project Manager: Frances Affleck
Designer: Stewart Larking
Illustration Manager: Bruce Hogarth

Davidson's

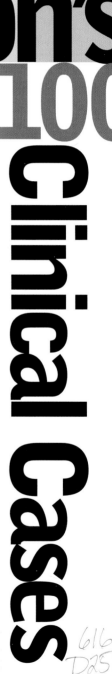

The Editors

Mark W.J. Strachan
BSc(Hons) MD FRCP Edin
Consultant in Diabetes and
Endocrinology Metabolic Unit,
Western General Hospital, Edinburgh;
Part-time Reader, University of Edinburgh, UK

Surendra K. Sharma
MD PhD
Chief, Division of Pulmonary,
Critical Care and Sleep Medicine;
Professor and Head, Department of Medicine,
All India Institute of Medical Sciences,
New Delhi, India

John A. A. Hunter
OBE BA MD FRCP Edin
Professor Emeritus of Dermatology,
University of Edinburgh, UK

CHURCHILL
LIVINGSTONE

ELSEVIER

Ed

CHURCHILL
LIVINGSTONE
ELSEVIER

© 2012 Elsevier Ltd. All rights reserved.

First edition 2008
Second edition 2012

ISBN 9780702044595
International ISBN 9780702044601

British Library Cataloguing in Publication Data
A catalogue record for this book is available from the British Library

Library of Congress Cataloging in Publication Data
A catalog record for this book is available from the Library of Congress

ELSEVIER your source for books,
journals and multimedia
in the health sciences

www.elsevierhealth.com

Working together to grow
libraries in developing countries

www.elsevier.com | www.bookaid.org | www.sabre.org

ELSEVIER   BOOK AID International   Sabre Foundation
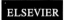

The publisher's policy is to use paper manufactured from sustainable forests

Printed in China

Contents

Preface

We were pleased with the favourable reception given to the first edition of our book and proud when it won first prize in the Medicine category of the 2009 British Medical Association Medical Book Competition. Indeed we feel that there has been more than enough support for our conviction that this text should be a welcome addition to the member of the Davidson family of books. Our original aim; that it should encourage and help students to approach clinical problems in a way similar to the contributors, all chosen because of their considerable clinical and teaching experience, appears to have been met. But medicine does not stand still and there have been ample advances and changes in the diagnosis and management of diseases to warrant an extensive update and revision of the text. We have dropped a few cases and added a number more to complete the century; hence the not so subtle change in the title of this edition!

Davidson's Principles and Practice of Medicine, now in its 21st edition, has stood the test of time because it continues to reflect Sir Stanley Davidson's determination to produce a book that was readable without ambiguity, uncertainty or wordiness. It attempts to provide an international perspective on disease, to reflect the huge success that the book has had in many parts of the world, especially in the Indian subcontinent.

In *Davidson's 100 Clinical Cases* we re-emphasise the value of interpreting available clinical and investigative information in a logical way before considering a definitive diagnosis. We asked our contributors to take the reader through their cases in a personal way and to avoid regurgitating long and all-embracing lists from larger textbooks! Our selection of cases continues to be based on the 'Presenting Problems' of the (21st) edition of *Davidson's Principles and Practice of Medicine* and illnesses that reflect an international outlook. We have remained strict in our editing in an effort to ensure uniformity in the layout and style of the many contributions.

We hope that our readers will continue to find that knowledge imparted in this manner is not only easy and painless to digest but useful in practice. Welcome to the second edition of *Davidson's 100 Clinical Cases*!

M.W.J.S., S.K.S. and J.A.A.H.
Edinburgh and New Delhi, 2011

Acknowledgements

Case 64: M Y Rao acknowledges assistance from Robert Rao MBBS, Nuffield Department of Surgery, John Radcliffe Hospital, University of Oxford, UK. Case 96: TAzhar acknowledges assistance from Suhaimi Ayoub MD MMED, International Islamic University of Malaysia, Pahang Darul Makmur, Malaysia. Case 4: Fig 24.1 supplied courtesy of A McMillan and G Scott, 2000, Colour Guide to Sexually Transmitted Infections, Churchill Livingstone, Edinburgh. Case 43: T Das acknowledges assistance from Dr Satinath Mukherjee, Department of Endocrinology, IPGMER, Kolkata, India. Case 50: The figure was reproduced with the kind permission of Dr Ian Penman, Department of Gastroenterology, Western General Hospital, Edinburgh. Case 60: The figure was provided courtesy of Dr Philip P. C. Ip, Department of Pathology and Clinical Biochemistry, Queen Mary Hospital, Hong Kong. Case 85: The figure was kindly provided by Prosessor Selim Benbadis, University of South Florida. Case 87: The figure was provided courtesy of Dr A. J. Farrell, SINAPSE Collaboration, University of Edinburgh. Case 98: The figure was reproduced from Hunter J H, Savin J A and Dahl M V, *Clinical Dermatology*, 3rd edn, 2002. With permission from Blackwell Publishing.

Contributors

T. Ahmed
MBBS FCPS (Bangladesh) FCPS (Pak) MRCP
FRCP Edin Glas Ire FACP FCCP
Professor of Medicine, Gono
Biswalidyalaya, Savar, Dhaka and
Ex Dean of Postgraduate Medicine,
Dhaka University, Bangladesh

I. D.-R. Arnott
BSc MBChB MD FRCP Edin
Consultant Gastroenterologist and
Honorary Senior Lecturer,
Gastrointestinal Unit, Western
General Hospital, Edinburgh, UK

T. Azhar
MBBS FRCP FFRRCS(I)
Deputy Rector, Academic and Planning,
International Islamic University Malaysia,
Kuala Lumper, Malaysia

S. Banerjee
MD
Professor, Department of Medicine,
Vivekananda Institute of Medical
Sciences, Kolkata, India

H. S. Bawaskar
Bawaskar Hospital and Research
Centre, Raigad Maharastra, India

P. Bloomfield
MD FRCP FACC
Consultant Cardiologist, Department of
Cardiology, Royal Infirmary of
Edinburgh, UK

J. D. Bos
MD PhD FRCP
Professor and Chairman, Department
of Dermatology, Academic Medical
Centre, University of Amsterdam,
the Netherlands

J. Collier
MD FRCP
Consultant Hepatologist, Department of
Gastroenterology and Hepatology, John
Radcliffe Hospital, Oxford, UK

J. I. O. Craig
MB ChB MD FRCP Edin FRCPath
Consultant Haematologist, Department
of Haematology, Addenbrooke's
Hospital, Cambridge, UK

A. Cumming
MBChB MD FRCP
Professor of Medical Education and
Consultant in Renal Medicine,
Department of Renal Medicine,
University of Edinburgh, UK

M. K. Daga
MD MNAMS
Director Professor of Medicine and Head
of Medical ITU, Department of Medicine,
Maulana Azad Medical College,
New Delhi, India

D. Dalus
MD FRCP PhD
Professor & Head, Department of
Internal Medicine, Medical College
Hospital, Trivandrum, India

T. Das
MD
Professor and Head, Department of
Medicine, Institute of Post-graduate
Medical Education and Research and
S.S.K.M. Hospital, Kolkata, India

R. J. Davenport
DM FRCP Edin BMBS BMedSci
Consultant Neurologist and Honorary
Senior Lecturer, Department of Clinical
Neurosciences, Western General
Hospital, Edinburgh, UK

J. M. Davies
MA MD FRCP FRCPath
Consultant Haematologist and Honorary
Senior Lecturer, Department of
Haematology, Western General Hospital,
Edinburgh, UK

A. Faiz
MBBS FCPS FRCP PhD
Professor of Medicine and Head, Department of Medicine, Dhaka Medical College, Dhaka, Bangladesh

M. J. Field
MD BS BSc FRACP
Professor of Medicine and Associate Dean, Northern Clinical School, Royal North Shore Hospital, University of Sydney, Australia

A. G. Frauman
Professor of Clinical Pharmacology & Therapeutics, Clinical Pharmacology & Therapeutics Unit, Department of Medicine, University of Melbourne, Austin, Victoria, Health Australia

B. M. Frier
BSc(Hons) MD FRCP Edin FRCPG
Consultant Diabetologist and Honorary Professor of Diabetes, Department of Diabetes, Royal Infirmary of Edinburgh, UK

J. Goddard
MBChB PhD FRCP Edin
Consultant Nephrologist, Department of Renal Medicine, Royal Infirmary of Edinburgh, UK

C. F. Gordon
MB ChB FRCP Edin
Consultant in Acute Medicine, Western General Hospital, Edinburgh, UK

H. A. Goubran
MBBCh MSc MD FACP FRCP Edin
Hematologist, Saskatoon Cancer Centre, Saskatchewan, Canada Emeritus Adviser to the Royal College of Physicians of Edinburgh, UK

N. Grubb
MD MRCP
Consultant in Cardiac Electrophysiology, Cardiovascular Research Unit, Royal Infirmary of Edinburgh and Honorary Senior Lecturer, University of Edinburgh, UK

S. B. Gunatilake
MD FRCP FCCP Hon FRACP
Consultant Neurologist, Professor of Medicine, Faculty of Medical Sciences, University of Sri Jayewardenepura, Sri Lanka

R. Gupta
MD DNB FRCP
Head, Rheumatology & Clinical Immunology, Medanta, The Medicaty, Gurgaon, India

P. Henriksen
Consultant Cardiologist
Western General Hospital
Crewe Toll Road
Edinburgh

A. T. Hill
MBChB MD FRCP Edin
Consultant in Respiratory Medicine and Honorary Senior Lecturer, Department of Respiratory Medicine, Royal Infirmary of Edinburgh, UK

J. A. A. Hunter
OBE BA MD FRCP Edin
Professor Emeritus of Dermatology, University of Edinburgh, UK

J. A. Innes
BSc MB ChB PhD FRCP Edin
Consultant Physician and Honorary Reader in Respiratory Medicine, Respiratory Unit, Western General Hospital, Edinburgh, UK

S. M. W. Jafri
MD FRCP Lond FRCPE FRCPG FACP FACG
Alicharan Professor and associate Dean Consultant Gastroenterologist, Chair, Department of Continuing Professional Education, Aga Khan University, Karachi, Pakistan

S. Jain
Professor of Internal Medicine, Postgraduate Institute of Medical Education and Research, Chandigarh, India

A. L. Jones
BSc MD FRCP Edin FRCP Fi Biol
Dean, Graduate School of Medicine, University of Wollongong, NSW; Conjoint Professor of Medicine and Clinical Toxicology, University of Newcastle, Australia

A. L. Kakrani
MD
Professor and Head, Department of Medicine, BJ Medical College and Sassoon General Hospitals, Pune (Maharashtra), India

L. Karalliedde
MBBS DA FRCA
Chairman, South Asian Clinical Research, South Asian Clinical Toxicology Research Collaboration (SACTRC), Sri Lanka;
Visiting Senior Lecturer, King's College Medical School, London

S. Keir
MD FRCP Edin
Consultant, Stroke Medicine, Western General Hospital, Edinburgh, UK

D. Kemmett
FRCP Edin
Department of Dermatology, Royal Infirmary of Edinburgh, Edinburgh, UK

J. A. Ker
MBChB MMed MD
Deputy Dean, Faculty of Health Sciences, Department of Internal Medicine, University of Pretoria, South Africa

M. King
FRCP MB ChB BSc
Consultant Acute Medicine, Western General Hospital, Edinburgh

B. Kumar
MD FRCP Edin FRCP Lord
Former Professor and Head, Department of Dermatology, Venereology and Leprology, Postgraduate Institute of Medical Education and Research, Chandigarh, India

P. Kuna
Division of Internal Medicine, Asthma and Allergy, Department of Medicine, Barlicki University Hospital, Lodz, Poland

C. L. Lai
MBBS(Hon) MD FRCP FRCP Edin FRCPG FRACP
Simon KY Lee Professor in Gastroenterology, Professor of Medicine and Hepatology, University Department of Medicine, Queen Mary Hospital, Hong Kong

C. A. Ludlam
MBChB BSc PhD FRCP FRCPath
Professor of Haematology and Coagulation Medicine, University of Edinburgh; Director, Haemophilia and Thrombosis Centre, Royal Infirmary of Edinburgh, UK

C. J. Lueck
PhD FRCP FRACP
Head, Department of Neurology, The Canberra Hospital, and Associate Professor, Australian National University Medical School, Canberra, Australia

G. Maartens
Division of Clinical Pharmacology, Department of Medicine, University of Cape Town, Cape Town, South Africa

A. M. J. MacLullich
BSc MBChB MRCP(UK) PhD
Professor of Geriatric Medicine, Edinburgh Delirium Research Group, Geriatric Medicine Unit, University of Edinburgh, UK

A. McMillan
MD FRCP FRCP Edin
Former Consultant Physician in Genitourinary Medicine, Department of Genitourinary Medicine, Royal Infirmary of Edinburgh, UK

E. R. McRorie
MB ChB FRCP
Consultant Rheumatologist and Honorary Senior Lecturer, Rheumatic Diseases Unit, Western General Hospital, Edinburgh, UK

G. K. Makharia
MD DM DNB MNAMS
Associate Professor, Department of
Gastroenterology and Human Nutrition,
All India Institute of Medical Sciences,
New Delhi, India

S. E. Marshall
FRCP FRCPath PhD
Professor of Clinical Immunology,
Department of Immunology, Ninewells
Hospital and Medical School, University
of Dundee, UK

A. Mohan
MBBS MD
Chief, Division of Pulmonary and
Critical Care Medicine;
Additional Professor and Head of
Department of Medicine, Sri
Venkateswara Institute of Medical
Sciences, Tirupati, Andhra Pradesh,
India

W. F. Mollentze
MD FCP (SA) MMed FACE FRCP
Head of Internal Medicine, Faculty of
Health Sciences, University of the Free
State, Bloemfontein, South Africa

A. Mubaidin
Department of Clinical Neurology,
King Hussein Medical Centre,
Amman, Jordan

D. E. Newby
BA BSc PhD BM DM DSc FRCP FRSE FMedSci
British Heart Foundation John Wheatley
Chair of Cardiology, Centre for
Cardiovascular Science, University of
Edinburgh, UK

D. Oxenham
MB ChB MRCP
Consultant in Palliative Care, Marie Curie
Hospice, Edinburgh, UK

P. L. Padfield
MB BCh FRCP
Associate Medical Director, Department
of Endocrinology, Metabolic Unit,
Western General Hospital,
Edinburgh, UK

P. Pais
MD
Dean and Professor of Medicine,
St John's Medical College, Bangalore,
India

I. D. Penman
BSc MD FRCP Edin
Consultant Gastroenterologist,
Centre for Liver & Digestive Disorders,
Royal Lufirmary of Edinburgh,
Edinburgh, UK

S. H. Ralston
MB ChB MD FRCP FMedSci FRSE
Arthritis Research UK Professor of
Rheumatology, Rheumatic Diseases
Unit, University of Edinburgh, Western
General Hospital, Edinburgh, UK

A. Ramachandran
MD PhD FRCP DSc MNAMS FICP
Chairman/Managing Director, Dr A
Ramachandran's Diabetes Hospitals;
President, India Diabetes Research
Foundation, Chennai, India

B. S. Ramakrishna
MD DM PhD FAMS
Department of Gastrointestinal Sciences,
Christian Medical College, Vellore
Tamilnadu, India

M. Y. Rao
MD PGDHHM
Associate Dean and Senior Professor of
Medicine, M.S. Ramaiah Medical
College, Bangalore, India

P. T. Reid
MD FRCP
Consultant in Respiratory Medicine and
Honorary Senior Lecturer, Respiratory
Medicine Unit, Western General
Hospital, Edinburgh, UK

V. Sakhuja
MD DM FAMS
Professor of Nephrology, Department of
Nephrology, Postgraduate Institute of
Medical Education and Research,
Chandigarh, India

R. Al-Shahi Salman
MA PhD FRCP Edin
MRC Senior Clinical Fellow and
Honorary Consultant Neurologist,
Division of Clinical Neurosciences,
Western General Hospital,
Edinburgh, UK

O. M. Schofield
MBBS FRCP Edin
Consultant Dermatologist, Department of
Dermatology, Royal Infirmary of
Edinburgh, UK

G. R. Scott
BSc MBChB FRCP
Consultant Physician, Chalmers Sexual
Health Centre, Royal Infirmary of
Edinburgh, UK

K. R. Sethuraman
MD PGDHE
Senior-Professor and Dean, Faculty of
Medicine and Deputy Vice-Chancellor
(International and Academic Affairs),
AIMST University, 08100, Malaysia

S. K. Sharma
MD PhD
Chief, Division of Pulmonary, Critical
Care and Sleep Medicine; Professor and
Head, Department of Medicine, All India
Institute of Medical Sciences,
New Delhi, India

P. Shepherd
MB BCh BAO FRCP FRCPath
Consultant Haematologist, Department
of Haematology, Western General
Hospital, Edinburgh, UK

J. S. T., Libya
I. Sherif's Professor of Medicine Tripoli
Medicine Centre Lidya

S. Singh
MMBS MD
Professor, Department of
Internal Medicine
Postgraduate Institute of Medical
Education and Research, Chandigarh,
India

J. Stone
MB ChB FRCP Edin PhD
Consultant Neurologist and Honorary
Senior Lecturer, Department of Clinical
Neurosciences, Western General
Hospital, Edinburgh, UK

M. W. J. Strachan
BSc(Hons) MD FRCP Edin
Consultant in Diabetes and
Endocrinology Metabolic Unit,
Western General Hospital, Edinburgh;
Part-time Reader, University of
Edinburgh, UK

S. Sundar
MD FRCP FNA
Professor of Medicine, Institute of
Medical Sciences, Banaras Hindu
University, Varanasi, India

M. J. Tidman
MD FRCP Edin FRCP Lord
Consultant Dermatologist, Department of
Dermatology, Royal Infirmary of
Edinburgh, UK

W. T. A. Todd
BSc MB ChB FRCP Edin FFTM
Consultant Physician, Lanarkshire Area
Infectious Diseases Unit, Monklands
Hospital, Airdrie, UK

M. L. Turner
MB ChB PhD FRCP FRCPath
Professor of Cellular Therapy and
Medical Director, Scottish National
Blood Transfusion Service,
Edinburgh, UK

A. N. Turner
PhD FRCP
Professor of Nephrology, Medical Renal
Unit, Royal Infirmary of Edinburgh, UK

S. Varma
MBBS MD
Professor and Head, Department of
Internal Medicine, Postgraduate Institute
of Medical Education and Research,
Chandigarh, India

S. W. Walker
MB BS MA DM
Senior Lecturer and Honorary
Consultant in Clinical Biochemistry,
University of Edinburgh, UK

L. Wall
BA MBBS MSc MD FRCP Edin
Consultant Medical Oncologist
Edinburgh Cancer Centre, Western
General Hospital, Edinburgh, UK

E. Wilkins
FRCP FRCPath
Consultant in Infectious Diseases,
Department of Infectious Diseases,
North Manchester General Hospital,
Manchester, UK

G. A. Wittert
MB BCH MD FRACP
Mortlock Professor and Head of School
of Medicine, University of Adelaide,
Australia

M. E. Yeolekar
MD MNAMS Med FICP
Director, North Eastern Iudia Gaudhi
Regional Institute of Health and Medical
Sciences (NEIGRIHMS), Shillong, India

Abbreviations

AIDS	Acquired immunodeficiency syndrome
ALT	Alanine aminotransferase
ANCA	Antineutrophil cytoplasmic antibodies
ANF	Antinuclear factor
APTT	Activated partial thromboplastin time
AST	Aspartate aminotransferase
BMI	Body mass index
CEA	Carcinoembryonic antigen
CRP	C-reactive protein
dsDNA	Double-stranded DNA
ECG	Electrocardiogram
ESR	Erythrocyte sedimentation rate
GGT (γ-GT)	Gamma-glutamyl transferase
GP	General practitioner
HBsAg	Hepatitis B surface antigen
HDL	High-density lipoprotein
HIV	Human immunodeficiency virus
LDH	Lactate dehydrogenase
LDL	Low-density lipoprotein
LFTs	Liver function tests
MCV	Mean cell volume
PCV	Packed cell volume
PT	Prothrombin time
RBC	Red blood cells
RF	Rheumatoid factor
SGOT	Serum glutamic oxaloacetic transaminase
SGPT	Serum glutamic pyruvic transaminase
TSH	Thyroid-stimulating hormone
U&Es	Urea and electrolytes
WCC	White cell count

1

Genital ulceration

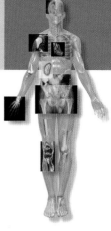

A. McMILLAN

Presenting problem

A 25-year-old white woman is referred to a genitourinary medicine clinic with a 2-day history of vulval pain and pain on passing urine. She has also noticed tender lumps in both groins. A few days before the onset of these symptoms, she had felt generally unwell with malaise and mild fever. She has no other symptoms and, other than using the combined contraceptive pill, she does not take any medication or use recreational drugs. The woman has not used any deodorants or similar chemical agents on the affected areas. Her last menstrual period was 8 days prior to the development of her symptoms and was normal. Using a mirror, she has noticed sores on her genitals. She has been married for 18 months to a businessman who travels frequently to Uganda. They had sexual intercourse 1 week previously, on the night he had returned from Africa. Intercourse was not traumatic. Her husband is in good health and has no genital symptoms or signs.

What would your differential diagnosis include before examining the patient?

The clinical features are suggestive of primary genital herpes, caused by herpes simplex virus (HSV). Candidiasis can cause superficial genital ulceration, but itch rather than pain is the principal symptom and lymph node enlargement is not a feature. Trauma secondary to intercourse seems unlikely, as is ulceration caused by drugs or chemicals. The patient's husband has travelled frequently to Africa, where ulcerative conditions such as syphilis, lymphogranuloma venereum (LGV) and chancroid are more prevalent than in the UK. If he has had sexual contact with a local person there, these conditions need to be considered.

Examination

The patient walks with some difficulty because of pain. Her temperature is 37.4°C. The inguinal lymph nodes are enlarged and tender bilaterally. On the mucosal surface of the vulva, there are multiple white plaques, and vesicles and shallow tender ulcers are noted on the labia, perineum and inner aspects of the upper thighs (Fig. 1.1). The ulcers are not indurated and do not bleed when touched. It is impossible to pass a vaginal speculum because of pain. Neither a rash nor oral ulceration is evident.

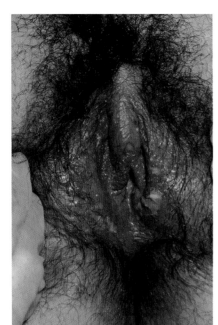

Figure 1.1 Primary herpes simplex of the vulva.

Has examination narrowed down your differential diagnosis?

The clinical appearance is consistent with genital herpes. Primary syphilis usually presents with a solitary, painless, indurated genital ulcer and, although atypical presentations are not uncommon, this seems an improbable diagnosis. Secondary syphilis is often associated with mucosal ulceration, but this is usually painless and in most cases a maculopapular or papular rash is also found. Lymphogranuloma venereum, caused by *Chlamydia trachomatis* serovar *lymphogranuloma venereum*, is unlikely. This condition is uncommon in women and is associated with transient painless genital ulceration followed several weeks later by unilateral lymph node enlargement. Chancroid, caused by *Haemophilus ducreyii* and common in Africa, is associated with multiple genital ulcers that bleed easily, and with inguinal lymphadenopathy. In the absence of other features, systemic conditions such as erythema multiforme and Behçet's syndrome are unlikely.

Has the diagnosis been clinched?

The clinical picture is almost diagnostic, but the diagnosis should always be confirmed so that the most appropriate management can be provided.

Further investigations

Herpes simplex virus type 1 DNA is detected in material obtained from one of the vesicles. Serological tests for syphilis, including an anti-treponemal IgM enzyme immunoassay to detect early infection, are negative. As culture for *H. ducreyii* and nucleic acid amplification methods for the detection of specific DNA sequences are only available in a limited number of centres, these tests are not undertaken in this case.

How will you treat this patient?

When the diagnosis is reasonably certain, antiviral therapy should be initiated before receiving the laboratory results. Aciclovir, given in an oral dosage of 200 mg five times per day for 5 days, is the most widely used and cheapest drug. It is well tolerated with few adverse effects, although a rash may occasionally complicate therapy. The use of aciclovir decreases healing time, new lesion formation and viral shedding; all symptoms are shorter than if the individual is untreated. Treatment, however, does not decrease the likelihood of subsequent recurrence. There is no place for topical aciclovir in the treatment of primary genital herpes. In addition to specific antiviral treatment, mild analgesics should be prescribed for pain, and the individual should frequently bathe the affected area with physiological 0.9% saline.

Oral valaciclovir and famciclovir are alternative antiviral agents that are as effective as aciclovir.

Counselling and support are essential in the management of the newly diagnosed individual with first-episode genital herpes. It is also helpful to give written information. Patients should be given the opportunity to return within a few days to discuss their anxieties and fears, and it is sometimes helpful to have a joint counselling session. In this case, the infection is likely to have been acquired from oral–genital contact with her husband, who is a symptomless excretor of the virus. There is no indication that he has been unfaithful.

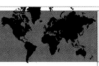

Key points and global issues

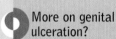

More on genital ulceration?

See Chapter 15 of
Davidson's Principles
& **Practice** of
Medicine (21st edn)

- In many countries an increasing proportion of cases of genital herpes is caused by herpes simplex virus type 1.

- Most new genital infections with herpes simplex virus have been acquired from symptomless excretors of the virus.

- Recurrent genital herpes is generally associated with mild clinical features. Individuals with mild recurrences can be educated to identify these so as to avoid sexual intercourse until symptoms resolve, thereby reducing the risk of onward transmission to an uninfected partner.

- An increasing proportion of genital ulcer disease in developing countries is caused by herpes simplex virus.

- Genital herpes is recognised as an important factor facilitating the transmission of the human immunodeficiency virus (HIV).

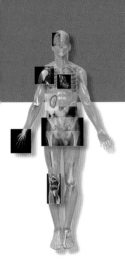

2

Urethral discharge

G. R. SCOTT

Presenting problem

A 34-year-old man presents in your GP surgery in the UK complaining of a urethral discharge that started the day before. He describes this as pus coming from the end of his penis, associated with severe pain when passing urine. You know he is married and that he works in the hotel trade.

What would your differential diagnosis include before examining the patient?

Chlamydia trachomatis is by far the most common sexually transmitted infection (STI) seen in men presenting with urethritis in the UK. However, the severity of this man's symptoms, also reflected in his rapid attendance for treatment, makes gonorrhoea a significant possibility. *Trichomonas* is a rare cause of urethral discharge in the UK and, although herpes simplex virus infection may present with urethritis, external genital ulceration is much more common. Non-specific urethritis, perhaps due to *Mycoplasma* or *Ureaplasma*, is also a possibility.

Further history and examination

You advise this man to attend the local genitourinary medicine (GUM) clinic but he asks you to manage him yourself. What essential questions must be asked? You must take a sexual history, perhaps prefacing this by saying, 'I understand you are married. When did you last have sex with your wife?'. The next question should be, 'When did you last have sex with anyone else?'. Let's say he answers somewhat gloomily, 'Last week'. The questioning should continue along the following lines: 'Is this a regular partner or was it more of a "one-off"?'; 'Was this local, within the UK or abroad?'; 'Did you use a condom?' and 'Was this partner female or male?'.

The last question is essential and should be asked in a neutral tone that does not infer one answer or the other. The fact that the patient is married does not exclude the possibility that he has had sex with a man. It transpires that he has had unprotected, insertive and receptive anal sex with another man 8 days ago.

General examination is unremarkable. Examination of the genitalia confirms the presence of a purulent urethral discharge (Fig. 2.1). Rectal examination is normal.

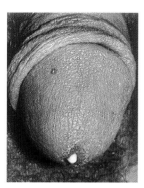

Figure 2.1 Urethral discharge.

Has examination narrowed down your differential diagnosis?

Gonorrhoea is relatively more common among men who have sex with men (MSM) than it is among heterosexual men in the UK, although chlamydia remains a distinct possibility. The findings on examination are consistent with either.

Many cities in the UK have seen increased numbers of cases of syphilis among MSM over the last 5 years. Hepatitis B is more common among MSM, and of course human immunodeficiency virus (HIV) infection is a major concern. It is important to remember that multiple concurrent STIs may be diagnosed.

Investigations

A urethral swab for culture of *Neisseria gonorrhoeae* is sent in the appropriate transport medium to the local laboratory. This must reach the laboratory on the day it is taken; otherwise any gonococci will die in transit. If there is any doubt about transport delay, a slide of the urethral discharge may be sent for microscopy, ensuring careful packaging. A first-voided urine (FVU) specimen is also sent for diagnosis of chlamydia by nucleic acid amplification test (NAAT). Increasingly in the UK, combined NAATs for gonorrhoea and chlamydia are coming into use, in which case a urethral swab will not be required and an FVU will suffice. There is an additional benefit in that sensitivity is not reduced if the sample takes 2 or 3 days to reach the laboratory.

Swabs from the rectum are sent for gonorrhoea and chlamydia testing because this man has had receptive anal sex; a pharyngeal swab is also sent for gonorrhoea testing.

Blood is taken for serological tests for syphilis and hepatitis B, with a view to vaccination against the latter if there is no evidence of current or past infection.

Blood is also taken for an HIV test, after an explanation of the procedure to be followed should the test be positive (pretest counselling), and arrangements are made to give the result in person.

How will you treat this patient?

Ideally, treatment should be given prior to confirmation of the microbiological diagnosis. However, there is no single agent that cures both gonorrhoea and chlamydia with sufficient certainty to be recommended, and gonococcal resistance is also emerging to the cephalosporins previously given as first line. Current UK guidance advocates culture of gonococci that includes assessment of antibiotic sensitivities piror to treatment with intramuscular ceftriaxone 500 mg, with azithromycin 1 g orally for possible chlamydial infection.

Managing confirmed or suspected gonococcal infection in primary care is therefore very difficult, and referral to GUM is strongly advised.

The urethral swabs grow gonococci. All other swabs are negative. He should be advised to abstain from sexual contact until cure has been confirmed, and sexual partners should be advised to attend for investigation. If he has had sex with his wife since acquiring gonorrhoea, she should be tested as well. Advice on safer sex would be particularly important in this case, and again referral to your local GUM service would be appropriate.

All serological tests are negative. These will need to be repeated in due course, as his most recent sexual contact was within the window period for these infections. His risk of HIV infection will depend on local prevalence of HIV, the number of (male) partners that he has had sex with and the type of sex. Anal sex carries the greatest risk of transmission, especially for the receptive partner. The presence of other STIs, such as gonorrhoea, increases risk of transmission. A single episode of insertive anal sex in a UK city with an HIV prevalence of ~5% would carry a relatively low risk, but a test for HIV should be recommended nevertheless.

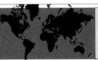

Key points and global issues

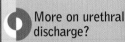

More on urethral discharge?

See Chapter 15 of **Davidson's Principles** & **Practice** of **Medicine (21st edn)**

- There is a wide range of human sexual expression in all parts of the world. Some married men will have sex with other men. This may range from low-risk sexual activity such as mutual masturbation, through oral sex to unprotected anal sex.

- A thorough risk assessment is essential in order to diagnose and treat infections for which a man is at risk, and to give advice and support in adhering to safer sexual practice in the future.

3

Proctitis in a man who has sex with men

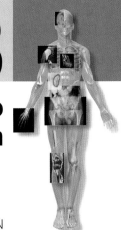

A. McMILLAN

Presenting problem

A 43-year-old white man presents to a genitourinary medicine clinic with a 10-day history of constipation, painful defaecation, streaking of the stools with slime, a feeling of incomplete emptying of his bowels, and the passage of blood anally to a degree that it splashes in the toilet pan. His health is otherwise good and he has not had previous bowel problems. At the age of 35 years he had acute hepatitis B, and 3 years before the current illness he was treated for urethral gonorrhoea and giardiasis. Otherwise he has had no significant illnesses in the past. He has never been tested for human immunodeficiency virus (HIV) infection. His most recent sexual contact was 3 weeks previously at a party in Amsterdam, when he had unprotected receptive anal intercourse with an unknown male.

What would your differential diagnosis include before examining the patient?

The clinical features are strongly suggestive of proctitis. As the onset was acute in an individual with no previous history of intestinal disease and, as there appears to be a temporal relationship between the onset of symptoms and the episode of unprotected anal intercourse, a sexually transmitted infection (STI) seems to be the most likely cause. Box 3.1 shows the STIs that can cause proctitis.

As the symptoms are severe, infection with *Chlamydia trachomatis* serovar *trachomatis* is unlikely. An outbreak of cases of severe proctitis caused by *C. trachomatis* serovar *lymphogranuloma venereum* (LGV), however, has been described recently among men who have sex with men (MSM) in industrialised countries, including the Netherlands. Primary syphilis usually has a pre-patent period of about 6 weeks, making this infection a less likely cause of this patient's symptoms. Primary herpetic proctitis is usually associated with perianal ulceration, but there is no history of this. Perirectal cellulitis following traumatic anal intercourse usually presents sooner, and there are often systemic features that are absent in this case.

> **BOX 3.1**
>
> **Sexually transmitted organisms causing proctitis**
>
> - *Neisseria gonorrhoeae*
> - *Chlamydia trachomatis*
>   Serovar *trachomatis*
>   Serovar *lymphogranuloma venereum*
> - *Treponema pallidum*
> - Herpes simplex virus

Examination

The patient looks well and is apyrexial. There is no abdominal tenderness or guarding, and no masses are felt; neither liver nor spleen is palpable. The perianal region appears normal with no ulceration. At sigmoidoscopy, the rectal mucosa is markedly oedematous and friable, with mucopus in the lumen. These inflammatory changes extend to about 12 cm from the dentate line, the more proximal mucosa appearing normal. Two ulcers, each about 1.5 cm in diameter, are noted within the inflamed mucosa.

Has examination narrowed down your differential diagnosis?

The diagnosis of distal proctitis is confirmed – the inflammatory changes do not extend beyond the rectosigmoid junction, unlike the appearance in proctocolitis. Although rectal gonorrhoea can produce acute proctitis, prominent ulceration is unusual. In most, but by no means all, cases of primary herpetic proctitis there is perianal ulceration and the patient is usually pyrexial. Infection with *C. trachomatis* serovar *trachomatis* usually causes minimal symptoms and signs, and is an unlikely cause of the proctitis in this case. The LGV serovar of *C. trachomatis*, however, is commonly associated with severe disease, and this must be high on the list of differential diagnoses. Primary syphilis also needs to be considered. The lack of abdominal tenderness and fever argues against a diagnosis of perirectal cellulitis.

Further investigations

A nucleic acid amplification test for *C. trachomatis* is positive, and genotyping shows infection with the LGV serovar, clinching the diagnosis of LGV proctitis. Negative culture and a negative nucleic acid amplification test for *Neisseria gonorrhoeae* and a negative polymerase chain reaction (PCR) assay for herpes simplex virus (HSV) DNA exclude concurrent infection with these organisms. A PCR for *Treponema pallidum* on a specimen taken from the ulcerated areas of the rectum, and syphilis serology, including an anti-treponemal IgM test to detect early infection, are negative. To exclude incubating syphilis, however, it would be necessary to repeat serological tests 1 and 3 months later.

Rectal biopsy is not likely to be helpful, as the histological changes associated with these infections are non-specific. The granulomatous changes found in LGV proctitis (Fig. 3.1) closely resemble those of Crohn's disease.

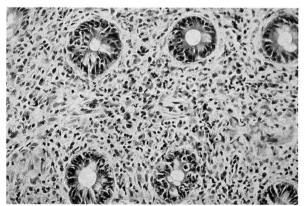

Figure 3.1
Granulomatous proctitis in *lymphogranuloma venereum*. There is infiltration of the lamina propria of the rectum with lymphocytes, histiocytes and plasma cells. Early granuloma formation is also shown.

Serological tests show that this patient is infected with HIV. He is only moderately immunocompromised, with a CD4$^+$ T-cell count of 387/mm^3 (normal range 500–1500/mm^3). Plasma hepatitis C RNA is not detected by a PCR, and an antibody test for hepatitis C virus is negative; to exclude infection acquired at the same time as LGV, however, serology should be repeated in 3 and 6 months' time.

How will you treat this patient?

As the proctitis is severe, treatment should not be withheld until laboratory test results are available. The most likely diagnosis from the history and examination is LGV proctitis, and doxycycline in an oral dosage of 100 mg 12-hourly for 3 weeks should be prescribed. Aciclovir, given orally in a dose of 200 mg five times per day for 5 days, should also be prescribed to treat possible HSV infection (while awaiting the results of the microbiological tests). As multiple rectal infections, including gonorrhoea, are common in MSM, it also seems prudent to treat this man with a single intramuscular injection of ceftriaxone (500 mg). He will require counselling regarding the new diagnosis of HIV and will clearly need long-term follow-up. Initiation of antiretroviral therapy is discussed, but is declined by the patient.

Key points and global issues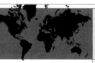

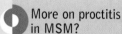
More on proctitis in MSM?

- *Lymphogranuloma venereum* should be considered in the differential diagnosis of acute onset severe proctitis in a MSM.

- Concurrent infection with HIV and hepatitis C are common in MSM with *lymphogranuloma venereum* proctitis.

- A 21-day course of doxycycline is the most effective treatment for *lymphogranuloma venereum* proctitis. Shorter courses of the drug are not curative.

- *Lymphogranuloma venereum* proctitis is being recognised with increasing frequency amongst MSM throughout the industrialised world.

- *Lymphogranuloma venereum* proctitis has been recognised for many years among women in developing countries, and has been associated with considerable morbidity.

See Chapter 15 of
Davidson's Principles & **Practice** of
Medicine (21st edn)

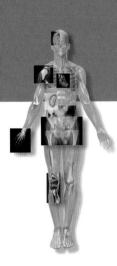

4

Vaginal discharge

G. R. SCOTT

Presenting problem

You are visiting a sub-Saharan African country to assist in the training of local staff in the delivery of antiretroviral therapy for human immunodeficiency virus (HIV). In a community-based clinic, a 23-year-old woman presents to you with a complaint of vaginal discharge and vulval itch. She is not known to have any ongoing health problems and does not take any regular medication.

What would your differential diagnosis include before examining the patient?

In the UK, the most likely diagnoses would be candidiasis or bacterial vaginosis, with the presence of itch making the former more likely. However, it is essential to assess the risk of a sexually transmitted infection (STI) by taking a sexual history. You quickly establish that this woman has had a regular male partner for several months. They are not using condoms, or indeed any form of contraception. In many parts of the world, condom use is not widespread among men. The patient should, therefore, be considered to be at risk of having an STI.

Trichomonas vaginalis (TV) is the most common treatable STI in the world with an estimated 170 million cases each year. The main symptom of TV is a vaginal discharge, often accompanied by vulval itch and/or irritation. Gonorrhoea and chlamydia are also common, with 62 and 90 million cases, respectively worldwide per annum, but vaginal discharge is a less common symptom with both.

Examination

General physical examination reveals no abnormal findings. Vaginal examination reveals a yellow discharge at the entrance to the vagina. You have a speculum but no light source; so ascertaining whether the discharge is vaginal or cervical is impossible.

Has examination narrowed down your differential diagnosis?

Not really! A discharge emanating from the cervix would make gonorrhoea or chlamydia more likely. A vaginal discharge would be more in keeping with TV, bacterial vaginosis and candidiasis. The only way to determine the underlying diagnosis is to examine a specimen of the discharge.

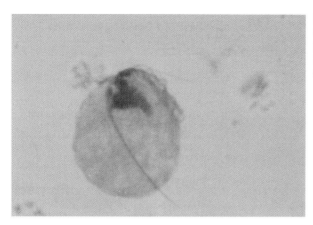

Figure 4.1 Wet mount of vaginal discharge demonstrating *Trichomonas vaginalis* organisms.

Investigations

Fortunately, there is a microscope to hand, along with facilities for carrying out simple Gram staining. Motile, flagellated organisms are identified in a wet-mount preparation (Fig. 4.1). Gram staining of the discharge reveals mixed organisms consistent with anaerobic infection.

Does this narrow down your differential diagnosis?

The organisms identified on the wet mount are typical of TV. Examination of *cervical* discharge for Gram-negative diplococci has a sensitivity of about 50% in the diagnosis of gonorrhoea, so the positive yield from a blind vaginal swab is going to be even lower. Culture of the discharge and automated nucleic acid amplification tests (NAATs) would increase the likelihood of detecting gonococci, but these facilities are not available. Both candida and bacterial vaginosis can be diagnosed accurately by microscopy of vaginal discharge.

How will you treat this patient?

Clearly, appropriate treatment should be given for any infection diagnosed by microscopy, in this case TV. However, multiple diagnoses are not uncommon. If local prevalence of gonorrhoea and chlamydia is known to be high, then effective antimicrobials for these infections should be given, even if the organisms are not identified. This woman should be prescribed metronidazole 2 g for TV, cefixime 400 mg or ciprofloxacin 500 mg for gonorrhoea, and either azithromycin 1 g stat or doxycycline 100 mg twice daily for 7 days for chlamydia; she should also be offered treatment for candida. Treatment would also be recommended for her partner, but persuading him to attend may be difficult.

A discussion about having an HIV test would also be routine practice in the UK for anybody diagnosed with an STI. Unhindered access to antiretroviral therapy (ART) makes a proactive approach easy to justify. Unfortunately, some parts of the developing world have limited programmes for delivering ART. As you are actively working with local staff to create treatment access, this woman should be offered an HIV test. Her partner should also be encouraged to attend the clinic for HIV testing.

Finally, the patient is not using any form of contraception. If she does not wish to become pregnant, long-acting injectable methods of contraception are more effective in preventing pregnancy than short-acting methods such as the oral contraceptive pill.

Key points and global issues

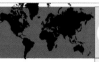

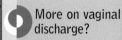
More on vaginal discharge?

See Chapter 15 of
Davidson's Principles
& **Practice** of
Medicine (21st edn)

- Accurate diagnosis is the bedrock of managing STIs, allowing precise treatment and informed tracing of sexual contacts.
- Laboratory support is taken for granted in the developed world, but routine culture or automated NAATs are rarely available in most countries.
- Affordable, accurate, rapid point-of-care tests, such as those now available for the diagnosis of HIV infection, would significantly improve management of STIs.

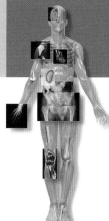

5

Fever in an individual with human immunodeficiency virus infection

E. WILKINS

Presenting problem

A previously well 35-year-old single white male resident in the UK is admitted with a 3-week history of fevers, sweats and pain on swallowing. He was diagnosed with HIV infection 1 month previously, following presentation with weight loss and chronic frequent watery diarrhoea. At that time, his CD4 count was found to be 24 cells/mm^3 and viral load >1 million copies/mL: a viral resistance test subsequently showed wild-type virus. He denied any history of travel outside Europe. Antiretroviral (ARV) combination therapy with lopinavir/ritonavir (Kaletra), tenofovir (TDF) and emtricitabine (FTC) was started and he is tolerating this well. Co-trimoxazole prophylaxis for *Pneumocystis* pneumonia was also commenced, but had to be discontinued because of a hypersensitivity rash and dapsone was substituted. He denies any other symptoms of note. His admission investigations are detailed in Box 5.1.

What would your differential diagnosis include before examining the patient?

PUO is the presenting feature of HIV in approximately 2% of patients with two-thirds having a CD4 count of <50 cells/mm^3 and 60% resulting from infection. The two most common causes of fever in later-stage HIV infection are mycobac-terial infection (either disseminated *Myco-bacterium avium intracellulare*, [MAI] or tuberculosis, [TB]) and lymphoma. The presence of frequent diarrhoea and weight loss in addition to this patient's fever may indicate a single aetiology (e.g. MAI, cytomegalovirus [CMV] or *Salmonella* infection) or reflect two or more coexisting causes (e.g. TB causing fever, and *Crypto-sporidium* or lopinavir/ritonavir causing diarrhoea). Similarly, his anaemia may indicate a disseminated process such as mycobacterial infection or lymphoma, but could also reflect Kaposi's sarcoma (KS) involvement of his gastrointestinal tract.

BOX 5.1	
Initial investigations	
Haemoglobin	70 g/L (7.0 g/dL)
Film	Hypochromic, microcytic
WCC	2.7×10^9/L (10^3/mm^3)
Differential count	
Lymphocytes	0.38×10^9/L (10^3/mm^3)
Neutrophils	1.91×10^9/L (10^3/mm^3)
Platelets	207×10^9/L (10^3/mm^3)
ALT	42 U/L
GGT	114 U/L
Albumin	17 g/L (1.7 g/dL)
Prothrombin ratio	1.0

Although not discriminatory features, they do identify potential investigations where the diagnosis may be confirmed (stool culture, endoscopy and bone marrow). Disseminated CMV infection is an infrequent but recognised cause of prolonged fever and needs to be considered as does multicentric Castleman's disease. Fever without breathlessness makes *Pneumocystis* pneumonia unlikely particularly as he is on prophylaxis, and without headache, cryptococcal infection is unlikely. Secondary syphilis is improbable but should be excluded. Finally, the recent commencement of ARV therapy raises the possibility of immune reconstitution syndrome (IRS), which occurs in approximately 15% of patients with mycobacterial co-infection. Although multiple aetiologies may exist, HIV alone will not be the cause.

Examination

The patient is febrile, but comfortable at rest. He is wasted, with lesions that resemble cutaneous and oral KS; he also has perianal herpes simplex and severe oropharyngeal candidiasis. He has two-finger breadth hepatosplenomegaly but no abdominal tenderness; rectal examination reveals an empty rectum. There is no lymphadenopathy and no localising signs for his infection. Dilated fundoscopy demonstrates no evidence of retinitis.

Has examination narrowed down your differential diagnosis?

Detailed examination in patients with HIV, particularly of the skin, mouth, genitals and perianal area, is often rewarding. The presence of lesions consistent with KS does not explain the fever but may explain the anaemia. The presence of oropharyngeal candidiasis makes oesophageal candidiasis a probable cause of his pain on swallowing. The hepatosplenomegaly is consistent with mycobacterial infection, visceral KS, Castleman's disease (also linked to HHV-8) and lymphoma, and is therefore not discriminatory in determining the aetiology of his fever, but it is a significant finding.

Further investigations

Blood and stool cultures at 48 hours are negative. The patient's CD4 count is 32 cells/mm^3 and viral load 1200 copies/mL. Cryptococcal antigen and treponemal antibody blood tests are negative, as is the CMV PCR. Induced sputa are negative on direct examination for *Pneumocystis jirovecii* and acid-fast bacilli, and there is no growth on standard culture. A chest X-ray is normal, but a computed tomogram (CT) of the chest reveals numerous enlarged lymph nodes 2–5 cm in diameter in the mediastinum. An upper gastrointestinal endoscopy demonstrates oesophageal candidiasis and gastric KS (Figs 5.1, 5.2).

Does this narrow down your differential diagnosis?

These results are consistent with the two most likely diagnoses, mycobacterial infection and lymphoma. CMV, cryptococcal infection and syphilis are now extremely unlikely but Castleman's disease is still possible as this may coexist with KS.

Definitive investigations

A bone marrow aspiration is performed and numerous acid-fast bacilli are identified on a Ziehl–Neelsen stain. Three weeks later, blood cultures grow mycobacteria.

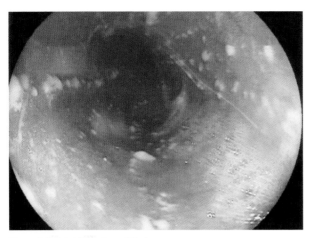

Figure 5.1 Oesophageal candidiasis.

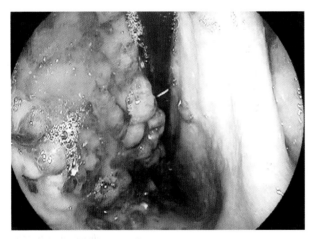

Figure 5.2 Kaposi's sarcoma of the stomach.

Does this further narrow down your differential diagnosis?

With the identification of mycobacteria, the differential lies between TB and MAI. His ethnicity, lack of history of travel outside Western Europe and the normal chest X-ray are all against this being TB. Nevertheless, the CXR may be normal in extrapulmonary and disseminated presentations of TB, which are far more common in HIV, especially in late-stage disease. Rapid distinction between the two mycobacterial species and detection of rifampicin resistance if *Mycobacterium tuberculosis* is confirmed will depend upon nucleic amplification techniques (e.g. polymerase chain reaction, PCR). Subsequent rapid sensitivity testing will allow rationalisation of therapy.

How will you treat this patient?

While awaiting identification of the species, it is important to consider choosing a combination of drugs that provides treatment for both mycobacterial species. It is also necessary to examine potential drug interactions with his antiretroviral agents. Ritonavir is a potent inhibitor of the cytochrome P450 complex and rifampicin a potent inducer. Because of this, rifampicin should not be prescribed with protease inhibitors and rifabutin, which has equal potency to rifampicin against *M. tuberculosis* but is also active against MAI, is the drug of choice. An alternative strategy, because his viral strain is fully sensitive to ARVs, is to switch him to efavirenz maintaining the TDF/FTC and give rifampicin. Pyrazinamide and isoniazid, although first-line anti-TB drugs, have no significant activity in clinical disease associated with MAI, whereas ethambutol and certain quinolones (e.g. ciprofloxacin) have proven activity against both mycobacteria. Lastly, both azithromycin and clarithromycin have activity against MAI and one should be included. Hence, although several combinations are possible, a suitable one would include rifabutin, azithromycin, ethambutol, ciprofloxacin and pyrazinamide. Treatment can then be modified when identification is established (dropping pyrazinamide if MAI is confirmed and switching to standard four-drug therapy if it is *M. tuberculosis*). His culture PCR confirms MAI, which is successfully treated, as is his KS, which is treated with cyclical liposomal doxorubicin. The oesophageal candidiasis is successfully treated with a 14-day course of fluconazole.

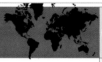

Key points and global issues

More on fever in HIV?

See Chapter 14 of **Davidson's Principles** & **Practice** of **Medicine (21st edn)**

- Except at seroconversion, prolonged fever will not be due to HIV alone.

- In known HIV patients with well controlled HIV on ARVs and a CD4 count >200 cells/mm^3, prolonged fever usually indicates a classical cause (e.g. deep bacterial infection), lymphoma, TB or immune reconstitution after commencing ARVs.

- In patients with late stage HIV, presentation is often atypical, focal disease less common, and multiple aetiologies often coexist. Prolonged fever is a presenting feature in 2–3% and is usually due to mycobacterial infection (MAI or TB), or lymphoma. Less frequent causes include salmonellosis, cryptococcal infection and Castleman's disease.

- Differential diagnosis must also include likely causes specific to that region, e.g. leishmaniasis (Central/South America, Asia and the Mediterranean).

- In identifying an infective cause, investigations may yield atypical results, serology is rarely helpful and demonstration of the organism through histology, antigen testing or nucleic amplification has a greater yield.

- Distinction between TB and MAI can often be difficult and treatment must cover both until speciation.

- Fever in late-stage HIV is highly likely to indicate TB in a person living in, or coming from, a TB-endemic area.

- Kaposi's sarcoma is uncommon in certain parts of the world (and extremely rare in India).

- The national AIDS control programmes of many countries do not include protease inhibitors in first-line antiretroviral therapy regimens and reserve them for patients who have failed either efavirenz or nevirapine based combinations.

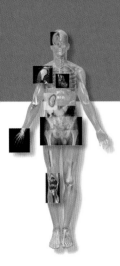

6

Adverse drug interaction

G. MAARTENS

Presenting problem

A 32-year-old man presents to the Emergency Department with profuse sweating and agitation. He had started antiretroviral therapy (tenofovir, emtricitabine and lopinavir/ritonavir) for HIV infection 2 days ago. He had no symptoms related to HIV infection and a moderately impaired CD4 lymphocyte count of 317 cells/μL. He has depression, which is well controlled on fluoxetine 40 mg daily that he has been taking for several years.

What would your differential diagnosis include before examining the patient?

Hypoglycaemia should always be ruled out first with acute neuropsychiatric presentations. Sepsis with delirium is an important consideration, particularly in a patient with impaired immunity. Thyrotoxic crisis or ingestion of stimulants, e.g. cocaine or amphetamines, could both present with these features. Mania from unrecognised bipolar disorder may be unmasked by antidepressants, but this normally occurs soon after starting antidepressants and diaphoresis (profuse perspiration) would be an unusual feature. An adverse drug reaction to one of the antiretrovirals should be considered because the problem occurred so soon after starting these, but agitation or mania are not associated with these drugs. The serotonin syndrome typically presents with agitation and diaphoresis. The serotonin syndrome develops when serotonergic drugs (such as fluoxetine) are taken in excessive doses, when two serotonergic drugs are taken together, or when a drug interaction from a co-administered drug results in increased exposure of a serotonergic drug. The protease inhibitor ritonavir is known to potently inhibit several cytochrome P450 enzymes, one of which metabolises fluoxetine. The onset of the presenting problem so soon after starting antiretroviral therapy is typical of this drug interaction.

Examination

Finger-prick glucose was normal. He is agitated and sweating profusely. His blood pressure is 174/106 mmHg, pulse 116/min and temperature 37.8°C. No focus of infection is apparent. Generalised hyperreflexia with clonus, dilated pupils and intermittent tremor are noted on neurological examination.

Has examination narrowed down your differential diagnosis?

Hypoglycaemia has been excluded. Sepsis is unlikely given the hypertension and neurological findings. Thyrotoxicosis should cause a wide pulse pressure, not hypertension, and would not explain the dilated pupils. The diaphoresis and neurological findings rule out mania. The neurological findings, hypertension and diaphoresis are all features of the serotonin syndrome, but could also be explained by ingestion of stimulants.

Initial investigations
Results of blood and urine tests are shown in Box 6.1.

Have examination and investigations clinched the diagnosis?

The investigations have ruled out thyrotoxicosis and ingestion of amphetamines or cocaine. Sepsis is unlikely with no obvious focus of infection, a normal white blood cell count and differential count, and can probably be ruled out given the clinical features. Therefore, the diagnosis is the serotonin syndrome caused by a drug interaction with fluoxetine's metabolism inhibited by the protease inhibitor ritonavir.

BOX 6.1	
Initial investigations	
Peripheral blood counts	Normal
Thyroid function tests	Normal
Urea and electrolytes	Normal
Urine for amphetamines and cocaine	Negative

How will you treat this patient?

He was admitted to hospital. Fluoxetine and the antiretroviral drugs were withdrawn. Diazepam was administered for the agitation and to reduce muscle activity. His symptoms and signs gradually settled over 48 h and he was discharged. A week later, a low dose of fluoxetine was started and the antiretroviral therapy recommenced without further incident.

General supportive care is important in the serotonin syndrome, especially cooling by evaporation if hyperthermia is present. Serotonin antagonists such as cyproheptadine or the atypical antipsychotic drug olanzapine should be used in severe disease. Fluctuations in blood pressure due to autonomic instability may be difficult to manage. Severe hypertension can be managed with short-acting β-blockers.

Key points and global issues

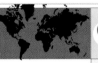

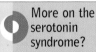

More on the serotonin syndrome?

See Chapter 9 of **Davidson's Principles & Practice** of **Medicine (21st edn)**

- The serotonin syndrome is often misdiagnosed, therefore, a high index of suspicion is required for diagnosis.
- Many drugs other than the selective serotonin reuptake inhibitors have serotonergic activity (e.g. pethidine, tramadol, monoamine oxidase inhibitors, valproate, sumatriptan, ondansetron, clomipramine).
- The serotonin syndrome may be precipitated by serotonergic drugs taken in excessive doses, by taking two serotonergic drugs together, or by a drug interaction from co-administering a drug resulting in increased exposure of a serotonergic drug.

- When prescribing drugs that are known to inhibit cytochrome P450 enzymes, it is important to check for potential drug interactions that may result in toxicity.

- In areas where antiretroviral and several other drugs are co-administered, it is imperative to check for drug–drug interactions.

- The serotonin syndrome may present with a clinical triad of changes in mental state, autonomic hyperactivity and neuromuscular abnormalities (tremor, hyperreflexia and clonus), but milder presentations with only one or two features are common. Life-threatening reactions with hyperthermia may occur.

7

Pyrexia of unknown origin

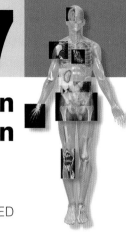

T. AHMED

Presenting problem

A 32-year-old man is readmitted to a tertiary care hospital because of persistent fever. The story is complicated. He was admitted to the same hospital 3 months ago with an evening rise of temperature of 2 months' duration. His temperature had risen to a maximum of 38.9°C and was associated with night sweats. He had lost 5 kg of body weight during the previous 2 months, but had no other symptoms except mild anorexia. He denied extramarital encounters. He said that there were no cats and dogs in the family. There were no positive findings on physical examination. Extensive investigations were carried out and these are summarised in Box 7.1.

The patient was treated empirically with a four-drug regimen of antituberculosis chemotherapy. Not only did the fever persist, but he also developed clinical jaundice after 6 weeks of anti-TB chemotherapy. The jaundice, however, disappeared after stopping the drugs. A detailed history taken on this admission does not reveal any additional information.

What would your differential diagnosis include before examining the patient?

The patient was extensively investigated on his initial admission. No cause for his fever was found and the scenario fits the definition of a pyrexia of

BOX 7.1	
Initial investigations	
Haemoglobin	100 g/L (10 g/dL)
WCC	20×10^9/L (10^3/mm³), 77% neutrophils
Blood film	No malarial parasites identified; no abnormal cells
ESR	110 mm/1st hour
U&Es, LFTs	Normal
Serum protein electrophoresis	Polyclonal gammopathy
Urinalysis	Normal
Blood and urine culture	No growth
Chest X-ray, upper and lower GI endoscopies, echocardiography, abdominal ultrasound, isotope bone scintigraphy and bone marrow examination	Normal
Tuberculin skin test (TST) with 5 tuberculin units (TU)	Negative

unknown origin (PUO). The causes of PUO vary with age, geography and subpopulations and the list is a very long one, although infections always top the list (Box 7.2). Among the infective causes, tuberculosis is the most common, particularly in this part of the world, followed by an occult abscess (which may not have been detected initially on abdominal ultrasound). But TB is unlikely in this case as the patient did not respond to standard antituberculous chemotherapy. Culture-negative bacterial endocarditis (due to previous use of antibiotics), fungal infections and sarcoidosis should also be considered. Among the malignant causes, lymphoma and renal carcinoma are possibilities. This patient's presentation and available investigations make a connective tissue disorder most unlikely.

Examination

Physical examination reveals that the patient is pale but not icteric. His axillary temperature is 38.1°C and he is sweating profusely; he appears chronically ill and thin. The liver edge is palpable 1 cm below the right costal border and is mildly tender; the spleen is also palpable 1.5 cm below the left costal margin. There are no peripheral lymph nodes. A grade 2/6 ejection systolic murmur is heard best at the lower left sternal border. The remainder of the examination is normal.

Has examination narrowed down your differential diagnosis?

Physical examination reveals hepatosplenomegaly as a new sign. The murmur may be either organic or functional. There are no other localising clues. Lymphoma and bacterial endocarditis are top of the list of possibilities but other infective conditions such as hepatosplenic abscesses, mycobacterial and fungal diseases, malaria and kala-azar should still be considered. Enteric fever should have been diagnosed by this time. For further narrowing down of the differential diagnosis, the focus of investigations should be the liver, spleen and cardiac murmur.

BOX 7.3

Further investigations on readmission

Haemoglobin	84 g/L (8.4 g/dL)
Total WCC	50.2×10^9/L (10^3/mm^3), 95% mature neutrophils
ESR	115 mm/1st hour
Blood film	No malarial parasites identified
Serological tests for Salmonella typhi, Brucella, Leptospira and Leishmania, HIV types 1 and 2, HBsAg, anti-HCV antibody	Negative
Blood and urine cultures	Negative
U&Es and calcium	Normal
LFTs (including LDH)	Normal, except for ALT 64 U/L

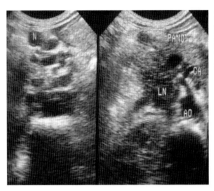

Figure 7.1 Multiple para-aortic, pre-aortic, precaval, retrocaval, mesenteric and peri-pancreatic lymph nodes on abdominal ultrasonography. N and LN, lymph nodes; CA, coeliac artery; AO, aorta; PANC, pancreas.

Further investigations

The results of blood tests are listed in Box 7.3. Chest radiography and transoesophageal echocardiography are normal. Abdominal ultrasonography reveals mild splenomegaly with a small rounded hypoechoic lesion (19 mm) within the spleen. The liver is also enlarged with multiple rounded hypoechoic lesions of varying sizes involving both lobes. There are also multiple para-aortic, pre-aortic, precaval, retrocaval, mesenteric and peri-pancreatic lymph nodes (Fig. 7.1). A rounded hypoechoic space-occupying lesion near the uncinate process of the head of the pancreas raises the possibility of a primary malignant tumour in the pancreas. A small amount of fluid is also seen in the pelvis. A contrast-enhanced computed tomogram (CT) of the abdomen and pelvis confirms the ultrasound findings, with peripheral enhancement of the lesions in the liver and spleen. A CT of the chest is normal.

Has the diagnosis been clinched?

Abdominal imaging with ultrasonography as well as CT in this young man with PUO reveals multiple hypoechoic lesions involving the liver and spleen, along with multiple enlarged para-aortic, mesenteric and peri-pancreatic lymph nodes. Ultrasonography may not be sufficient in the evaluation of structural lesions of various organs and the use of CT provides additional information, such as the presence of necrosis and calcification in TB and fungal infections. The differential diagnosis at this stage should include TB, fungal infections, sarcoidosis, lymphoma and metastatic carcinoma, as all these conditions can produce hypoechoic lesions in the liver and spleen and have associated lymphadenopathy. This patient has been treated with anti-TB drugs without a significant response, thus TB is unlikely; drug-resistant TB (DR-TB), however, cannot be excluded. A chest X-ray reveals classical bihilar lymphadenopathy and right paratracheal lymphadenopathy in most patients with sarcoidosis. A normal chest X-ray in this patient makes the diagnosis of sarcoidosis unlikely. TB, fungal infections and lymphoma can also produce mediastinal lymphadenopathy on the chest X-ray. The neutrophil leucocytosis makes the diagnosis less clear-cut and raises the possibility of leukaemia and lymphoma. The normal bone marrow findings, however, exclude the possibility of leukaemia, but not lymphoma. A tissue specimen from the liver or spleen or any of the lymph nodes, under image guidance, should reveal the definitive diagnosis. Ideally, this would be a core biopsy, but fine-needle aspiration cytology (FNAC) is an alternative if the necessary expertise to perform the former is not available.

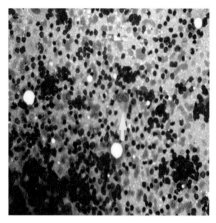

Figure 7.2 Ultrasound-guided fine-needle aspiration cytology (FNAC) from the retroperitoneal lymph nodes showing a Reed–Sternberg cell on Giemsa stain.

Definitive diagnosis

An ultrasound-guided FNAC from a retroperitoneal lymph node reveals predominantly small lymphocytes admixed with binucleate Reed–Sternberg cells, which have enlarged vesicular nuclei and prominent nucleoli (Fig. 7.2), Therefore, the cytomorphological features in this patient are those of Hodgkin's lymphoma and imaging investigations indicate stage IV B disease.

How will you treat this patient?

This patient requires combination chemotherapy with 6–8 cycles of either ChIVPP (chlorambucil, vinblastine, procarbazine and prednisolone) or ABVD (Adriamycin, bleomycin, vinblastine and daunorubicin). The latter regimen is more potent, but is also more expensive. The patient should be informed about the side-effects of this chemotherapy. The stage of the disease, along with the presence or absence of systemic symptoms, influences the response to treatment. In the UK, a young man such as this, with extensive disease at presentation and treated with an ABVD regimen, would have a >80% 5-year survival. The treatment response should be evaluated by clinical criteria, as well as by repeat CT examination. Positron emission tomography (PET), if available, is the most sensitive means of documenting remission.

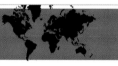

Key points and global issues

More on py of unknown origin?

See Chapter 13 of **Davidson's Principle** & **Practice** of **Medicine (21st edn**

- PUO is more likely to be caused by an uncommon presentation of a common problem than by a rare disorder.

- The first step in the evaluation of a patient with PUO for the physician, who has not seen the case previously, is to elicit the history carefully and to repeat the physical examination and investigations if necessary.

- Causes of PUO vary in different geographical areas and also depend on the extent of the initial investigations.

- TB is the most common cause of PUO worldwide, particularly in the developing world and immigrants from those countries.

8

Fever with jaundice and a purpuric rash

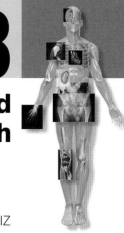

A. FAIZ

Presenting problem

A 35-year-old farmer from a rural area is admitted to the medical unit with a history of fever for 5 days and yellowish discoloration of the eyes. He has noticed darkening of the urine for 2 days and over the last 24 h has developed red spots over his body. The fever is high-grade and continuous; the patient is mentally alert. He does not take any regular medication. Prior to referral, a private practitioner carried out some routine blood tests. The results of these tests are detailed in Box 8.1.

BOX 8.1

Initial investigations

WCC	16×10^9/L (10^3/mm³)
Bilirubin	105 µmol/L (5 mg/dL)
AST	120 U/L
Urea	13.5 mmol/L (81 mg/dL)
Creatinine	159 µmol/L (1.8 mg/dL)
Urine examination	
Albumin	+
RBC	+
Cast	+

What would your differential diagnosis include before examining the patient?

This combination of the presenting problems: fever, jaundice and rash, warrants the consideration of a wide range of diseases in the differential diagnosis, depending on place, period and prevalence. This is a particularly common problem in the tropics, although it may occur anywhere in world. The possibilities are *falciparum* malaria, leptospirosis, dengue, viral hepatitis and septicaemia. Severe *falciparum* malaria and leptospirosis should always be borne in mind in endemic areas. Jaundice and renal involvement are recognised complications in both conditions but a rash is unusual in malaria. However, patients with *falciparum* malaria can develop purpuric spots due to thrombocytopenia. A patient with acute viral hepatitis or dengue may present with this type of picture. In acute viral hepatitis, the fever is low-grade and usually precedes jaundice and bleeding, though this is not an absolute rule. Similarly, in dengue haemorrhagic fever (DHF), bleeding usually occurs once the febrile episode is over; hepatic involvement may complicate the initial febrile phase and renal involvement is rare. Septicaemia culminating in disseminated intravascular coagulation is also a strong possibility. Rickettsial diseases should also be considered in areas where such infections are prevalent. Patients may have a tell-tale eschar and brain involvement. Yellow fever should also be considered in areas where the disease is endemic; it does not occur in Asia. Bradycardia and leucopenia are observed.

The initial investigations in this patient show leucocytosis and mild renal impairment. These two features favour the diagnosis of leptospirosis, but may

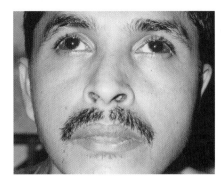

Figure 8.1 Bilateral conjunctival haemorrhages and scleral jaundice in a patient with leptospirosis.

also occur in septicaemia and severe malaria. A leucocytosis is unlikely in dengue and viral hepatitis.

Examination
The patient is slightly pale and icteric. He has a widespread purpuric rash with conjunctival haemorrhages (Fig. 8.1). His pulse and blood pressure are normal. The liver is enlarged but there is no splenomegaly. The lungs are clear.

Has examination narrowed down your differential diagnosis?
Anaemia, jaundice, renal dysfunction and hepatomegaly are common in leptospirosis and severe malaria. A purpuric rash and conjunctival congestion are features of both leptospirosis and DHF.

Dengue infections are a major cause of morbidity and mortality in the tropical and subtropical regions of the world. Although sporadic cases of dengue can occur, disease outbreaks or epidemics are much more common. The patient may have back pain and severe myalgia ('break-bone fever'). The illness may be mild and self-limiting, but severe forms of disease such as DHF or dengue shock syndrome (DSS) can occur. The severe form is characterised by hypovolaemia, raised haematocrit and low platelet counts. Endothelial permeability and subsequent plasma leakage are important pathological features of DHF. Patients may develop unilateral or bilateral pleural effusions, ascites or a perihepatic collection of fluid. Typically, gallbladder wall thickening occurs. These findings can be detected on ultrasonography of the abdomen and chest. The exact cause for the drop in the platelet count is not known. Mechanisms include transient suppression of haematopoiesis and immune-mediated platelet clearance. Bleeding can occur from several sites, such as the gastrointestinal tract, lungs and nose. Intracranial haemorrhage can be fatal. Hypotension or shock occurs in severe cases.

Leptospirosis requires serious consideration in this patient because he has a leucocytosis and hepatic and renal dysfunction, in addition to a purpuric rash. Leptospirosis is common in the tropics. Recent large outbreaks have been described in Asia, Central and South America and the USA. The disease appears to be ubiquitous in wildlife and in many domestic animals. The most frequent host is a rodent, especially the common rat. The organisms persist indefinitely in the convoluted tubules of the kidney without causing apparent disease, and are shed into the urine periodically. Leptospires can enter human hosts through intact skin or mucous membranes, but entry is facilitated by cuts or abrasions. This spirochaete can survive in water for months. Our patient is a farmer; certain occupational groups are at high risk and these include agricultural workers, sewage workers, veterinarians, workers in abattoirs and those in the fishing industry. People engaged in recreational water activities are also likely to acquire the infection. After a brief period of bacteraemia, leptospires are distributed throughout the body. The main organs affected in humans are the kidneys, liver, meninges and brain. Leptospires damage the wall of small vessels, leading to vasculitis, which is ultimately responsible for several manifestations of the disease, including haemorrhages and hypovolaemia. In some patients, a non-oliguric hypokalaemic renal failure can occur at an early stage of leptospirosis. Moderate to severe hypokalaemia, if present, is a useful laboratory parameter to differentiate leptospirosis from other infectious causes of acute renal failure. Our patient has a purpuric rash and hepatic and renal dysfunction. Leptospirosis does not usually cause marked hepatocellular necrosis. However, it can produce severe disease, known as Weil's syndrome, characterised by hepatic and renal dysfunction with bleeding manifestations. Centrilobular necrosis with Kupffer cell hyperplasia is seen in the liver histopathology.

Hepatic involvement in leptospirosis requires differentiation from acute viral hepatitis. In leptospirosis, fever and jaundice occur concomitantly, whereas in acute viral hepatitis, fever is frequently low-grade and is followed by the onset of jaundice. In contrast to acute viral hepatitis, leptospirosis produces large increases in serum bilirubin and alkaline phosphatase, and a modest increase in hepatic enzymes (up to 200 U/L), whereas viral hepatitis causes a several-fold increase in the hepatic enzymes (often >1000 U/L) and a modest increase in serum bilirubin. In addition, creatine phosphokinase may be elevated during the first week in nearly half of the cases of leptospirosis. In severe cases, rhabdomyolysis occurs and contributes to renal dysfunction. Rarely, a fatal pulmonary syndrome may occur in severe leptospirosis due to haemorrhage in the lungs. This syndrome may produce acute respiratory failure. Narrowing down of the differential diagnosis requires further investigations.

 Further investigations

The results of further investigation are provided in Box 8.2.

Does this narrow down your differential diagnosis?

The negative results of thick and thin films, as well as the 'dipstick' test for malaria, make it most unlikely that the patient is suffering from severe malaria. Dengue and rickettsial fever have also been excluded. Leptospirosis remains a

---

BOX 8.2

Further investigations

Thick and thin peripheral blood film for malarial parasites	Negative
Immunochromatographic 'dipstick' test for *falciparum* malaria	Negative
Bilirubin	105 μmol/L (5 mg/dL)
ALT	170 U/L
AST	240 U/L
Prothrombin time	12 s (control 12 s)
Haemoglobin	90 g/L (9 g/dL)
Platelets	150×10^9/L (10^3/mm^3)
Blood culture	Negative
Blood tests for dengue antigen and antibody	Negative
Rickettsia group-specific microscopic agglutination test	Negative

strong possibility in this case, but definitive diagnostic tests are required for its confirmation.

The definitive diagnosis of leptospirosis depends upon the isolation of the organism, serological tests or detection of specific DNA. Blood cultures may be positive if taken before the 10th day of the illness and leptospires appear in the urine during the second week of illness. The serological investigation of choice is the microscopic agglutination test (MAT). Enzyme-linked immunosorbent assay (ELISA) and immunofluorescent assays are also available. Polymerase chain reaction (PCR) shows great promise in detecting leptospiral DNA in blood in early symptomatic disease; it is positive in the urine from the 8th day onward and remains positive for many months afterwards.

Definitive investigations

Leptospires are isolated from a urine specimen and so the final diagnosis is leptospirosis.

How will you treat this patient?

Intravenous benzylpenicillin is administered as 1.5 mega-units 6-hourly for 1 week or doxycycline in oral doses of 100 mg 12-hourly for 1 week. Parenteral ceftriaxone 1 g daily or cefotaxime 1 g 6-hourly is equally as effective as penicillin. Rarely, a Jarisch Herxheimer reaction can occur during initiation of antibiotic treatment. The patient's renal failure should be monitored closely; if deterioration occurs, peritoneal or haemodialysis may be life-saving. The general care of the patient is critically important. Blood should be taken early for grouping and cross-matching. Episodes of bleeding should be treated by prompt blood transfusion. Higher mortality rates have been reported in elderly patients, those with Weil's syndrome and severe pulmonary haemorrhage syndrome.

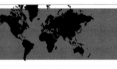

Key points and global issues

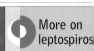

More on leptospiros

See Chapter 13 of **Davidson's Princip** & **Practice** of **Medicine (21st ed**

- Dengue is endemic in South-east Asia and India, and is also seen in Africa.

- Viral haemorrhagic fever produces a non-specific syndrome and can be caused by several different viruses. It should be included in the differential diagnosis because of the increase in international travel.

- African haemorrhagic fever due to Marburg and Ebola viruses can present with haemorrhage and hepatitis but renal involvement is absent.

- Malaria occurs throughout the tropics and subtropics at altitudes below 1500 metres.

- Leptospirosis is one of the most common zoonotic diseases, favoured by a tropical climate and flooding during monsoons.

- Leptospirosis control measures should consist of avoidance of exposure to infected urine/tissues, rodent control and vaccination of animals. Vaccination of humans (against a specific serovar) has been successful in some Asian and European countries.

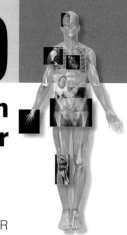

9

Short duration high-grade fever

S. SUNDAR

Presenting problem

A 30-year-old farmer is brought to an Emergency Department in Delhi on a hot July afternoon with a high-grade fever and altered conscious level. He was found in a disoriented state by co-workers in the field. His wife reports that he is normally very fit and well, but that he has had a very high temperature for the past 8 days and was febrile when he went out to work this morning. She gives no history of severe headache, loss of consciousness or seizures.

What would your differential diagnosis include before examining the patient?

This patient presented with a very high temperature and reduced conscious level, with a history of manual labour under the hot tropical sun. Heat stroke is very high up the list of potential differential diagnoses and must be treated immediately. However, the preceding history of fever should arouse suspicion of other potential causes.

The differential diagnosis of short duration high-grade fever in the tropics is extensive. Malaria is one of the most common infections, and so cerebral malaria, which is a medical emergency, has to be considered. Enteric fever usually presents with altered consciousness by the end of the second week. Encephalitis and meningitis (tuberculous, other bacterial and viral) are other possibilities, although extreme elevation of temperature is uncommon in meningitis. Japanese B encephalitis is endemic in India, South-east Asia, Japan and China. It has a case fatality of 25–50%, and survivors are left with disabling neurological sequelae. Other common causes of fever in the tropics, like dengue and leptospirosis, should also be considered while examining this patient, although the level of consciousness is seldom affected in these conditions.

Examination

The patient's rectal temperature is recorded to be 40°C and his skin is hot and dry. His Glasgow Coma Scale (GCS) is 7, but there is no meningism and no focal neurological signs. Pulse rate is 120/min and blood pressure is 94/52 mmHg. The spleen is palpable 2 cm below the costal margin. The rest of the examination is normal.

The patient's clothes are removed, his entire body is sprayed with water in front of a fan and ice packs are applied. After a venous blood sample is taken, intravenous fluids are started. With this treatment, the patient's temperature normalises in 45 min, but there is only mild improvement in his conscious level (GCS 10).

Has examination narrowed down your differential diagnosis?

The failure of the farmer's conscious level to improve significantly following cooling makes heat stroke unlikely. The absence of conjunctival haemorrhage, icterus and signs of meningeal irritation makes leptospirosis or meningitis less probable. Dengue usually presents with a transient morbilliform rash, severe aches ('break-bone fever') and circulatory failure, or with haemorrhagic signs like petechiae, ecchymosis or gastrointestinal bleeding in its infrequent haemorrhagic form. The absence of any of these features practically rules out dengue. The presence of splenomegaly makes malaria and enteric fever more likely possibilities. The sequelae of viral encephalitis are so serious that it must be formally excluded.

Investigations

Initial blood test results are shown in Box 9.1. Blood cultures and a Widal test are negative. Magnetic resonance imagining (MRI) of the brain and cerebrospinal fluid (CSF) examination are normal. CSF testing for Japanese B encephalitis virus is negative. Thick and thin peripheral blood smears show high levels (>5% infected red blood cells) of ring forms of *Plasmodium falciparum* (Fig. 9.1).

Does this narrow down your differential diagnosis?

MRI findings of bilateral thalamic lesions are quite characteristic of Japanese B encephalitis. The absence of these features and the negative antigen tests exclude this important diagnosis. The presence of ring forms of *Plasmodium falciparum* in the peripheral smear of a patient with impaired consciousness, where other encephalopathies have been ruled out, clinches the diagnosis of cerebral malaria.

BOX 9.1	
Initial investigations	
Haemoglobin	70 g/L (7 g/dL)
WCC	16.4×10⁹/L (10³/mm³)
Platelets	167×10⁹/L (10³/mm³)
Urea	36 mmol/L (100 mg/dL)
Creatinine	120 µmol/L (1.36 mg/dL)
Glucose	4.5 mmol/L (81 mg/dL)
Bilirubin	34.2 µmol/L (2 mg/dL)
AST (SGOT)	75 U/L
ALT (SGPT)	92 U/L
Alkaline phosphatase	200 U/L

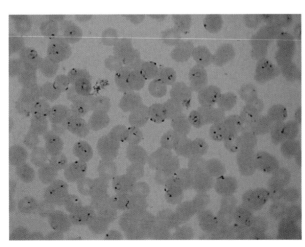

Figure 9.1 Peripheral blood smear of the patient showing numerous erythrocytes infected with ring forms of *Plasmodium falciparum*. The size of the erythrocytes is normal, with several of them infected with multiple parasites; this is characteristic of *falciparum* infection.

How will you treat this patient?

As cerebral malaria is associated with significant mortality and persistent neuro-cognitive impairments in survivors (especially children), it is a medical emergency and requires careful and urgent management with parenteral antimalarial therapy. The airway should be maintained, dehydration should be corrected with intravenous fluids and the patient should be nursed on his side. Intravenous artesunate should be commenced: artesunate should be given as 2.4 mg/kg i.v. at 0, 12 and 24 hours and then once daily for 7 days. However, as soon as the patient has recovered sufficiently to swallow tablets, oral artesunate 2 mg/kg once daily is given instead of i.v. therapy, to complete a total cumulative dose of 17–18 mg/kg. Hypoglycaemia is an important and serious complication of cerebral malaria and occurs as a result of malaria itself or its treatment with quinine. This complication is more common in children and pregnant women. Since artesunate is contraindicated in the 1st trimester of pregnancy, quinine should be used and is given as an intravenous infusion over 4 h. Treatment should be started with a loading dose infusion of 20 mg/kg quinine *salt* – up to a maximum of 1.4 g quinine can be given over 4 h. Then every 8–12 h, a maintenance dose of 10 mg/kg quinine *salt* is given (up to a maximum of 700 mg/dose), until the patient can take drugs orally. Once the patient is able to take oral medication, mefloquine 25 mg/kg (total dose) should be added. Alternatively, doxycycline 100 mg daily could be administered for 7 days. Clindamycin should be substituted for doxycycline during pregnancy. Fresh blood should be transfused if the patient has a severe anaemia.

Blood pressure, urine output, blood glucose, parasite count and haematocrit should all be monitored regularly so that other complications of severe *falciparum* malaria (hypoglycaemia, severe anaemia, acute renal failure, acute respiratory distress syndrome, peripheral circulatory failure and shock) can be detected and managed early.

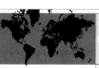

Key points and global issues

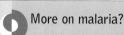
More on malaria?

See Chapter 13 of
Davidson's Principles
& **Practice** of
Medicine (21st edn)

- Infection with *Plasmodium falciparum* can lead to life-threatening complicated malaria with multi-organ involvement.

- In residents of the tropics or travellers returning from endemic countries, fever with an altered conscious level should arouse suspicion of complicated malaria.

- Malarial retinopathy, characterised by whitening of the macula (sparing of the central fovea), peripheral retina, retinal vessels, papilloedema and haemorrhages occurs more commonly in children with cerebral malaria (>60%) and indicates a poor prognosis.

- A high incidence of both transient and permanent neurological deficits in children with cerebral malaria produces a huge socioeconomic burden in countries with limited resources. Therefore, early diagnosis and treatment are crucial.

- As chloroquine resistance is quite common in malaria-endemic regions of the world, treatment of complicated malaria should only be initiated with either quinine or artemisinin derivatives and it is usually prudent to add a second antimalarial drug. Steroids should not be administered, as they are harmful.

- Prevention of malaria should be a priority and diligent efforts must continue to develop efficient insecticides and vaccines.

10

Weight loss

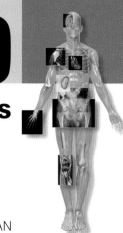

A. MOHAN

Presenting problem

A 74-year-old woman presents with anorexia and weight loss of 15 kg over the preceding 3 months. There is no history of fever or diarrhoea. She is an otherwise healthy woman who has never visited a hospital until the present episode of ill-health. She does not smoke or drink alcohol and is not taking any medication.

What would your differential diagnosis include before examining the patient?

When an elderly woman presents with gradual onset of anorexia and weight loss without accompanying fever, the differential diagnosis (Box 10.1) would include organic causes such as underlying malignant disease, chronic infections, gastrointestinal disorders, chronic obstructive pulmonary disease, diabetes mellitus, hyperthyroidism, chronic renal failure, depression and dementia. Although not applicable to this case, alcoholism and drug-induced weight loss would also have to be considered as causes in the appropriate setting.

Examination

Physical examination reveals a frail, pale-looking, emaciated elderly woman whose body mass index (BMI, kg/m^2) is 13. She is well-oriented in time, place and person, and her mini-mental status examination (MMSE) score is 26. She can clearly understand her problem and is worried as to why she is losing weight. There is no evidence of peripheral lymphadenopathy or hepatosplenomegaly. Pelvic examination is normal. The rest of the physical examination is also unremarkable.

Has examination narrowed down your differential diagnosis?

Other than evidence of wasting and pallor, there are no clues to help in the localisation of this patient's weight

BOX 10.1

Causes of weight loss in an elderly patient

Physiological causes
- Anorexia of ageing

Organic causes
- Underlying malignant disease (primary or metastatic)
- Endocrine disorders (hyperthyroidism, diabetes mellitus, Addison's disease)
- Renal failure
- Chronic infections such as tuberculosis, HIV/AIDS, brucellosis and parasitic infestations
- Gastrointestinal problems (e.g. malabsorption syndrome, inflammatory bowel disease, pernicious anaemia, cirrhosis)
- Chronic obstructive pulmonary disease
- Chronic congestive cardiac failure
- Parkinsonism

Other causes
- Alcohol and drugs (metformin, levodopa and angiotensin-converting enzyme (ACE) inhibitors)
- Psychiatric problems (e.g. depression, dementia)
- Unknown

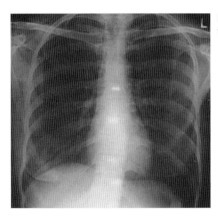

Figure 10.1 A normal X-ray (postero-anterior view) on the patient's admission.

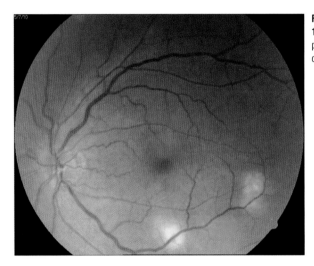

Figure 10.2 Ophthalmoscopic picture showing multiple choroidal tubercles.

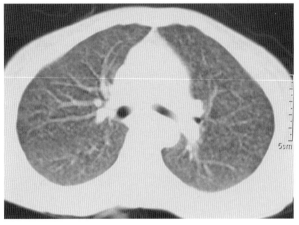

Figure 10.3 High-resolution CT of the chest of the same patient, showing a classical miliary pattern.

loss. This is often the case. Given that she is well-oriented and has clear thinking, depression, dementia and other psychological problems and physiological anorexia of ageing seem unlikely. Even although fever is absent, infection cannot be excluded, as fever sometimes may not be evident in elderly individuals with chronic low-grade infections.

Investigations

The following blood results are obtained: haemoglobin 72 g/L (7.2 g/dL), a total leucocyte count of 2.8×10^9/L (10^3/mm^3) and a platelet count of 90×10^9/L (10^3/mm^3). Peripheral smear examination shows a normocytic normochromic picture and pancytopenia. The erythrocyte sedimentation rate (ESR) is elevated (80 mm at the end of the 1st hour, Westergren method). Serum biochemistry, including electrolytes and urine examination, are normal. Urine culture is sterile. An oral glucose tolerance test rules out diabetes mellitus. Stool examination for parasites and occult blood is negative on three occasions. A tuberculin skin test (TST) with 5 tuberculin units (TU) of purified protein derivative (PPD) is negative. She is human immunodeficiency virus (HIV)-seronegative. The thyroid profile is within normal limits. The chest X-ray on admission (Fig. 10.1) is reported to be normal. Abdominal ultrasonography reveals kidneys with normal size and echo texture and no intra-abdominal lymphadenopathy or focal lesions in liver, spleen or other viscera. The patient undergoes upper gastrointestinal endoscopy and colonoscopy and these tests are also unremarkable.

In view of the pancytopenia, trephine biopsy of the bone marrow is performed. It reveals granulomas with caseous necrosis and acid-fast bacilli (AFB). Subsequently, a fundus examination performed following mydriatic administration reveals choroidal tubercles (Fig. 10.2). A high-resolution computed tomography (HRCT) of the chest (Fig. 10.3) reveals a classical miliary pattern. Lumbar puncture is also performed and the cerebrospinal fluid analysis is documented as normal.

Does this narrow down your differential diagnosis?

The patient has 'cryptic miliary tuberculosis'. Unlike in classical miliary tuberculosis, fever may sometimes be absent, especially among the elderly, and patients may present with progressive wasting, mimicking a metastatic carcinoma. In these patients, the chest X-ray may be normal and the TST is often negative. Blood dyscrasias such as pancytopenia may sometimes be evident. This constitutes a valuable diagnostic clue and would call for bone marrow examination, which may confirm the diagnosis as in this case. In earlier days, cryptic miliary tuberculosis was often diagnosed at autopsy. However, with the availability of HRCT, many of these cases are now diagnosed during life.

How will you treat this patient?

Miliary tuberculosis is fatal if untreated and antituberculosis treatment remains the essential treatment strategy. In the absence of associated meningeal involvement, 6 months of treatment (a 2-month intensive phase with isoniazid, rifampicin, pyrazinamide and ethambutol, followed by a 4-month continuation phase with isoniazid and rifampicin) appears to be adequate. In the presence of associated tuberculosis meningitis, treatment needs to be given for at least 12 months. In view of the high frequency of associated tuberculosis meningitis in miliary tuberculosis, all patients with miliary tuberculosis should undergo a lumbar puncture so that they receive treatment of the optimum duration. The World Health Organization endorses the use of directly observed treatment, short-course (DOTS) therapy for all patients with tuberculosis.

Key points and global issues

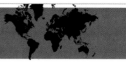

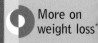

More on
weight loss

See Chapter 22 of
Davidson's Principl
& **Practice** of
Medicine (21st edn

- Miliary tuberculosis is a potentially lethal disease with varied clinical manifestations and is uniformly fatal if not treated. A high index of clinical suspicion and systematic diagnostic evaluation directed at establishing an early diagnosis will facilitate early institution of specific antituberculosis treatment that can be life-saving.

- Clinical presentation of miliary tuberculosis in the elderly can be misleading. Absence of fever and the presence of anorexia and weight loss mimicking metastatic carcinoma all delay the diagnosis of miliary tuberculosis.

- Miliary tuberculosis is increasingly being encountered in elderly patients. The HIV/AIDS pandemic, widespread use of immunosuppressive drugs, the modulating effect of BCG (bacille Calmette–Guérin) vaccination, increasing use of CT, and a wider application of invasive diagnostic methods may all be relevant in explaining some of this demographic shift.

- Choroidal tubercles, if present, are pathognomonic of miliary tuberculosis and offer a valuable clue to the diagnosis. Therefore, systematic ophthalmoscopic examination after mydriatic administration must be performed in every patient in whom the diagnosis is suspected.

- Disseminated histoplasmosis, especially in HIV/AIDS patients, can also produce a similar appearance on HRCT of the chest.

- Several other diseases can produce a miliary pattern on HRCT of the chest. These include miliary metastasis from thyroid malignancy and pneumoconiosis.

11

Acute diarrhoea

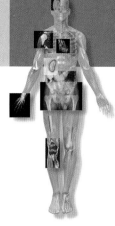

W. T. A. TODD

Presenting problem

A 68-year-old Caucasian woman is admitted to hospital 2 weeks after returning from a Spanish holiday. While she was there, she had symptoms of a urinary tract infection and at a local clinic was given a 5-day course of co-amoxiclav, which she completed while she was away. For 1 week, she has had intermittent fevers and shivers accompanied by profuse diarrhoea. Her bowels have been opening 8–10 times daily and the diarrhoea is watery with some fresh blood staining in the last 72 h. She also complains of colicky lower abdominal pain relieved by defaecation. Her GP sent a stool sample for bacterial culture and the patient was given a 3-day course of ciprofloxacin, but she remains symptomatic despite having completed this. She is normally well, smokes 10 cigarettes/day, drinks only social alcohol and her only regular medication is omeprazole for reflux oesophagitis. Her partner had loose stools for 3–4 days on return from holiday, but is now better.

What would your differential diagnosis include before examining the patient?

There are numerous potential causes of blood-stained diarrhoea, but the history of fever and rigors, the recent holiday abroad and similar symptomatology in a family contact all suggest an infective cause. The most likely culprits would be: *Campylobacter*, non-typhoidal salmonellae, verocytotoxigenic *Escherichia coli* (VTEC), e.g. *E. coli* O157, *Shigella* (rare) and *Clostridium difficile*. The possibility of non-infectious diarrhoea must also be considered, with, diverticular disease, inflammatory bowel disease and new-presentation of bowel malignancy as possibilities.

Examination and initial investigations

On examination, the woman is pyrexial, with a temperature of 38.1°C, and is clinically dehydrated. Pulse is 112/min, respiratory rate 20 breaths/min and blood pressure 110/67 mmHg. Her abdomen is not distended, but she is tender in the infra-umbilical region and there are active bowel sounds. A rectal examination reveals loose brown liquid stools with admixed fresh blood. Initial blood test results are shown in Box 11.1. Chest and abdominal X-rays are normal. The stool culture from the sample sent from the GP surgery grows a *Salmonella* species.

Have examination and initial investigations narrowed down your differential diagnosis?

Clinical examination is notoriously unhelpful in differentiating infective from other causes of acute diarrhoea. The lack of definitive surgical features on abdominal examination is reassuring. The stool culture, however, has confirmed *Salmonella* gastroenteritis. In view of the patient's age and ongoing fever, plus her medication with a proton pump inhibitor, the possibility of *Salmonella* bacteraemia must be considered.

She may still have background diverticular disease, although this is less likely to be implicated in her presentation on this occasion. Infective gastroenteritis from any cause can produce symptoms and signs of colonic inflammation, but salmonellae tend to produce predominantly small bowel disease.

Further investigations

Blood cultures reveal *Salmonella* species in the aerobic bottles. A transthoracic echocardiogram is normal and, in particular, the aortic root dimension is normal. An ultrasound examination of the abdomen is unremarkable. Plain X-rays of the cervical, thoracic and lumbar spines are normal. Erythrocyte sedimentation rate (ESR) is 49 mm/h and C-reactive protein (CRP) is 65 mg/L.

Does this narrow down your differential diagnosis?

This woman has *Salmonella* bacteraemia; at her age this can have serious consequences, with possible endovascular and distant bone infection. Blood cultures are positive in 1–5% of those with salmonella gastroenteritis. Risk factors for bacteraemia are extremes of age, gastric hypoacidity, immunocompromise both acquired and secondary to conditions such as rheumatoid arthritis and TNF blockade with agents such as infliximal. *Salmonella* bacteraemia is particularly associated with metastatic infection.

Endovascular infection occurs in 10–20% of persons over 50, and usually involves the aorta. Any cause of hypochlorhydria, including proton pump inhibitor therapy, removes the body's primary defence against food poisoning bacteria, including Salmonellae. Antimicrobial therapy, particularly with aminopenicillins can prolong faecal carriage of *Salmonella* species.

How will you treat this patient?

Initially, she needs adequate fluid to replace both her established losses and, additionally, to cover for ongoing fluid loss from persistent diarrhoea. If she can take oral fluid, then she should have 1–2 L of oral rehydration solution (ORS), followed by 200 mL per each loose stool; this is in addition to her normal maintenance fluid requirements. If she cannot take oral fluid, then intravenous fluid replacement with predominantly normal saline should be given to replace established losses rapidly (1–2 L in the first 4 h), then fluid maintenance should continue, with additional allowance for any ongoing diarrhoeal losses.

The microbiology laboratory must be asked to confirm antimicrobial susceptibility of this isolate since, notoriously, *Salmonella* originating from the Mediterranean and Asia has increased levels of ciprofloxacin resistance. The antibiotics

BOX 11.1	
Initial investigations	
Haemoglobin	142 g/L (14.2 g/dL)
WCC	12.5×10^9/L (10^3/mm^3)
Platelets	410×10^9/L (10^3/mm^3)
Sodium	134 mmol/L (mEq/L)
Potassium	3.4 mmol/L (mEq/L)
Chloride	103 mmol/L (mEq/L)
Bicarbonate	18 mmol/L (mEq/L)
Urea	9.7 mmol/L (27.17 mg/dL)
Creatinine	100 µmol/L (1.13 mg/dL)
AST	29 U/L
ALT	43 U/L
LDH	396 U/L
Alkaline phosphatase	104 U/L
GGT	71 U/L
Bilirubin	13 µmol/L (0.78 mg/dL)

required for *Salmonella* eradication are frequently associated with *C. difficile* infection, so must be used with caution. Although high-dose ciprofloxacin remains the treatment of choice, the increasing resistance to this antibiotic in Europe and Asia must be considered. Oral therapy is sufficient, unless there is persistent vomiting or evidence of ongoing sepsis or endovascular/bony infection. A prolonged (2–3-week) course should be prescribed. The i.v. fluoroquinolones or ceftriaxone are alternatives, as is azithromycin. Endovascular or bone infections require surgical intervention and prolonged therapy, guided by microbiological and clinical expertise.

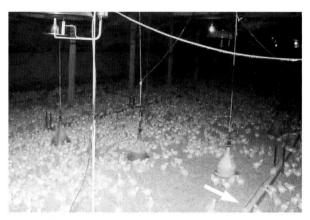

Figure 11.1 Intensive rearing in sheds with thousands of birds together promotes the spread of Salmonellae. The continuous feed belt (arrow) is open to faecal contamination.

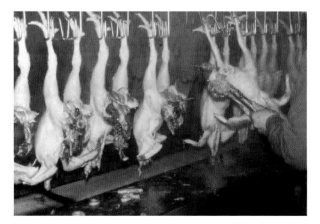

Figure 11.2 Mass slaughter operations clearly add to the potential for cross-contamination of carcasses.

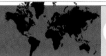
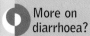
See Chapter 13 of
Davidson's Principles
& **Practice** of
Medicine (21st edn)

- Non-typhoidal (or food poisoning) *Salmonella* remains, worldwide, a very common cause of food-borne disease.

- Many different foods are implicated, ranging from faecal contaminated vegetables and crops to dairy products. Meat products, particularly those containing chicken or uncooked eggs, are the most important and the serotypes most often involved are *S. typhimurium*, dt.104 and *S. enteritidis*, phage type 4.

- The spread of these serotypes has been facilitated by both intensive rearing conditions (Fig. 11.1) and mass production of broiler chickens (Fig. 11.2) prevalent in parts of the developed world. Free-range birds found throughout the world in smallholdings pose a much-reduced risk in this respect.

- An embargo on uncooked egg dishes, coupled with an aggressive culling and vaccination policy in the UK and Scandinavia, has significantly reduced the incidence of *Salmonella* food poisoning over the last decade. This is not so in parts of the world where no such action has been undertaken.

- Quinolone resistance is widespread in Asia, Southern Africa and parts of Europe where these drugs are often freely available as over-the-counter preparations (without prescription) and consequently used with indiscretion.

12

Eosinophilia

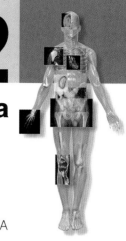

S. VARMA

Presenting problem

A 32-year-old man of Indian origin is referred to the chest clinic with a 6-month history of progressive breathlessness and dry cough that is worse at night. There is no history of fever, chest pain, haemoptysis or wheezing. The patient complains of anorexia and weight loss, but was apparently normal 6 months ago. He is not on any medication. He denies any associated joint pain or swelling, focal sensory or motor symptoms, rashes or the passage of worms in his stools. There is no family history of atopy or asthma. A chest X-ray, performed on the advice of his GP, was normal. Sputum smears for acid-fast bacilli have been negative on three occasions. A complete blood count is subsequently carried out and an increased eosinophil count is identified (Box 12.1).

BOX 12.1	
Initial investigations	
Haemoglobin	110 g/L (11 g/dL)
WCC	28.8×10⁹/L (10³/mm³)
Differential count	
Polymorphs	36%
Lymphocytes	12%
Monocytes	1%
Eosinophils	51%
Absolute eosinophil count	14.7×10⁹/L (10³/mm³)
Peripheral blood film	No atypical cells

What is your differential diagnosis before examining the patient?

The patient has eosinophilia (peripheral blood eosinophil count $>5.0\times10^9$/L (10^3/mm^3); this is common in many settings such as parasitic infections, drugs (sulphonamides, penicillins, cephalosporins, etc.), allergies (hay fever, asthma, allergic bronchopulmonary aspergillosis, etc.) and malignancies (chronic myeloid leukaemia, Hodgkin's disease, etc.). Peripheral blood eosinophilia can be classified into secondary (cytokine-driven reactive phenomenon), clonal (presence of a bone marrow histological, cytogenetic or molecular marker of a myeloid malignancy) and idiopathic (neither secondary nor clonal) categories (Box 12.2). However, a moderate ($1.5–5.0\times10^9$/L (10^3/mm^3)) to marked ($>5.0\times10^9$/L (10^3/mm^3)) increase in the eosinophil count is often associated with Loeffler's syndrome, idiopathic hyper-eosinophilic syndrome, tropical pulmonary eosinophilia, eosinophilic pneumonia, allergic bronchopulmonary aspergillosis (ABPA) and clonal eosinophilic disorders, such as eosinophilic leukaemia.

Loeffler's syndrome is a benign disorder characterised by transient migratory pulmonary infiltrates and peripheral blood eosinophilia, generally lasting for 3 weeks and associated with the passage of larvae during the life cycles of *Ascaris lumbricoides*, hookworms (*Necator americanus* and *Ancylostoma duodenale*) and *Strongyloides stercoralis* through the lungs. Marked eosinophilia with pulmonary symptoms is also known to occur in association with visceral or cutaneous larva migrans, infection with lung flukes and haematogenous spread of *Trichinella spiralis* or schistosomal infections.

ABPA is characterised by bronchial hyperreactivity, pulmonary infiltrates and central bronchiectasis in a patient with long-standing asthma or cystic fibrosis and hypersensitivity to the conidial colonisation of *Aspergillus fumigatus*. The Churg–Strauss syndrome is a systemic antineutrophil cytoplasmic antibody (ANCA)-associated vasculitis that involves small- and medium-vessel arteries and is characteristically accompanied by asthma and peripheral blood eosinophilia. Eosinophilic pneumonias (acute and chronic) are a rare group of steroid-responsive pulmonary eosinophilic disorders.

The idiopathic hyper-eosinophilic syndrome represents a heterogeneous group of disorders with the common feature of prolonged eosinophilia of unknown cause and multi-organ dysfunction, including the heart, central nervous system, kidneys, lungs, gastrointestinal tract and skin. Tropical pulmonary eosinophilia is a symptom complex of dyspnoea, fever, intense eosinophilia, pulmonary infiltrates, with or without wheezing, and weight loss. Characteristics of tropical eosinophilia include an extreme degree of peripheral blood eosinophilia (generally $\geq 30 \times 10^9/L$), high titres of antifilarial antibody and extreme elevation of serum immunoglobulin (Ig) E, typically more than 1000 IU/mL. Classically, there is an absence of circulating microfilariae in the presence of high antifilarial antibody titres. Eosinophilic leukaemia is now considered a chronic myeloproliferative disorder and is grouped with chronic myeloid leukaemia. It may occur as part of an established chronic myeloproliferative disorder such as chronic myeloid leukaemia; at times it accompanies acute leukaemia or it may be unclassified.

Examination

Physical examination does not reveal any skin lesions, lymphadenopathy or hepatosplenomegaly. Examination of the chest and cardiovascular and other systems is unremarkable.

Has examination narrowed down your differential diagnosis?

No, not at all! In some haematological abnormalities such as eosinophilia, there are no characteristic physical signs or so-called 'easy spot' diagnoses (e.g. a patient with acromegaly or Cushing's syndrome). Further diagnosis, as in this case, will often depend on investigations directed towards common conditions such as parasitic infestations, ABPA and so on. Also, unlike many other disorders, there are no initial key discriminatory tests and a battery of investigations has to be performed before the diagnosis can actually be 'hit'.

Further investigations

A stool examination is normal and an immediate hypersensitivity skin test against *Aspergillus fumigatus* is negative. Echocardiography is normal and so is an ultrasound examination of the abdomen. Spirometry is suggestive of mild airflow obstruction without any significant bronchodilator reversibility. High-resolution computed tomography (HRCT; Fig. 12.1) shows randomly scattered 'miliary' nodular opacities distributed throughout the lung fields with areas of patchy ground-glass opacities. The patient undergoes a fibreoptic bronchoscopy. A differential cell count in the bronchoalveolar lavage fluid reveals an eosinophil count of 35%; bronchoscopic lung biopsy reveals a bronchocentric eosinophilic infiltrate. The total serum IgE level is significantly elevated at 4500 IU/mL (normal 0–300 IU/mL). An enzyme-linked immunosorbent assay (ELISA) for antifilarial antibody (antibodies against *Wuchereria bancrofti*) is positive.

Does this narrow down your differential diagnosis?

A diagnosis of tropical pulmonary eosinophilia is made.

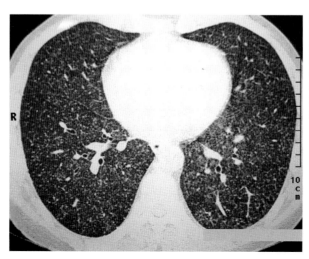

Figure 12.1 High-resolution computed tomography shows bilateral, randomly scattered, miliary nodular opacities and patchy ground-glass opacities.

How will you treat this patient?

This young man is started on diethylcarbamazine at a dosage of 6 mg/kg per day for 3 weeks. With this, he shows complete resolution of symptoms. HRCT of the chest is repeated after 4 weeks and shows almost complete clearance of the lesions. Repeat spirometry, performed 6 weeks after treatment, is reported to be normal. The response to treatment confirms the final diagnosis of tropical pulmonary eosinophilia.

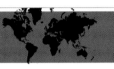

Key points and global issues

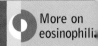

More on eosinophili

See Chapter 13 of **Davidson's Principl & Practice** of **Medicine (21st ed**

- Parasitic infections, especially by tissue-dwelling helminths, are the most common cause of marked eosinophilia in endemic areas. Elsewhere, allergic phenomena and drug hypersensitivity are frequent causes. Other causes include connective tissue diseases, neoplasia, idiopathic hyper-eosinophilic syndrome and primary bone marrow disorders like chronic myeloproliferative disorder or leukaemia.

- A travel history, as well as epidemiological information about parasitic infection, is important in all patients with eosinophilia. In persons with a history of travel to tropical countries, parasitic diseases should be actively pursued.

- Eosinophilia is more marked in patients with tissue-dwelling helminths. Stool examination is generally non-informative in such cases. Serological or molecular tests are needed to confirm the diagnosis.

- Relapses after successful treatment may occur in tropical pulmonary eosinophilia. Re-treatment with diethylcarbamazine is usually successful in such cases.

13

Snake bite

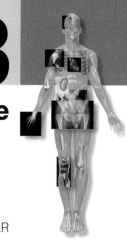

H. S. BAWASKAR

Presenting problem

A 65-year-old woman is admitted at 6.00 a.m. to a general hospital in India. A relative reports that the patient is unable to open her eyes, lift her neck from pillow, has slurred speech and difficulty in swallowing. She was well the previous day and had worked on a farm as usual. At 3.30 a.m., the patient had arisen from her floor-bed with abdominal pain and had vomited. She also complained of mild pain and heaviness in her left calf, where she thought she had been bitten, possibly by a rat. There is no history of hypertension, transient ischaemic attacks, use of pesticides, headache or recurrent abdominal colic. A 1 metre long krait was seen under piles of firewood stored in the corner of the family hut and was killed by a member of the family (Fig. 13.1).

What would your differential diagnosis include before examination?

Pain in the abdomen and vomiting commonly occur in acute appendicitis, but do not progress to paralysis. Progressive weakness in all limbs, which is increased toward the end of the day, is seen in myasthenia gravis. Sudden onset of weakness, sweating, vomiting and extensive fasciculation are seen in a myasthenia crisis due to excessive dosing of anticholinesterases and in organophosphorus poisoning, but there is no history to suggest either of these possibilities. Absence of headache, transient ischaemic attack, hypertension and asymmetrical weakness make a stroke unlikely.

The finding of the snake in the home is certainly suspicious! The krait is nocturnal and on its way to hunt rats, lizards and mice it may enter a floor-bed and bite an individual. The majority of cases are reported between midnight and 6.00 a.m. The fangs of a krait are short (2–4 mm) and it injects a venom into the skin that is more poisonous than cobra venom. The victim usually gets minor pain at the bite site with no swelling or other manifestations. Hence, many cases give a history of 'unknown' bite, rat bite, ant bite or indeed no bite! A cobra bite would typically cause sudden severe pain, swelling, ecchymosis, local necrosis and neuroparalysis. There is also a rapid onset of local swelling and pain following a bite from a Russell's viper, but in addition, there is uncontrolled bleeding from the fang marks, with development of tense blisters and gangrene with systemic bleeding. An Echis bite causes swelling at the site of the bite, which develops slowly, and systemic bleeding may be seen after 1 week.

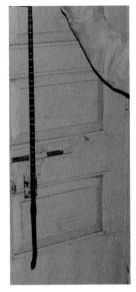

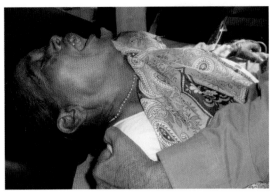

Figure 13.2 Bilateral ptosis and broken necks sign following krait bite.

Figure 13.1 The krait was found in the corner of the hut.

Examination

The patient is fully conscious, but has bilateral complete ptosis (Fig. 13.2), external ophthalmoplegia and dilated pupils which react poorly to light. Muscle power in the neck is grade 3/5 and in the limbs is 4/5. She is unable to count up to 10 in one breath and there is pooling of saliva in the mouth; she cannot open her mouth fully and is unable to protrude her tongue beyond the teeth margins. No fasciculations are seen. Plantar reflexes are flexor and tendon reflexes are present and symmetrical.

Her extremities are cold, the pulse is regular at 118 beats/min and her blood pressure is 170/110 mmHg. The respiratory rate is 6/min with intercostal muscle contraction and abdominal respiration (paradoxical respiration). Her expiratory nasal blow is poor and oxygen saturation on room air is 82%. There is no unusual odour of her breath or clothes. Her abdomen is soft with no tenderness in the iliac fossae. There is a small pin-head bite mark with minimal surrounding erythema and swelling seen over the middle of the left calf.

No abnormality is seen in peripheral blood. An electrocardiogram shows T-wave inversion in the precordial leads. Random blood sugar is 5.8 mmol/L (106 mg/dL). Whole blood clots within 20 min.

Have examination and initial investigations narrowed down your differential diagnosis?

Examination confirms the initial suspicions of a krait bite. There is no garlic odour, miosis and fasciculations to suggest organophosphorus poisoning and no features of an acute abdomen or acute stroke. Krait venom is a β-bungarotoxin, which initially promotes release of acetylcholine, resulting in abdominal pain, vomiting, sweating and raised blood pressure. Thereafter, it blocks predominately pre-synaptic acetylcholine receptors at the neuromuscular junction. Progressive neuromuscular blockade results in quadriplegia, ophthalmoplegia, bulbar palsy

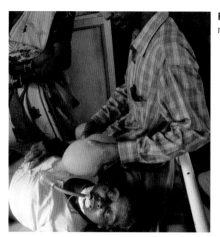

Figure 13.3 Transient improvement after neostigmine.

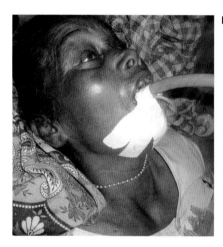

Figure 13.4 Complete recovery after 72 h.

and respiratory paralysis; reflexes are preserved and initially, the patient will be fully conscious. Raised blood pressure and abdominal pain are due to autonomic stimulation by krait venom. The dilated, poorly-reacting pupils suggest venom action on ciliary muscles.

Further investigations

There is a transient positive response (increased muscle power, reduction in ptosis, improvement in nasal blow) to intravenous neostigmine (Fig. 13.3).

How will you treat this patient?

Reassure the victim and anxious relative that with modern treatment total recovery is possible (Fig. 13.4). The patient requires respiratory support and ideally should undergo endotracheal intubation and assisted ventilation with a manual ventilator or mechanical ventilator. She should be transferred to an intensive care unit, if the facility is available. Anti-snake venin (ASV) should be administered – the precise form depends on local circumstances. In some areas, a polyvalent ASV is used, in others ELISA testing of urine and blood may be performed to confirm the type of snake bite and then a monospecific antivenin may be administered. In this instance, a polyvalent ASV, prepared by the Haffkine Institute, Mumbai, is used; this contains antivenin against cobra, krait, Russell's viper, and *Echis carinatus*. 100 mL of polyvalent snake antivenin is added to 100 mL of normal saline and infused at 2 mL (10–15 drops) per minute for 15 min, then the rate of infusion is increased to 3 mL/min. There is a risk of anaphylaxis, and the patient should be carefully monitored for signs of this; if there is no adverse reaction, the infusion should be continued and run-through over 1 hour; 25 µg/kg neostigmine should also be given by the intravenous route in the first hour and this must be preceded by 0.6 mg atropine to counteract the muscarinic actions of neostigmine. Anaphylaxis is managed in the conventional way with parenteral adrenaline, antihistamine and steroids and nebulised bronchodilators.

If there is no improvement within 1 hour, a further 50 mL of antivenin is added to 50 mL normal saline and is administered over 20 min. Then 20 mL of ASV, 1 mg neostigmine and 0.6 mg atropine are added to 500 mL of normal saline (elapid cocktail) and given 4-hourly for 24 h. Hypertension is controlled with 10 µg/min intravenous nitroglycerine given by infusion pump and assisted ventilation is continued until the victim is self-ventilating satisfactorily and starts pulling at the endotracheal tube. The patient should be followed-up regularly for 6 weeks in an outpatient department to rule out late serum sickness (lethargy, fever, lymphadenopathy and arthralgia) and neuropathy.

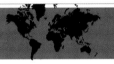

Key points and global issues

More on snake bites

See Chapter 9 of **Davidson's Princip & Practice** of **Medicine (21st ed**

- Snake bite is an occupational hazard and a disease of poverty and farmers and labourers.

- Worldwide, 3.4–5.5 million people are bitten by snakes each year, resulting in about 400 000 amputations and 20 000–125 000 deaths.

- The incidence and number of deaths from snake bites are higher than that seen individually from Chagas' disease, cholera, dengue haemorrhagic fever, leishmaniasis, Japanese encephalitis and yellow fever.

- The vast majority of snake-bite deaths occur in Asia (estimates range from 15 400–57 600 per annum) and sub-Saharan Africa (estimates range from 3500–32 100 deaths per annum).

- India has a higher mortality rate (>50 000/year) from snake bites than any other country.

- An ELISA test to detect krait antigen in the blood and urine samples can be used to confirm the diagnosis in doubtful cases, but is not widely available in India.

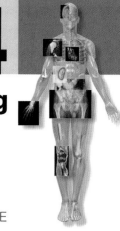

14

Unknown sting

L. KARALLIEDDE

Presenting problem

A 25-year-old woman, who lives in a small village in the south of India, is rushed to the Accident and Emergency Department of her local hospital. She was gathering firewood in the forest behind her cottage when she was stung on her right index finger by a scorpion hiding in the dead wood. She has been in good health until this incident and is not on any medication.

What would your differential diagnosis include before examining the patient?

Scorpions are nocturnal animals; their natural habitat is under stones or dead wood. In areas where scorpions are found, however, it is necessary to watch out for dark hiding places indoors, e.g. in cupboards, under the duvet and bed, in baseball gloves, in caps and in shoes. In general, scorpions are not aggressive and they do not hunt for prey; they wait for them. Scorpions do not attack human beings spontaneously, but sting when they feel trapped or are stepped on or disturbed. Thus, most stings occur on the hands or feet. Out of 1500 scorpion species, 50 are dangerous to humans. This woman comes from a part of the world where scorpions live, and if she says that she has been stung by a scorpion, then there should be no cause to doubt her as scorpion stings are familiar or known to the community.

Examination

On examination, the patient is restless and agitated – she is visibly in pain. Her right hand is very tender to the touch, and on tapping the affected finger, there is excruciating pain. Her pupils are dilated, and she is sweating profusely and is vomiting. Her pulse is 130 beats/min and blood pressure is 179/112 mmHg. In the short time that she has been in the Accident and Emergency Department, her condition has deteriorated rapidly. She becomes increasingly tachypnoeic, her oxygen saturation (on high-flow oxygen) falls to 89% and widespread crepitations are heard in the chest.

Has examination narrowed down your differential diagnosis?

There are 46 known species of scorpion in India, and unless the patient (or relatives) brings the offending scorpion into hospital with them, it is usually impossible to know which particular species was responsible. Stings from some of these species simply cause minor skin irritation, akin to a sting from a bee or wasp. As with stings from insects, scorpion stings can cause anaphylactic reactions in susceptible individuals.

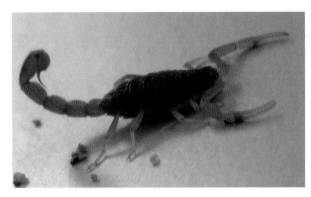

Figure 14.1 The Indian red scorpion.

Some species of scorpions, however, have a highly toxic venom that can be fatal. *Mesobuthus tamulus* (Indian red scorpion) is the most lethal species in the Buthidae family of scorpions (Fig. 14.1). Indian red scorpion venom contains neurotoxins that block sodium channels and thus cause spontaneous depolarisation of parasympathetic and sympathetic nerves. This results in an 'autonomic storm', characterised by transient cholinergic symptoms (vomiting, sweating, salivation, priapism (persistent and painful erection of the penis) in males, bradycardia and ventricular ectopics) and then sustained sympathetic stimulation (hypertension, tachycardia, pulmonary oedema, hyperglycaemia and shock), which is usually fatal. This woman is clearly extremely unwell and is deteriorating fast. This does not look like an anaphylactic reaction – there is no urticarial rash or wheeze. Unfortunately, it seems as though she is having a major toxic reaction to the scorpion sting.

Investigations

A 12-lead ECG shows sinus tachycardia and a chest X-ray reveals changes consistent with pulmonary oedema. Blood gas results are shown in Box 14.1. Routine biochemistry is normal and there is no coagulopathy. Blood glucose is 14.4 mmol/L (259 mg/dL).

Does this clinch the diagnosis?

This woman has all the hallmarks of an 'autonomic storm' response to the scorpion sting – most probably from an Indian red scorpion. Her prognosis is not good. She has a metabolic acidosis, which will almost certainly be a lactic acidosis – a direct consequence of tissue hypoxia. The pulmonary oedema is most likely due to acute left ventricular failure from myocardial toxicity and profound vasoconstriction and hypertension.

How will you treat this patient?

This woman is in extremis and requires urgent action to save her life. If the necessary facilities and expertise are available, she should be transferred to an intensive care unit where facilities for monitoring and assisted ventilation are available. Antivenin for a red scorpion sting is available in some parts of India. This is a solution of enzyme-digested, refined antibodies prepared from equine blood; 1 mL of the reconstituted serum neutralises 1 mg of dried red scorpion

BOX 14.1

Blood gas results on 60% oxygen

PO_2	6.9 kPa (52 mmHg)
PCO_2	3.1 kPa (23 mmHg)
H^+	64 nmol/L (pH 7.19)
HCO_3	19 mmol/L (mEq/L)

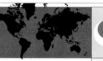

venom. However, there are problems with scorpion antivenin that limit its clinical use. Antivenins themselves can cause serious anaphylactic reactions; moreover, they are species-specific and, as has already been noted, in most instances, the precise species of scorpion causing the sting is not known. An alternative to administering antivenin is to give the α-blocker prazosin (0.5 mg 8-hourly orally or through a nasogastric tube, until all symptoms subside); indeed, randomised controlled studies have not proved that antivenin is more efficacious than prazosin in the management of Indian red scorpion stings.

Prazosin is a vasodilator and this should help the pulmonary oedema. Short-acting intravenous β-blockers (e.g. esmolol or metoprolol) may be used cautiously to control the tachycardia. Loop diuretic treatment will also be required and there is the option of additional vasodilator therapy such as nitrates or sodium nitroprusside. The next 24 h will be critical; the patient's relatives will need support and counselling, and will need to know that the outlook is grave, even with the best possible supportive therapy.

Key points and global issues

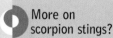

> **More on scorpion stings?**
>
> See Chapter 9 of
> **Davidson's Principles & Practice of Medicine (21st edn)**

- Scorpions are found in South, West and North Africa; North, Central and South America; India; the Middle East; and the Caribbean. The world's most dangerous scorpions live in North Africa, from Spain to the Middle East (species in genera *Androctonus, Buthus, Buthotus, Leiurus*), Central and South America, Caribbean (*Tityus*), India (*Mesobuthus*), Southern USA, Mexico, Central America, Caribbean (*Centruroides*), China (*Buthus*), Western and Southern Africa (*Parabuthus, Hottentotta*). For every person killed by a poisonous snake, 10 are killed by a poisonous scorpion in Mexico. They can also be transported from their natural habitats to foreign countries with foodstuffs and other cargo.

- Scorpion venom may contain multiple toxins, e.g. neurotoxins, cardiotoxins, nephrotoxins, haemolytic toxins, phosphodiesterases, hyaluronidase, histamine, serotonin, tryptophan and cytokine releasers.

- Local tissue effects vary among species. Effects are minimal with *Centruroides*, while scorpions from the Middle East (particularly the *Hemi Scorpius* genera found in Iraq and Iran) can cause severe local reactions, including necrosis.

- Most deaths occur during the first 24 h after the sting.

- Caribbean scorpions cause severe abdominal pain, vomiting and even haematemesis following envenoming.

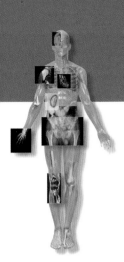

15

Organophosphorus poisoning

A. FAIZ

Presenting problem

A 30-year-old man is admitted to hospital in a state of reduced consciousness (Glasgow Coma Scale 9) with froth coming out of his mouth and laboured respiration. According to his family members, he was found collapsed in his room 1 h ago. He is an otherwise healthy man taking no regular medication. The accompanying person also brought an unlabelled empty container, found in the same room, which is reported to store pesticides. The man's clothing is soaked with vomitus. A strong pungent garlic-like odour is apparent and is found to come from the patient's body; the container also has a similar smell. Further questioning reveals a family dispute the previous night. The patient has no past history of psychiatric illness.

What would your differential diagnosis include before examining the patient?

With the background of a family quarrel, self-poisoning is definitely at the top of the list in an otherwise healthy young man, but in view of altered consciousness, laboured breathing and froth coming out of mouth, a post-epileptic state should also be considered. However, the history and presenting features of acute illness are suggestive of a deliberate suicidal attempt, most likely with some kind of organophosphorus (OP) compound. Other agents like organochlorines are not available nowadays. Pyrethroid insecticides rarely cause severe poisoning. Aluminium phosphide ingestion should be considered in areas where it is common (e.g. Northern India). It has a characteristic odour of rotten fish.

Examination

The patient is found to be cyanosed and dyspnoeic, with small pinpoint pupils. There are muscle fasciculations and reduced tendon jerks. His pulse is 102/min and blood pressure is 80/60 mmHg. He has bilateral crepitations.

Has examination narrowed down your differential diagnosis?

The findings of typical garlic odour, miosis and muscle fasciculations are so pathognomonic that there should be no doubt about OP poisoning. Altered consciousness, muscle fasciculations and cyanosis stratify the case as severe. The accompanying persons should be interrogated about the amount and the brand ingested. Lung crepitations can be attributed to bronchorrhoea and aspiration of secretions from salivation due to the muscarinic effects of an acute cholinergic syndrome. Bradycardia is typical (due to muscarinic features) but tachycardia may occur in 20% of cases (due to nicotinic effects, hypoxia and hypotension).

Following aluminium phosphide poisoning, the patient is generally fully conscious, despite the presence of shock. Pyrethroids rarely cause severe poisoning but convulsions can occur following their ingestion.

Further investigations

Laboratory confirmation of OP poisoning is neither necessary nor always possible before starting treatment. In doubtful cases, a test dose of atropine (1 mg i.v.) may be helpful. (A marked increase in heart rate and skin flushing eliminate the possibility of OP poisoning.) Pulse oximetry and cardiac status should be monitored. An electrocardiogram may demonstrate prolonged QTc and other arrhythmias. Urea and electrolytes are unremarkable. Arterial blood gases on high-flow oxygen are shown in Box 15.1. Blood should also be sent for cholinesterase estimation, although its levels correlate poorly with the severity of the clinical features.

BOX 15.1

Arterial blood gas results on high-flow oxygen

PaO_2	7.4 kPa (55 mmHg)
$PaCO_2$	3.1 kPa (23 mmHg)
H^+	34 nmol/L (pH 7.47)
HCO_3^-	24 mmol/L (mEq/L)

How will you treat this patient?

The patient is hypoxic despite high-flow oxygen and should be managed in an intensive care unit. Establishment of an airway is the priority. Suction and endotracheal intubation, followed by assisted ventilation with a high concentration of oxygen, will be necessary. Atropine should be started immediately at a dose of 1.8–3 mg i.v. bolus and doubled every 5 min, until atropinisation (clear lungs, dry tongue, normal heart rate and blood pressure) has occurred. Following atropinisation, an atropine infusion is given every hour at 20–30% of the dose required for atropinisation (~5 mg/h). The patient should be observed frequently and the atropine dose titrated. At times large doses of atropine are required and may produce anticholinergic effects. Pralidoxime chloride (which reactivates acetylcholinesterase and prevents muscle weakness, convulsions or coma) should be given as a 1 g i.v. bolus in 15–30 min, followed by an infusion of 0.5 g/h in adults. Convulsions should be controlled with intravenous diazepam. Meticulous nursing care is mandatory. After the initial resuscitation, decontamination should be undertaken by changing the clothing and washing the skin with soap and water. While decontaminating the eyes and skin, the healthcare worker should protect himself from secondary contamination. The eyes should be irrigated; gastric lavage with charcoal may be tried at this stage. The patient should be observed regularly and carefully for early detection of the intermediate syndrome (IMS; Fig. 15.1); this is rapidly progressive weakness from the ocular muscles to the neck, proximal limbs and respiratory muscles, typically occurring between 24–96 h, and develops in 20% of the patients. Early recognition and intervention with endotracheal intubation are required. Recovery from IMS is complete. Organophosphate-induced delayed polyneuropathy (OPIDN), characterised by cramping, numbness and paraesthesia in distal limbs, with weakness, gait apraxia and foot or wrist drop, is a recognised late complication. It usually occurs about 2–3 weeks after acute exposure due to degeneration of long myelinated nerve fibres. Recovery from OPIDN is incomplete. Before discharge, this patient should have psychiatric evaluation to identify any underlying psychiatric illness.

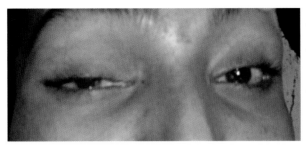

Figure 15.1 A young woman with intermediate syndrome following organophosphorus poisoning. She is unable to keep her eyes open due to muscular weakness.

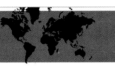

Key points and global issues

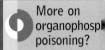

More on organophosph▊ poisoning?

See Chapter 9 of
Davidson's Principles
& **Practice** of
Medicine (21st edn)

- Pesticides or insecticides used by victims differ in various parts of the world according to local use and availability.

- Worldwide, the incidence of OP pesticide poisoning is estimated at 3 million/year, with approximately 300 000 deaths.

- Case fatality varies and is higher in developing countries. In Asia, it ranges from 20% to 70%, depending on the season and availability of health services.

16

Paracetamol (acetaminophen) overdose

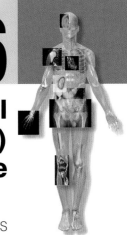

A. L. JONES

Presenting problem

A 23-year-old woman, who is 34 weeks pregnant with her first child, is seen in the Emergency Department after taking 28 paracetamol (500 mg) tablets 2 h ago. She is 62 kg in weight. She did not co-ingest any other drug or alcohol. She complains of nausea and intermittent vomiting, but this has been consistent throughout her pregnancy.

What would your differential diagnosis include before examining the patient?

There is no real diagnostic difficulty in this case. The issue of greatest concern is that she has probably ingested 225 mg/kg of paracetamol, i.e. more than 150 mg paracetamol per kg of body weight. Hence, she is at risk of developing hepatotoxicity and/or (more rarely) nephrotoxicity. The additional risk is that paracetamol can cross the placenta and this places the baby at risk. The onset of vomiting in this case is too early to be due to paracetamol-induced liver damage if, as she states, the timing of ingestion was only 2 h ago. Paracetamol overdose *per se*, as well as pregnancy itself, can cause early-onset vomiting.

Examination

All her clinical observations (heart rate, blood pressure, etc.) are within normal limits. She has no renal angle tenderness and no right upper quadrant tenderness. (Such signs might occur if she had taken the overdose at an earlier time than stated, or in a staggered way, and was beginning to develop signs of renal or hepatic injury, respectively.) Her uterus is of a size that is in-keeping with her stated gestation. She has a very low mood and odd affect.

Has examination narrowed down your differential diagnosis?

Examination of the patient reveals no evidence of current hepatotoxicity or nephrotoxicity, in-keeping with the patient's history of *recent* ingestion of paracetamol. However, if left untreated, she would be expected to develop liver damage from paracetamol within the next 24–36 h. Her low mood indicates the need to apply the Beck's depression scale (or to undertake some other form of immediate mood assessment), in order to determine her risk on the ward and the appropriate degree of nursing/psychiatric support. In view of the fact that she is pregnant, she may also have obstetric needs.

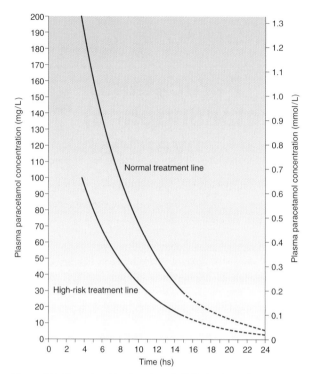

Figure 16.1 Paracetamol treatment graph. Patients whose plasma paracetamol concentration is above the normal treatment line should receive antidote. The high-risk treatment line is used in individuals who may develop paracetamol toxicity at lower levels (see text). After 15 h (dotted lines) the prognostic accuracy is uncertain. (*Source*: University of Wales College of Medicine Therapeutics and Toxicology Centre).

Initial investigations

Paracetamol levels in the blood are checked 4 h after ingestion and the concentration plotted on a paracetamol treatment normogram (Fig. 16.1). Prothrombin ratio, liver function tests and venous bicarbonate concentrations are normal (Box 16.1). Serum paracetamol concentrations should be measured in any patient who admits to taking excess paracetamol, anyone who has ingested white tablets and any patient with unexplained coma. Blood paracetamol concentrations taken within 4 h of ingestion are not interpretable. Prothrombin ratio (PTR) is the most sensitive marker of ensuing liver dysfunction in paracetamol poisoning; it becomes elevated at 18–24 h after significant ingestion, with ensuing hepatotoxicity. Prothrombin ratio is checked in this case, because of the need to be certain that ingestion has not taken place earlier than the patient states, i.e. to establish that there is no evidence of liver damage from paracetamol at her time of presentation. Plasma venous bicarbonate is a useful early screening test for metabolic acidosis and can warn of impending liver damage from paracetamol.

BOX 16.1	
Initial investigations	
Paracetamol level at 4 h after ingestion	350 mg/L
Urea and electrolytes (U&Es)	Normal
Liver function tests (LFTs)	Normal
Prothrombin time/ratio	Normal
Plasma venous bicarbonate	Normal

How will you treat this patient?

This patient requires a full course ($20\frac{1}{4}$ h) of the antidote for paracetamol poisoning, because her blood paracetamol level at 4 h is above the normal treatment line (Fig. 16.1). She is not glutathione-deplete (e.g. due to alcoholism, anorexia or known human immunodeficiency (HIV) disease) or on enzyme-inducing agents (e.g. carbamazepine, phenobarbital, phenytoin or rifampicin) and so the lower, 'high-risk' treatment line is not used.

The antidote, intravenous *N*-acetylcysteine, will protect her liver and kidneys from paracetamol-induced hepatotoxicity. The dose is 150 mg/kg over 15 min, then 50 mg/kg over 4 h and then 100 mg/kg over 16 h. During infusion of the first two bags of *N*-acetylcysteine, up to 5% of patients develop an anaphylactoid reaction (flushing and wheezing). Watch out for this, and if it occurs, stop the infusion for at least 30 min and give an antihistamine drug. At the end of the $20\frac{1}{4}$ h infusion, the patient needs to be clinically examined for upper quadrant tenderness or renal angle pain; if she is clinically well, however, she does *not* require further blood tests because *N*-acetylcysteine given within 10 h of paracetamol ingestion offers virtually 100% protection from liver/renal injury.

There are, of course, two patients here: mother and fetus. Both paracetamol and *N*-acetylcysteine cross the placenta, and fortunately the fetus is fully protected by treating the mother with the antidote. Neither *N*-acetylcysteine nor paracetamol is known to be teratogenic (harmful) to the fetus. The mother will require a treatment for nausea that will not harm the baby – such as cyclizine. She also needs psychiatric evaluation to assess her ongoing suicidal risk. If you are in doubt about the care of a poisoned or potentially poisoned patient, doctors at a poisons information centre are there to help guide you on such issues. Keep a note of the poisons centre number with you.

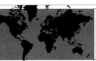

Key points and global issues

More on paracetamol poisoning?

See Chapter 9 of
Davidson's Principles
& **Practice** of
Medicine (21st edn)

- Paracetamol poisoning is extremely common in the UK but also occurs in other parts of the world; paracetamol is called acetaminophen in the USA and Canada.

- Availability of the antidote *N*-acetylcysteine is not global. Up to 10 h after an overdose, oral methionine (12 g orally 4-hourly, to a total of four doses) is a suitable alternative antidote for paracetamol poisoning if intravenous *N*-acetylcysteine is neither available nor affordable.

- The incidence of acute liver failure developing from paracetamol does not appear to be the same in every country. In Australia, acute liver failure from paracetamol is rare but in the UK it is much more common; many factors dictate this risk.

- Do not forget the potential of drowsy patients having ingested a paracetamol/opioid combination. Check the paracetamol level in such patients.

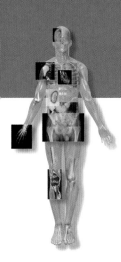

17

Aluminium phosphide poisoning

S. SINGH

Presenting problem

A 28-year-old unemployed man is seen in the Emergency Department about 5 h after ingestion of aluminium phosphide (ALP). According to his relatives, he was found collapsed in his room near an empty tube containing 'QuickPhos' tablets (3 g ALP tablets; 10 in one container) (Fig. 17.1). Immediately after ingestion, he had started vomiting, complaining of abdominal pain. He passed a loose stool. There is no previous history of any illness and he is otherwise well adjusted. His clothes are soaked with vomitus and there is a pungent rotten smell in his breath. The 'QuickPhos' container has a similar odour.

What would your differential diagnosis include before examining the patient?

Aluminium phosphide is a fumigant used to control insects and rodents in a variety of settings. The history and presenting features of this patient suggest ingestion of ALP tablets with suicidal intent. Pain in the abdomen, vomiting and diarrhoea are generally the initial complaints. Patients continue to remain conscious, though anxious and confused, until coma develops as a result of cerebral hypoxia due to shock. Other pesticides like organophosphorus compounds and endosulfan could lead to similar symptoms. However, they are not available in tablet form and loss of consciousness and respiratory failure develop early after their ingestion. Although a pungent garlic-like odour is not uncommon with these pesticides, the rotten fish-like odour is observed generally with ALP poisoning. Our patient's persistent inability to find any suitable work is most probably the reason for his suicidal attempt.

Examination

The patient is confused with a GCS of 10. His BP is 80/60 mmHg, pulse 116/min and RR 24/min. His temperature is 37°C and pupils are normal. Peripheral cyanosis is present with cold extremities. His chest is clear and his abdomen is soft with normal bowel sounds.

Has examination narrowed down your differential diagnosis?

The finding of a rotten fish-like odour in the breath, shock, normal pupils, cold peripheries with cyanosis, absent fasciculation and a clear chest rules out other

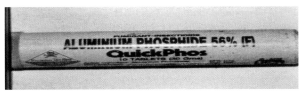

Figure 17.1 Aluminium phosphide tablets.

pesticide poisoning and is consistent with severe ALP poisoning. The discovery of an empty tube of ALP nearby confirms this.

Investigations

Haemoglobin is 14 g/L (14.8 g/dL); total and differential cell counts are normal. The arterial blood gas (ABG) analysis reveals a severe metabolic acidosis with hypoxia (Box 17.1). An electrocardiogram shows a sinus tachycardia and occasional ventricular ectopics. Serum sodium 140 mmol/L (mEq/L); potassium 3.9 mmol/L (mEq/L); urea 6.8 mmol/L (19 mg/dL); creatinine 88.4 µmol/L (1 mg/dL) and blood glucose 3.9 mmol/L (70 mg/dL). To confirm ALP poisoning, the presence of phosphine can be detected by using a filter paper impregnated with freshly prepared silver nitrate solution and holding it close to mouth or dipping it in gastric contents. The colour will change to black if phosphine is present in the breath or in stomach contents. Similarly, phosphine can be detected by collecting breath in a breathing bag and using a specific phosphine detector tube. The most sensitive test is gas chromatography, although this is not feasible in most emergency settings.

BOX 17.1	
Arterial blood gas analysis while breathing room air	
H^+	102 nmol/L (pH 6.99)
PO_2	7.6 kPa (57 mmHg)
PCO_2	3.7 kPa (27.8 mmHg)
HCO_3	6.6 mmol/L (mEq/L)
Sat.O_2	85%

How will you treat this patient?

There is no specific antidote and the treatment is supportive. The patient should be managed, preferably in an intensive care unit, with careful monitoring of vital parameters including arterial blood gas analysis. Immediate therapy of this patient entails management of shock and the severe metabolic acidosis. Two i.v. lines should be secured, one for infusion of saline (0.9% sodium chloride) and the other for sodium bicarbonate. A recent study suggests that careful correction of the acidosis leads to a reduced mortality, but this needs to be confirmed in further investigations. As our patient is in shock, administration of inotropic agents (generally dopamine along with dobutamine) should be started. However, if the shock is severe, noradrenaline may also be administered. Urinary output should be measured hourly. Glucocorticoids (100 mg hydrocortisone i.v. every 6 h) have been tried with little success. Magnesium is a membrane stabiliser and improves cardiac arrhythmias, but has not been found to reduce mortality. Gastric lavage, although regularly undertaken in the Indian subcontinent due to legal reasons, should preferably be avoided, as there is the possibility of increased liberation of phosphine and a risk of aspiration. There are no randomised trials to suggest that it benefits patients. The prognosis is poor, with a survival rate as low as 30%. Unfortunately, renal failure (acute tubular necrosis) and hepatic damage (hepatic necrosis due to shock) are common in survivors. Patients generally remain conscious until shock leads to hypoxic brain damage. Hypoglycaemia is not uncommon and, rarely, becomes severe. Acute respiratory distress syndrome is another complication which requires assisted ventilation in the ICU.

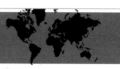

Key points and global issues

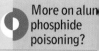

More on alum phosphide poisoning?

See Chapter 9 of **Davidson's Principles** and **Practice** of **Medicine (21st edn)**

- Aluminium phosphide poisoning, although predominantly a problem in rural northern India, is now being reported frequently in Iran. Sporadic cases have been reported from several other countries.

- There is no specific antidote and aggressive supportive measures, preferably in an intensive care unit, should be provided.

- There is a need to strictly control the supply of ALP tablets which, in several countries including India, is too readily available.

18

Disseminated malignancy

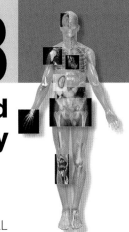

L. WALL

Presenting problem

A 45-year-old woman is referred following an ultrasound scan showing multiple hepatic metastases. She had sought medical care with a 48-h history of abdominal pain, diarrhoea and vomiting. These symptoms have now resolved. She has had several similar episodes over the past 5 years. Between episodes she is well. Her bowels open three times per day and are soft to watery. She has no significant previous medical history. She is taking hormone replacement therapy for flushing, but symptoms remain poorly controlled. She takes no other medication. She has relevant family history. She works full time.

What would your differential diagnosis include before examining the patient?

This woman has disseminated malignancy. The history might suggest a gastrointestinal origin of disease, with intermittent episodes of partial intestinal obstruction. It is important not to focus on one system too early in the investigation of advanced malignancy. In view of this patient's age, we must also consider the prospect of a hereditary element to her disease, although even in young patients, sporadic tumours predominate.

Examination

She is flushed. Cardiovascular and respiratory examinations are normal. She has no palpable cervical or axillary lymphadenopathy. Breast examination is normal. Abdominal examination shows a non-tender liver palpable down to the level of the umbilicus. Rectal and pelvic examinations are normal. Skin examination is also normal.

Has examination narrowed down your differential diagnosis?

While the clinical examination findings might appear not to have provided any new information, there are important negative findings. Breast cancer is a relatively common malignancy in young women, and patients can be systemically well, even in the presence of metastatic disease. This diagnosis is unlikely with a normal breast examination.

At present, the findings suggest an abdominal malignancy. This degree of hepatomegaly is not common among cancer patients, and implies a relatively slow growing tumour. When tumours progress slowly, hypertrophy of the

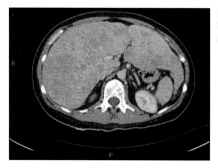

Figure 18.1 CT scan of the liver showing gross hepatomegaly and multiple metastatic deposits in the liver.

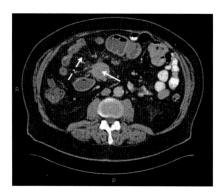

Figure 18.2 CT scan of the abdomen showing a carcinoid tumour in the small bowel (solid arrow); the associated desmoplastic reaction in the mesentery is drawing in loops of small bowel (broken arrow).

unaffected liver can maintain good hepatic function, despite extensive disease. The differential diagnoses include a slow growing colorectal cancer, an abdominal sarcoma such as a gastrointestinal stromal tumour and a neuroendocrine tumour, although we cannot exclude other diagnoses at this time.

Initial investigations

Full blood count, hepatic and renal function and magnesium levels are all normal. There is no role for checking tumour markers at this time. A computed tomography scan of the thorax, abdomen and pelvis demonstrates multiple hepatic lesions consistent with metastases (Fig. 18.1). It also shows a mesenteric, desmoplastic lesion (characterised by the overgrowth of fibrous tissue causing adhesions) suggestive of a nodal mass related to a small intestinal neuroendocrine (carcinoid) tumour (Fig. 18.2).

Does this narrow down your differential diagnosis?

The history, clinical and radiological findings are consistent with a primary small intestinal neuroendocrine tumour. Flushing and loose bowels also suggest the diagnosis of carcinoid syndrome. These diagnoses both need confirmation.

Definitive investigations

The diagnosis of carcinoid syndrome can be confirmed by hormonal assessment. The commonest way to do this is to measure the excretion product of hormones in the urine, 5-hydroxyindoleacetic acid (5-HIAA).

For the majority of cancer types, a tumour biopsy is required to confirm the diagnosis. If the biopsy is of the liver, it should first be assessed whether the hepatic disease is amenable to curative surgical resection, as following a biopsy there is a risk of disseminating tumour cells down the biopsy tract. Curative hepatic surgery will not be an option for this patient, so she has a liver biopsy to confirm the diagnosis. With the possible history of carcinoid syndrome, a biopsy may trigger hormonal release and a carcinoid crisis, so she is pre-treated with octreotide prior to the biopsy.

How will you treat this patient?

The definitive investigations confirm a well-differentiated neuroendocrine tumour with a proliferation index of 1%. These tumours usually progress slowly with an average survival of a few years. This woman also has a significantly elevated 5-HIAA consistent with the diagnosis of carcinoid syndrome.

The carcinoid syndrome should be managed with somatostatin analogue therapy. This has a very good chance of controlling hormonal symptoms, and may also slow down growth of the tumour. Patients with a long history of hormonal symptoms are at risk of cardiac valvular problems, so an echocardiogram should also be performed.

Some clinicians advocate resection of primary neuroendocrine tumours within the GI tract, even in the presence of metastatic disease. This reduces the risk of further obstructive episodes, and may also affect the natural history of the disease. Surgery can be challenging, as hormonal release from the tumour can result in considerable peritumoral fibrosis. The decision as to whether to go down this path needs to be made in a multidisciplinary forum considering disease extent, patient symptoms, comorbidity and patient preference.

Classical anti-cancer chemotherapy drugs target proliferating tumour cells. Given the low proliferation of these tumours, it may not be surprising that chemotherapy has not been demonstrated to affect survival in this disease. Current research into treatments targeting facets of tumours other than proliferation may offer more therapeutic options in the future.

Standard, external-beam radiotherapy has not been demonstrated to affect the natural history of these tumours, but can be a useful palliative option, particularly in patients with bony metastatic disease. The systemic use of hormonal analogues attached to radioactive isotopes (e.g. ^{131}I-mIBG) to target tumour cells more accurately has been demonstrated to help hormonal symptoms in some patients and may also affect tumour growth.

Key points and global issues

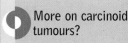
More on carcinoid tumours?

See Chapter 20 of
Davidson's Principles
& **Practice** of
Medicine (21st edn)

- Many patients present with disseminated malignancy without having been previously diagnosed with a primary tumour. Although the pathway of investigation will not be the same for all patients, there are principles that apply to all.

- Investigations should depend on symptoms and clinical findings rather than a predefined list of possible tests.

- Early biopsy is often preferable to multiple imaging investigations.

- While for an individual with well preserved organ function and good performance status extensive investigation is appropriate, for patients presenting in the terminal stages of their disease extensive investigation is of no prognostic or therapeutic benefit.
- In all patients, management of the presenting symptom(s) should occur alongside investigation.

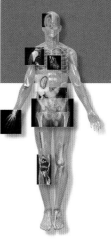

19

Spinal cord compression

D. OXENHAM

Presenting problem

A 40-year-old man presents to hospital, having not passed urine for the previous 24 h. He is acutely uncomfortable and has a large suprapubic mass. A urinary catheter is inserted and drains 1200 mL of clear urine. He was diagnosed 1 year ago with non-small cell lung cancer, which was initially treated with radical radiotherapy. At diagnosis there was no evidence of metastases and initial treatment appeared successful. Over the last 4 months, he has developed increasingly severe lower back pain, which has been partially controlled with codeine, paracetamol and diclofenac.

What would your differential diagnosis include before examining the patient?

Any patient presenting with back pain and known or suspected metastatic cancer should be presumed to have spinal cord compression until proved otherwise. The presence of sphincter disturbance makes cord compression the most important diagnosis to exclude. Non-oncological causes of spinal cord compression (rheumatoid arthritis, osteoporosis, Paget's disease of bone) should also be considered, although they are unlikely in this patient.

The other possible explanation for urinary retention in this situation would be constipation or a side-effect of medications (e.g. amitriptyline or opioids). Urinary retention may also be caused by diabetes, stroke, heavy metal poisoning or multiple sclerosis. It would be foolish to assume these diagnoses in a patient with previous cancer and back pain; if you fail to investigate this patient adequately, he may develop an avoidable paralysis.

Examination and initial investigations

On examination, the man has some tenderness over his first lumbar vertebra. Neurological examination is entirely normal with no areas of sensory deficit or signs of motor weakness. There is no loss of perineal sensation or reduction in anal tone.

The lumbar spine X-ray is normal. A full blood count reveals a mild anaemia of chronic disease (104 g/L or 10.4 g/dL) and biochemistry is normal, except for a low albumin (31 g/L or 3.1 g/dL).

Have examination and initial investigations narrowed down your differential diagnosis?

In this situation, a normal neurological examination should not reduce your suspicion of cord compression. If you wait until the cord compression has

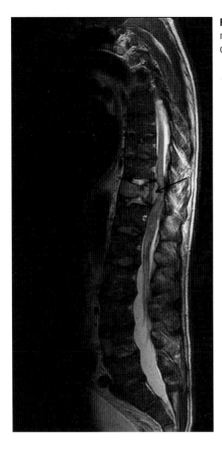

Figure 19.1 MRI of the spine demonstrating a metastasis at the level of L1 (arrow), which is causing compression of the spinal cord.

progressed to produce a classic clinical picture of flaccid lower limb paralysis and loss of sensation below the level of compression (a 'sensory level'), you will have failed your patient miserably! Treatment is likely to preserve function but unlikely to reverse significant neurological deficit. A normal plain X-ray of the lumbar spine does not exclude either bone metastases or cord compression. On the other hand, an abnormal X-ray would make the diagnosis almost certain.

Further investigations

The investigation of choice is magnetic resonance imaging (MRI) of the spine; this will demonstrate any significant cord compression. In this patient, there is a metastasis protruding into the spine at the level of L1 (Fig. 19.1).

How will you treat this patient?

Spinal cord compression is a medical emergency and treatment should be started quickly to avoid unnecessary neurological damage. All treatment should balance potential benefit and harm, but in most situations where metastatic spinal cord compression is suspected, the correct initial therapy would be 16 mg intravenous or oral dexamethasone.

Further management would depend on local services, but options would be either radiotherapy or surgical decompression. This should be discussed urgently with local specialists and managed according to their advice.

Key points and global issues

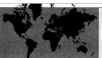

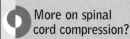
More on spinal
cord compression?

See Chapter 11 of
Davidson's Principles
and **Practice** of
Medicine (21st edn)

- CT and MRI are important diagnostic tools for an early diagnosis; however, access to these investigations may be limited in developing nations.

- Except for breast and prostate cancer, cord compression is generally a late complication of advanced metastatic disease. The level of investigation and intervention should be appropriate to the stage of disease and prognosis.

- All treatments are a balance of risk (including cost and access) versus benefit. Some patients may be appropriately managed with steroids and good analgesia.

- Tuberculosis is a significant cause of cord compression in developing nations. Lower thoracic and lumbar vertebrae are commonly involved. Early diagnosis and treatment are rewarding, but often the diagnosis is made at a stage when the patient has developed paralysis.

- Spinal epidural abscess commonly occurs in the thoracic or lumbar spine. Patients usually have comorbid conditions such as diabetes mellitus or HIV infection. Early diagnosis and treatment with antibiotics and surgical drainage can prevent neurological sequelae.

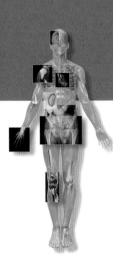

20

Central chest pain

P. BLOOMFIELD

Presenting problem

A 55-year-old man of Asian origin presents to a small rural hospital 50 miles from the nearest city with a new onset of chest pain. The pain is severe, is located in the centre of his chest and radiates into his left arm. The pain has come on suddenly and the man reports feeling very sick and sweaty. It has lasted more than an hour and at one point, the man thought he was going to die. He gives a history of breathlessness and some chest discomfort when moving heavy boxes in his shop over the last few months. He admits to taking little exercise outside his work, and has gained weight in recent years. He has smoked 15 cigarettes a day since he left school. He had his blood pressure taken once at a visit to his doctor a year or so ago, was told it was high but has been too busy to go back and have it measured again. There is a strong family history of diabetes mellitus and his older brother has had a heart attack.

What would your differential diagnosis include before examining the patient?

The most common cause of chest pain with characteristic features of myocardial ischaemia is an acute coronary syndrome. Other possible causes would include: acute aortic dissection in which the pain is often very sudden in onset and may be intrascapular – it commonly occurs in those with hypertension; acute pericarditis in which the pain is often sharp and eased by sitting forward; musculoskeletal pain, which is not usually associated with nausea and vomiting. This man has important risk factors for the development of ischaemic heart disease: hypertension, smoking and family history. The features of autonomic upset here, i.e. sweating and nausea, suggest possible myocardial infarction.

Examination

The patient looks unwell and sweaty. He is overweight (98 kg) with significant central obesity. Pulse is 104 beats/min and blood pressure is 190/105 mmHg in both arms. All peripheral pulses are present and equal. The heart sounds are normal and there are no murmurs or added sounds. His respiratory rate is 20/min and there are bilateral crepitations in both lung bases.

Has examination narrowed down your differential diagnosis?

The physical examination has revealed signs of pulmonary oedema. Heart failure is a common accompaniment of myocardial infarction and reflects a significant

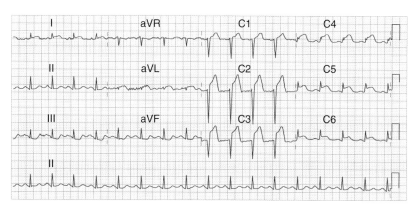

Figure 20.1 A 12-lead ECG showing an acute anterior myocardial infarction.

degree of myocardial damage; hence it is associated with a worse prognosis. Rarely, acute pulmonary oedema may be a consequence of rupture of a papillary muscle (of the mitral valve) or of rupture of the interventricular septum. Both would tend to be associated with a murmur and with significant haemodynamic compromise, which is not the case here. Acute coronary syndrome is often not accompanied by any physical signs; pallor and sweating are part of the autonomic upset that may be a feature of myocardial infarction. Peripheral pulses may be lost with aortic dissection but the presence of all peripheral pulses does not exclude aortic dissection, which is commonly accompanied on presentation by hypertension.

Further investigations

The most important immediate bedside test in the evaluation of chest pain is a 12-lead electrocardiogram (ECG) and should be done immediately in the evaluation of patients with chest pain. The ECG in this man is shown in Figure 20.1. Chest X-ray is normal.

Does this narrow down your differential diagnosis?

The ECG is diagnostic of an acute ST-elevation anterior wall myocardial infarction. The ECG is the most important bedside investigation in patients presenting with chest pain. It can lead to a prompt diagnosis and avoid the need for unnecessary investigations. In this case, the diagnosis is immediately established.

How will you treat this patient?

The patient needs treatment for pain with morphine and an antiemetic. He should be given aspirin (300 mg) and clopidogrel (600 mg) to swallow. Intravenous access should be promptly established and high-flow oxygen given. The patient should be monitored (ECG), as ventricular fibrillation may occur. The patient should be considered for acute reperfusion therapy with percutaneous coronary intervention (PCI) or thrombolytic treatment. Treatment should be given promptly as delay in opening the infarct-related artery leads to further loss of myocardial tissue. '*Minutes mean muscle*.' If the patient had been in a hospital where PCI was available, the team should be immediately alerted. This patient, however, is in a rural hospital 50 miles from a hospital with PCI. What action should be taken? Should he be treated transferred or treated locally?

PCI is superior to thrombolytic therapy only if it can be administered promptly; for this man, thrombolytic drugs should be given. Treatment should be given to lower blood pressure before thrombolytic drugs are given, and this can usually be achieved with sublingual or intravenous nitrates. All patients, except those with a bradycardia (<65/min), hypotension (systolic blood pressure <105 mmHg) or pulmonary oedema, should be given intravenous β-blockade (metoprolol 5–15 mg); in this patient, pulmonary oedema would preclude the use of a β-blocker. If PCI is not performed, coronary angiography should be carried out in the days following the event to determine the need for revascularisation therapy.

After the acute episode has settled, attention should turn to interventions that might improve this man's prognosis and reduce the morbidity associated with the myocardial infarction. Aspirin therapy should be continued long-term. Clopidogrel should be continued for a year. Angiotensin-converting enzyme (ACE) inhibitors reduce ventricular remodelling and the risk of subsequent heart failure and should be commenced in all patients, especially if there is evidence of left ventricular impairment at echocardiography, which should be carried out before this man leaves hospital. Patients with acute myocardial infarction complicated by heart failure and left ventricular dysfunction appear to benefit from additional aldosterone receptor antagonism (e.g. eplerenone 25–50 mg daily). Beta-blockade reduces mortality in the weeks following a myocardial infarction, and again should be instituted in the absence of any contraindications.

Modification of risk factors is also crucial. The patient should be advised to stop smoking in the strongest possible terms, to lose weight and to take regular exercise. Statin therapy reduces the risk of further cardiovascular events by 25% over a 10-year period and should be commenced in all patients following a myocardial infarction, irrespective of total cholesterol concentration, unless there is a significant contraindication. Blood pressure should be treated aggressively.

Simple clinical tools can predict outcome in myocardial infarction. This man on presentation had tachycardia and pulmonary oedema. The GRACE score uses these and other clinical features such as ST segment change on the ECG, age and serum creatinine to calculate early mortality in acute coronary syndrome. Prognosis is additionally related to the degree of myocardial damage, as estimated by echocardiography.

Finally, the psychological morbidity of this event should not be overlooked. This man has had a life-threatening illness that is likely to reduce his life expectancy and may affect his ability to work and perform other activities of daily living. Psychological support should be offered and often patients find value from attending rehabilitation classes where they can receive advice on lifestyle and exercise from trained practitioners.

Key points and global issues

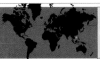

More on myocardial infarction?

See Chapter 18 of **Davidson's Principles & Practice of Medicine (21st edn)**

- The 12-lead ECG is the most important initial investigation of patients with chest pain and may lead to an immediate diagnosis. If the ECG does not show diagnostic changes and acute coronary syndrome is suspected, the ECG should be repeated after 30–60 min.

- ST elevation MI requires prompt treatment with reperfusion therapy; PCI if available promptly, if not intravenous thrombolytic therapy.

- Cardiovascular disease is the most frequent cause of death in the Western world and its incidence is increasing in many other parts of the world. It may soon become the most common cause of death on all continents.

- Ischaemic heart disease commonly affects those with diabetes, the incidence of which is increasing throughout the world, especially as obesity becomes more common.

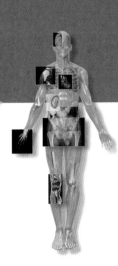

21

Breathlessness and peripheral oedema

D. E. NEWBY

Presenting problem

A 56-year-old man presents with a 6-month history of exertional breath-lessness and fatigue. There is no associated chest pain or chest tightness. Over the last 2 months, he has noticed progressive swelling of his ankles and recently describes three-pillow orthopnoea and abdominal bloating. He is now limited to walking 200–300 m on the flat.

He has no history of hypertension, diabetes mellitus or hypercholesterolae-mia. He admits to drinking 40 units of alcohol per week and smokes 20 ciga-rettes per day. He had tuberculosis and rheumatic fever as a child. He also reports a cough productive of sputum for 2 months during the winter.

What would your differential diagnosis include before examining the patient?

Breathlessness as a symptom is predominantly caused by cardiac or respiratory disease, although occasionally metabolic acidosis or anaemia may present in this way. The most likely differential diagnoses here are congestive cardiac failure (with many potential causes), progressive chronic obstructive pulmonary disease or a combination of the two factors (cor pulmonale). The differential diagnosis would also include chronic pulmonary thromboembolism, interstitial lung disease, chronic bronchial asthma, angina equivalent and bronchogenic carcinoma.

Examination

The patient is mildly dyspnoeic on moving to the examination couch. He is pink with no evidence of central cyanosis. The pulse is weak and fast with a blood pressure 95/60 mmHg. The jugular venous pressure is markedly ele-vated up to the level of the ear lobes. Heart sounds reveal an added sound. The lung bases have reduced breath sounds and there is marked pitting peripheral oedema up to the knees. On abdominal examination, there is shifting dullness and hepatomegaly.

Has examination narrowed down your differential diagnosis?

The clinical features are more suggestive of congestive cardiac failure with pre-dominantly right-sided signs of fluid retention. Cor pulmonale remains a possi-bility. However, it must be remembered that congestive heart failure is not a diagnosis in itself. The underlying cause should be identified; coronary heart disease is a common aetiological factor.

Investigations

Serum biochemistry demonstrates a marginally elevated serum urea and creatinine concentration, normal serum bicarbonate concentration and deranged liver function tests.

The electrocardiogram (ECG) shows no evidence of myocardial ischaemia or prior infarction. There is a sinus tachycardia, low-voltage QRS complexes and T wave flattening.

The chest X-ray shows small bilateral pleural effusions and upper lobe venous diversion. The cardiothoracic ratio is at the upper limit of normal.

Echocardiography demonstrates good left ventricular function with no left ventricular dilatation, hypertrophy or regional wall motion abnormality. The heart valves function normally and there is a trivial pericardial effusion. The motion of the septum appears unusual and the Doppler velocities across the aortic valve are reduced. The right ventricle is not dilated and there is no evidence of pulmonary hypertension.

Spirometry demonstrates a forced expiratory volume in 1 s (FEV_1) of 2.0 L/min and forced vital capacity (FVC) of 3.0 L/min. Pulse oximetry records an oxygen saturation of 97% on air.

Have examination and initial investigations narrowed down your differential diagnosis?

The clinical features demonstrate a patient with symptomatic congestive cardiac failure and the associated examination findings of a raised jugular venous pressure and peripheral oedema. The three most common causes of heart failure are coronary artery disease, hypertension and valvular heart disease. These are unlikely, given the clinical findings and investigations. Although mild airways obstruction is present, the patient has no cyanosis and is well oxygenated on room air; there is no suggestion of cor pulmonale or pulmonary artery hypertension. This makes a respiratory cause for the patient's breathlessness unlikely.

Although alcoholic and viral cardiomyopathies are potential causes, echocardiography has demonstrated a normal-sized left ventricle with good systolic function. Further investigation of the patient's diagnosis should therefore focus on the causes of heart failure in the presence of good left ventricular function and including diastolic dysfunction and high-output cardiac failure. The latter is usually associated with a hyperdynamic circulation and is unlikely, given the low-volume pulse and hypotension.

Definitive investigations

Causes of diastolic heart failure include restrictive cardiomyopathies (including amyloidosis, myocardial fibrosis and left ventricular hypertrophy), constrictive pericarditis and pericardial effusions. Given the echocardiographic appearances, the differential diagnosis focuses on the presence of a restrictive cardiomyopathy or constrictive pericarditis. Causes of restrictive cardiomyopathy include amyloidosis and sarcoidosis. The former can be confirmed by histological examination of a fat, rectal or myocardial biopsy. Such patients should also be investigated for the presence of multiple myeloma.

Severe constrictive pericarditis can sometimes be detected on the chest X-ray by the presence of pericardial calcification. The patient therefore undergoes computed tomography (CT) of the chest. This demonstrates marked pericardial thickening and calcification (Fig. 21.1). Pericardial calcification can

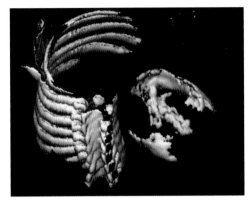

Figure 21.1 Three-dimensional reconstruction of CT of a patient with constrictive pericarditis. Ribs and spine are to the left and the calcified shell of pericardium to the right.

occur in the absence of constrictive pericarditis and the diagnosis is made at cardiac catheterisation. The final, definitive investigation is cardiac catheterisation and this shows high filling pressures as well as equalisation of the diastolic pressures in all chambers of the heart.

How will you treat this patient?

Breathlessness and peripheral oedema are treated with loop diuretic therapy. This will reduce the fluid retention and filling pressures of the heart. However, over-vigorous diuresis may lead to hypotension and pre-renal failure, and this limits the ability to relieve the symptoms completely.

Patients with constrictive pericarditis should undergo surgical removal of the pericardium—pericardiectomy. This removes not only the parietal, but also the visceral pericardium and can cause considerable cardiac damage, especially to the right ventricle. Although symptoms are improved, patients are often left with significant peripheral oedema, breathlessness and right heart failure postoperatively. This limits their symptomatic recovery and they often remain chronically disabled by their condition.

> **BOX 21.1**
>
> **Causes of constrictive pericarditis**
>
> - Tuberculous pericarditis
> - Haemopericardium
> - Viral pericarditis
> - Rheumatoid arthritis and systemic lupus erythematosus
> - Post-pericardotomy syndrome
> - Purulent pericarditis, such as is caused by *Staphylococcus aureus*
> - Neoplastic infiltration
> - Polyserositis
> - Idiopathic

Key points and global issues

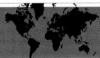

More on constrictive pericarditis?

See Chapter 18 of **Davidson's Principles & Practice of Medicine (21st edn)**

- Although it is often impossible to identify the original insult, causes of constrictive pericarditis (Box 21.1) have marked geographical variability.

- Tuberculous pericarditis is the most common cause in Asia and Africa, and arises as a complication of pulmonary tuberculosis.

- In Africa, a tuberculous pericardial effusion is a common feature of the acquired immunodeficiency syndrome (AIDS).

22

Hypertension in a young adult

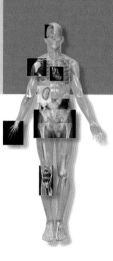

P. L. PADFIELD

Presenting problem

A 28-year-old man with no previous health problems decides to join a local health club. As part of his initial assessment for a fitness programme, he has his blood pressure (BP) measured. The reading is 182/106 mmHg and he is advised to call and see his GP, who discovers that the young man's father is on drug treatment for hypertension, which was picked up when he was in his 50s. There is no other relevant family history. The young man is well, although anxious about the implications of having hypertension. He is a non-smoker, drinks 18 units of alcohol per week, takes no prescribed or self-administered medications, and admits to enjoying salt on his food. He has no knowledge of any childhood illnesses such as urinary infections. On direct questioning, he describes no headaches, palpitations or sweating attacks, and appears truly asymptomatic.

What would your differential diagnosis include before examining the patient?

Hypertension is relatively uncommon in young people. Systolic BP increases with age in Western society and individuals destined to become hypertensive in later life tend to have BPs in the higher centiles at all ages. It is worth considering 'white coat hypertension' (high BP in a clinic setting with normal BP at home or outside hospital) in all apparently hypertensive individuals; there is no reliable way of identifying this without some form of 'out of office' measurement (ambulatory or self-monitored BP) and possible causes of secondary hypertension should be on every physician's mind (Box 22.1). It is difficult to know the true prevalence of secondary hypertension, but the younger the patient, the more likely a specific disorder will be present. Most guidelines suggest investigation for a cause if hypertension is detected before the age of 30 years, but the pick-up rate of correctable conditions is small above the age of 20 years.

BOX 22.1
Causes of hypertension
• Renal
Any chronic renal disease
Polycystic kidneys
Renovascular disease
• Adrenal
Phaeochromocytoma
Primary hyperaldosteronism
Cushing's syndrome
Some congenital adrenal enzyme defects
• Coarctation of the aorta
• Takayasu's aorto-arteritis
• Drug effects
NSAIDs
Liquorice
Combined oral contraceptive pill (women)

Examination

There is no obvious suggestion of an endocrine disease such as Cushing's syndrome or acromegaly (both of which can cause hypertension), although the patient is a little overweight with a body mass index of 27. All peripheral pulses are present and synchronous, there are no abdominal bruits and the kidneys are not palpable. Auscultation of the heart is normal and funduscopy is also unremarkable. BP is recorded as 168/100 mmHg (mean of two readings after 5 min rest).

Initial investigations

Urinalysis is negative and reveals no overt proteinuria or microalbuminuria. Renal function is normal, as are plasma electrolytes. The full blood count and erythrocyte sedimentation rate are likewise unremarkable. An electrocardiogram shows no evidence of left ventricular hypertrophy (best assessed by adding up the depth of the S wave in chest lead V2 and the height of the R wave in chest lead V5, which should come to <35 mm).

Have examination and initial investigations narrowed down your differential diagnosis?

Coarctation of the aorta and polycystic kidney disease might have been picked up if present. In someone of this age, an abdominal bruit would have suggested renal artery stenosis (less discriminatory in older people with an increased likelihood of aortic turbulence), but the absence of a bruit means nothing. A normal level of plasma potassium makes primary aldosteronism less likely, though not impossible. Funduscopy is a poorly practised art, but the presence of haemorrhages and 'exudates' (with or without papilloedema) would have increased the likelihood of renovascular disease (a prevalence rate of 40% in some series with grade III retinopathy). It remains most likely that this young man has primary hypertension.

Further investigations

There is no generally agreed list of investigations but it would be prudent to perform a 24-h urine collection for metadrenaline and normetadrenaline (to exclude a phaeochromocytoma), and to obtain blood in the supine or seated position for plasma renin activity (PRA) and aldosterone. (A low renin with a high aldosterone means primary hyperaldosteronism, whereas a high PRA might suggest renovascular disease.) How far one should go to exclude a diagnosis of renovascular disease is debatable. A renal ultrasound will pick up a disparity in kidney size (and would also diagnose polycystic kidneys) and might be carried out in such a person. Doppler ultrasound to measure renal blood flow is very observer-dependent and magnetic resonance imaging (MRI) of the renal arteries is expensive, but either may be indicated if a high index of suspicion arises from other tests. Before life-long medication is decided upon, either ambulatory BP monitoring (Fig. 22.1) might be performed or, more cost-effectively, the patient might be given an electronic self-monitoring device to use for several days (Fig. 22.2).

The young man is fitted with an ambulatory monitor and the day-time average BP is recorded as 158/96 mmHg. A 24-h urine collection shows no evidence of catecholamine excess, and supine PRA and aldosterone are within the normal range. An MR angiogram shows no evidence of renal artery stenosis.

Does this narrow down your differential diagnosis?

The ambulatory monitor confirms that the young man has sustained hypertension and investigations have revealed no evidence of a secondary cause. Therefore, he has primary hypertension.

How will you treat this patient?

Hypertension is an undeniable risk factor for cardiovascular disease but is not an illness in its own right. People should be discouraged from considering themselves unwell. There is good evidence that salt restriction will lower BP, and weight reduction with exercise should also help. If BP remains in excess of 160/100 mmHg, then British guidelines recommend drug therapy. If BP is lower, then treatment decisions are guided by whether or not the 10-year cardiovascular risk is in excess of 20%. One of the difficulties in interpreting such guidance is that 10-year risks are vanishingly low in young people, but many take the view that treatment is needed to prevent the long-term damage to blood vessels that may become less reversible by the time someone reaches 40 or 50 years of age.

Assuming the young man accepts the need to take life-long medication that will not make him feel better (a great deal of skill in communication is needed for such discussions), then current advice would recommend starting him on an angiotensin-converting enzyme (ACE) inhibitor (or an angiotensin receptor antagonist if he develops a cough with the ACE inhibitor, of which there is a 10% chance); these classes of drug are most suited to young men (best avoided in young women if pregnancy is likely). Goal BP would be 140/90 mmHg and it is unlikely that a single agent will achieve this; the second stage would be to add a calcium channel blocker or thiazide diuretic. The best third drug (if necessary) is uncertain, but most likely one would add a thiazide or a calcium channel blocker (depending upon the second choice).

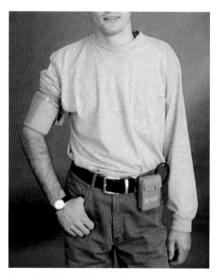

Figure 22.1 An ambulatory BP monitor.

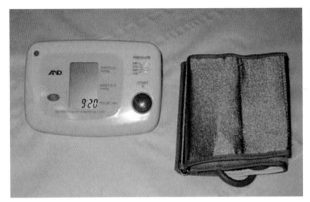

Figure 22.2 A home BP monitor. Data can be downloaded directly to a PC.

Key points and global issues

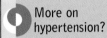
More on hypertension?

See Chapter 18 of **Davidson's Principles & Practice of Medicine (21st edn)**

- Hypertension is among the commonest disorders recognised by the World Health Organization as a cause of premature deaths – both in the developed and developing worlds.

- Many countries cannot afford the cost of drugs to treat hypertension effectively.

- Takayasu's aorto-arteritis is a rare but an important cause of hypertension, especially in young Asian females.

23

Syncope

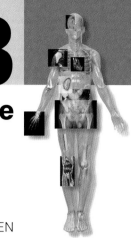

P. HENRIKSEN

Presenting problem

A 75-year-old woman is admitted following an episode of collapse. She was crossing the road and describes 'just going down' with no warning symptoms. She sustained some facial bruising and witnesses who attended her suggest that she was unconscious for up to 1 min. There did not appear to be evidence of seizure activity and, although slightly dazed, her recovery was quick within a few minutes. She is taking ramipril and bendroflumethiazide for hypertension and is generally fit and independent, enjoying a good exercise capacity.

What would your differential diagnosis include before examining the patient?

The differential diagnosis for transient loss of consciousness includes both syncope and seizure. Syncope is defined as a transient loss of consciousness due to global cerebral hypoperfusion, characterised by rapid onset, short duration and spontaneous complete recovery. Syncope may be further divided

---

BOX 23.1		
Features in the history suggesting a cause of loss of consciousness (LOC)		
	Syncope likely	**Seizure likely**
Pre-LOC	Nausea, vomiting, light-headed, sweating Blurred vision	Aura
During LOC	Short duration tonic-clonic movement (<15 s) occurring after LOC	Prolonged tonic-clonic movement commencing with LOC LOC for >5 min Automatisms (chewing)
After LOC	Rapid recovery Nausea and vomiting Lethargy	Prolonged confusion Unusual behaviour Aching muscles

into cardiac causes (with important prognostic implications when due to an arrhythmia or structural heart disease), neurally-mediated reflex syncope and postural or orthostatic hypotension. The history is pivotal in determining the diagnosis and an account of events immediately before, during and after the episode of loss of consciousness is required. The patient often has incomplete recall and collateral history from a witness may prove invaluable. Box 23.1 lists factors in the history that suggest syncope or seizures. The patient's age, together with the fact that the episode occurred during exertion and resulted in injury with rapid recovery, raise concern about cardiac syncope. Examination and initial investigations should be directed towards identifying an underlying cardiac rhythm disturbance or structural heart disease.

Examination and initial investigations

The patient is orientated and has some bruising on her face. The blood pressure is 162/85 mmHg and there is no postural drop. Her pulse is 54/min, regular, and she has a soft ejection systolic murmur audible over the aortic valve area. Neurological examination is normal.

An ECG demonstrates right bundle branch block, together with a prolonged PR interval (1st-degree block). An echocardiogram demonstrates good systolic function with no left ventricular hypertrophy. There is some thickening of the aortic valve, but it is not stenosed. Full blood count and urea and electrolytes are within normal limits.

Have examination and initial investigations narrowed down your differential diagnosis?

Yes. The resting ECG abnormalities indicate conduction disease and suggest arrhythmic syncope and the possibility of intermittent heart block. The echocardiogram has excluded aortic stenosis which may present with exertional syncope. In patients with cardiac syncope, the 12-lead ECG should be examined closely for repolarisation abnormalities pointing to possible ventricular tachycardia. These include prolongation of the QT interval or ST elevation in chest leads V1–3 in association with right bundle branch block, indicative of the Brugada syndrome in younger patients. The ECG may also reveal evidence of myocardial ischaemia and previous infarction. These findings, together with left ventricular impairment on echocardiography, also raise the possibility of ventricular tachycardia. Documentation of the supine and erect blood pressure following a 2 min period of standing is part of the initial evaluation. Although the presentation is not suggestive in this case, postural hypotension is common in the elderly. A drop in systolic pressure on standing of 20 mmHg is diagnostic. If present, culprit medications such as antihypertensives or underlying conditions associated with autonomic neuropathy, including diabetes mellitus and neurodegenerative disease, should be considered.

Given the serious presentation of exertional syncope resulting in injury this patient should be admitted for a period of heart rhythm monitoring, looking for evidence of heart block and bradycardia. If no abnormality is detected, further ambulatory rhythm recordings should be conducted. In patients with

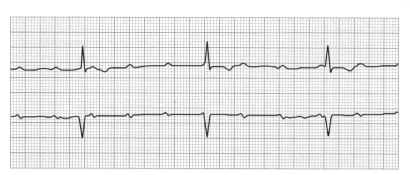

Figure 23.1 The Holter ECG demonstrated evidence of intermittent complete heart block.

recurrent syncope the goal is to capture the cardiac rhythm during an episode. Conduction disease can be intermittent and if syncopal episodes recur, but are not captured by Holter recording, then an implantable loop recorder can be used to facilitate prolonged periods of rhythm monitoring. Patients with no evidence of cardiac disease, but recurrent syncope suggestive of vasovagal or neurally-mediated syncope, may be further evaluated by tilt table testing and carotid sinus massage. These patients may have a long history of fainting with precipitating factors such as unpleasant stimuli, cough or micturition. Information from provocation testing is helpful where the episodes are recurrent and diagnostic doubt about seizures remains or when the patient's occupation is affected.

Further investigations
The results from a period of ambulatory ECG recording are shown in Figure 23.1.

Does this narrow down your differential diagnosis?
There is a transient complete heart block on the ambulatory ECG recording. Although this was asymptomatic, it confirms the suspicion that conduction disease, with intermittent periods of heart block and bradycardia, is responsible for the patient's symptoms.

How will you treat the patient?
If bradycardia is suspected, heart rate slowing medication should be stopped. Patients who are being evaluated for syncope should receive advice about driving. The patient should be considered high risk if there is evidence of cardiac disease or an abnormal ECG. This is particularly so where syncope has occurred without warning and resulted in injury. Current UK driving legislation would mandate a 6-month break from driving in this patient. The identification of intermittent heart block is an indication for implantation of a permanent dual chamber pacemaker.

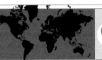
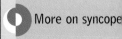
See Chapter 18 of
Davidson's Principles
& **Practice** of
Medicine (21st edn)

- Cardiac syncope has a 25% 1-year mortality. Neurally-mediated syncope is not associated with an excess mortality.

- Initial assessment is therefore directed towards identifying underlying structural heart disease or a cardiac rhythm disturbance.

- Implantable loop recorders are helpful in patients with infrequent episodes where concern about a cardiac rhythm disturbance remains.

- Patients presenting with syncope should be given advice about driving.

- Patients in resource-limited settings generally have poor access to healthcare facilities due to lack of availability of infrastructure and expertise. These patients should be investigated in hospitals with well-equipped diagnostic facilities.

24

Palpitation

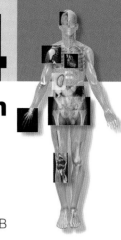

N. GRUBB

Presenting problem

A 19-year-old student with no prior medical history is referred to a cardiology clinic with a history of intermittent palpitation. Since the age of 16, she has been aware of sudden episodes of a rapid, regular, forceful heart rhythm but these always stopped within 15 min. Sometimes she was able to terminate the palpitation by holding her breath. She has not identified any specific triggers for episodes, although they are more likely to occur when she is tired. In between episodes she feels completely well. In the past few months, prior to university examinations, she has had two episodes of dizziness associated with very rapid and irregular palpitation and during one of these she blacked out. Her GP ordered some blood tests, which are unremarkable (Box 24.1).

What would your differential diagnosis include before examining the patient?

Palpitation is a common symptom in young people. Sinus tachycardia can cause palpitation, and may be triggered by anxiety or by external factors such as alcohol, caffeine or some recreational drugs (e.g. amphetamines, ecstasy). Thyrotoxicosis and anaemia can also cause a sinus tachycardia, but have been excluded here. In this case, the sudden onset and recurring pattern would be unusual for sinus tachycardia, and suggests a paroxysmal tachyar-

BOX 24.1	
Initial investigations	
Haemoglobin	125 g/L (12.5 g/dL)
TSH	1.4 mU/L
Free T$_4$	16 pmol/L (800 pg/dL)

rhythmia. Supraventricular tachycardia (SVT) is the most likely diagnosis in a young patient with no cardiac history, whereas ventricular tachycardia would be more likely in an older patient with a history of cardiovascular disease. The history of syncope is worrying and suggests that this patient requires urgent investigation.

Examination

The patient appears well and relaxed. Radial pulse is 65/min and regular. The young woman is normotensive and there is no clinical evidence of cardiac failure. Precordial examination is normal and she has no added heart sounds or murmurs. There are no abnormal cardiorespiratory findings.

Has examination narrowed down your differential diagnosis?

Examination is done principally to identify structural heart disease and heart failure. Palpitation and syncope occurring in the presence of cardiomyopathy, heart failure or valve disease may signal a tendency to malignant ventricular arrhythmia. The normal examination findings here are reassuring, but do not help to discriminate the underlying cause of the patient's palpitation.

Further investigations

A 12-lead ECG shows sinus rhythm, with a short PR interval and abnormal QRS complexes (Fig. 24.1). The upstroke of the QRS complex is slurred and there are associated T-wave abnormalities. An ambulatory electrocardiogram (ECG) recording shows sinus rhythm and, during symptoms of regular palpitation, a narrow-complex tachycardia, rate 190/min, suggestive of SVT. There is one episode during which she felt dizzy, associated with an extremely rapid, broad-complex tachycardia. Transthoracic echocardiography shows a structurally normal heart.

Does this narrow down the differential diagnosis?

The combination of a short PR interval and a 'delta wave' (slurred upstroke to the QRS complex) is diagnostic of the presence of an accessory atrioventricular pathway. If this is associated with palpitation, the condition is known as the Wolff–Parkinson–White (WPW) syndrome. Usually, WPW syndrome causes paroxysms of SVT characterised by regular, rapid palpitation. These episodes are caused by atrioventricular re-entry, in which anterograde conduction usually proceeds via the atrioventricular node and retrograde conduction proceeds via the accessory pathway. The ECG typically shows a regular tachycardia with narrow QRS complexes. The occurrence of syncope in a patient with WPW syndrome should immediately raise suspicion of pre-excited atrial fibrillation, in which atrial fibrillation waves conduct extremely rapidly to the ventricles via the accessory pathway, producing a very fast, irregular, broad-complex tachycardia. In some cases, the ventricles are stimulated so rapidly that ventricular fibrillation and sudden death occur. Ambulatory ECG monitoring is used to confirm the nature of the rhythm during symptom episodes. This is important in directing

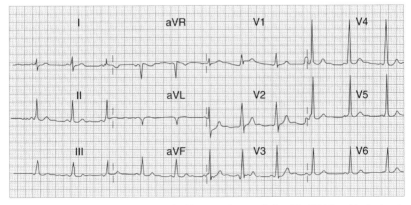

Figure 24.1 A 12-lead ECG showing classical features of pre-excitation. The PR interval is short and the onset of the QRS complex is characterised by a 'delta wave' or slurred upstroke.

treatment, since patients with WPW syndrome may experience palpitation unrelated to their accessory pathway (e.g. from extrasystoles or sinus tachycardia).

How will you treat this patient?

Episodes of SVT can be terminated by triggering vagal reflexes, which inhibit the tachycardia by causing transient atrioventricular nodal block. Patients can be taught the Valsalva manoeuvre and carotid sinus pressure, although these are not always effective. Persistent episodes may require hospital treatment. For patients known to have WPW syndrome, an intravenous flecainide infusion is probably the safest way to terminate the SVT. Flecainide blocks sodium channel conduction in accessory pathway tissue. Intravenous adenosine, while indicated for SVT management in general, should be avoided in known WPW syndrome because there is a small risk of it precipitating pre-excited atrial fibrillation. Digoxin is contraindicated because it promotes accessory pathway conduction.

First-line treatment for patients with WPW syndrome is catheter ablation therapy. This involves a procedure carried out under light sedation, in which catheter electrodes are introduced into the heart via the femoral vein. These are used to help locate the accessory pathway, which is then ablated using radiofrequency energy. Success rates exceed 95% and the risk of major complication is very small. Rarely, the accessory pathway is located close to the atrioventricular node; if damaged, permanent pacing may be required. Catheter ablation therapy eliminates the risk of death from pre-excited atrial fibrillation.

Long-term drug therapy tends to be used only in patients awaiting catheter ablation or in rare cases where the accessory pathway cannot be eliminated by catheter ablation. Sodium channel blockers such as flecainide or propafenone reduce the risk of SVT and pre-excited atrial fibrillation but do not eliminate it. The small procedural risk associated with catheter ablation is, for most patients, offset by eliminating the risk of pre-excited atrial fibrillation and the need for life-long drug prophylaxis.

Key points and global issues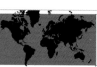

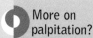 More on palpitation?

- Wolff–Parkinson–White syndrome is associated with some structural cardiac diseases, e.g. hypertrophic cardiomyopathy, mitral valve prolapse and Ebstein's anomaly. An echocardiogram should be performed in all cases.

  See Chapter 18 of
  Davidson's Principles
  & **Practice** of
  Medicine (21st edn)

- Catheter ablation facilities are not available in all centres. Where catheter ablation is not feasible, patients should be referred to an electrophysiology centre or, less ideally, treated with a class Ic anti-arrhythmic drug, such as flecainide.

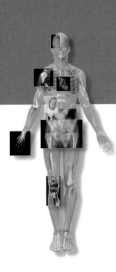

25

Infective endocarditis

M. E. YEOLEKAR

Presenting problem

A 14-year-old boy is admitted to a tertiary care hospital for evaluation of a prolonged fever. The history is given by his mother, who says that his symptoms began at the age of 6 weeks, when he started having difficulty in breast-feeding, with increased sweating and frequent crying episodes. He has never appeared blue. The boy has required frequent hospitalisations for repeated respiratory infections and one of these admissions prompted referral to a cardiac specialist. After initial evaluation, a transthoracic echocardiogram demonstrated a large ventricular septal defect (VSD) and early surgery was advised. Due to financial constraints, surgery was deferred and the boy continued with conservative medical treatment, avoiding any form of exertion. For the last 3 months, he has had a low-grade fever, increasing breathlessness, exertional palpitations, a poor appetite, muscle pains and weight loss (about 5 kg). He also has vague pains involving all joints of his hands and feet, although there is no joint swelling or restriction of movements. He denies having paroxysmal nocturnal dyspnoea (PND) or orthopnoea. There is no history of any chest pain, syncope or pedal swelling.

What would your differential diagnosis include before examining the patient?

This young boy has a large VSD. Difficulty in breast-feeding with increased sweating and frequent crying episodes are suggestive of congestive cardiac failure during infancy. His current symptoms of prolonged fever, weight loss, anorexia and polyarthralgia, on the background of congenital heart disease, would put infective endocarditis (IE) at the top of the differential diagnosis list. IE is a well-known precipitating factor for the worsening of stable congenital heart disease, and VSD is the most common congenital heart disease to be complicated by IE. The clinical course of IE is variable and dependent on numerous factors, including the causative pathogen, the nature and extent of underlying valvular disease and the status of prior health.

Other causes of such a prolonged fever include infections (tuberculosis, fungal infections, occult abscess), malignancy (lymphomas, leukaemias), connective tissue disorders and sarcoidosis, but they all seem unlikely. Fever is the most common symptom of IE and is present in 85–90% of patients, although rarely it may be absent in elderly patients, immunocompromised individuals and those with cardiac or renal failure. Fever with polyarthralgia, dyspnoea and palpitations would also raise the possibility of acute rheumatic fever in this age group, but a duration of 3 months and the absence of a preceding sore throat make this unlikely.

Examination

This patient is thin and febrile. He is pale and has clubbing of all fingernails and toenails. His vital signs are stable, except for a pulse rate of 110/min. All peripheral pulses are felt equally. There are subconjunctival haemorrhages in his right eye, and splinter haemorrhages (dark red linear subungual streaks located proximally; an embolic phenomenon) are noted in the nail beds of many fingers. His oral hygiene is poor and he has caries in a left upper molar.

Examination of the cardiovascular system reveals a grade 3/6 high-pitched pansystolic murmur, best heard in the third and fourth left intercostal spaces close to the sternum; these are consistent with a large VSD. The spleen is palpable 2 cm below the left costal margin and is non-tender. The remainder of the examination is normal.

Has examination narrowed down your differential diagnosis?

The presence of a prolonged history of pyrexia, pallor, clubbing, subconjunctival and splinter haemorrhages and splenomegaly is highly suggestive of IE. The other peripheral manifestations of IE that may be encountered include: petechiae (the most common one); Osler's nodes (painful, pea-sized, purplish nodules on the pulp of the fingers); Janeway lesions (non-tender erythematous macules over palms and soles); Roth's spots (oval retinal haemorrhages with a pale centre) and arthritis. Most of these signs are seen after 6 weeks and are characteristic of subacute bacterial endocarditis caused by *Streptococcus viridans*. Poor oro-dental hygiene in this patient has probably predisposed to the development of IE by causing intermittent bacteraemia.

Investigations

The patient's haemoglobin is 100 g/L (10 g/dL), with a peripheral smear showing normocytic normochromic anaemia. The total white cell count is 15×10^9/L (15×10^3/mm³) with 80% polymorphs. The erythrocyte sedimentation rate (ESR) is 60 mm at the end of 1st hour and the platelet count is normal. Urinary examination reveals numerous red blood cells and casts. Renal and liver function tests are normal. The chest X-ray shows cardiomegaly and a prominent pulmonary vasculature. A 12-lead ECG reveals evidence of biventricular hypertrophy (large equiphasic QRS in the midprecordial leads).

Blood cultures result in a significant growth of *Strep. viridans* after 48 h of incubation, and the growth is sent

---

BOX 25.1

Common causes of culture-negative endocarditis

- Prior administration of antibiotics (most common cause)

- *Abiotrophia* species of streptococci which are nutritionally deficient

- HACEK organisms (*Haemophilus species*, *Actinobacillus actinomycetem-comitans*, *Cardiobacterium hominis*, *Eikenella corrodens* and *Kingella kingae*)

- Right-sided endocarditis

- Fungi

- *Bartonella* species

- *Coxiella burnetii* (Q fever)

- *Legionella* species

- *Chlamydia psittaci*

- *Brucella* species

- *Tropheryma whippelii*

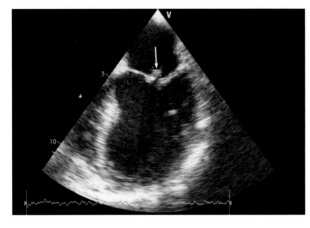

Figure 25.1
Transoesophageal
echocardiography
reveals a vegetation on
the anterior mitral
leaflet (arrow).

for sensitivity testing. Two-dimensional transthoracic and transoesophageal echocardiography (Fig. 25.1) reveals a large VSD with a 6×10 mm vegetation attached to the anterior mitral valve leaflet.

Has the diagnosis been clinched?

Yes. The positive blood culture for *Strep. viridans* and the echocardiographic evidence of a vegetation confirm infective endocarditis. The presence of a mild normocytic normochromic anaemia, poly-morphonuclear leucocytosis, a raised ESR and an active urinary sediment (due to the immune complex glomerulonephritis) all support the diagnosis. A VSD increases the risk of IE on both right- and left-sided valves; in this patient, the vegetation is present on the mitral valve due to increased blood flow across the valve. Blood culture is a crucial investigation (even although it is negative in about 14% of all cases – Box 25.1), which helps not only in diagnosis but also in guiding antibiotic therapy. Therefore, in all suspected cases of IE, three sets of blood cultures must be drawn 1 h apart under strict aseptic precautions before starting antibiotic treatment. The most common organism identified, as in this case, is *Strep. viridans*, second to follow being *S. aureus*. Electrocardiography rarely shows diagnostic findings. Transoesophageal echocardiography (TEE), particularly with biplane probes, has led to improvement in the rate of detection of vegetations.

How will you treat this patient?

If left untreated, IE has a high mortality (20–40%) due to its inherent complications (Box 25.2). Therefore, empirical treatment must be started with a synergistic combination of bactericidal antibiotics effective against *Strep. viridans* (pending the sensitivity report). Typically,

---

BOX 25.2

Complications of infective endocarditis

Cardiac complications

- Congestive cardiac failure (leading cause of death)
- Abscess (pericardial, aortic annular or myocardial)
- Conduction abnormalities (due to invasive disease)
- Coronary artery embolism
- Valvular regurgitation (cusp/leaflet flail or perforation)
- Valvular obstruction
- Prosthetic valve dehiscence
- Ventricular septal perforation

Extracardiac complications

- Systemic embolisation (stroke, renal or splenic infarction or ischaemic limb)
- Mycotic aneurysm (<5%)
- Abscesses
- Immune complex glomerulonephritis

this would involve intravenous benzyl penicillin and gentamicin for 2 weeks, with intravenous benzyl penicillin continued for a further 2 weeks. Vancomycin may be substituted for benzyl penicillin in penicillin-allergic patients or when staphylococcal infection is suspected. Improvement usually follows 3–7 days of successful antimicrobial therapy. A shorter course of treatment may be considered in 'low-risk' patients, including those with a rapid clinical response, small vegetations and infection of a native valve with a sensitive organism (low minimum inhibitory concentration). Persistent or recurrent fever may be a manifestation of treatment failure, drug fever, secondary nosocomial infection or abscess (intracardiac or extracardiac) formation. Surgery for IE (most common indication being congestive heart failure with left-sided endocarditis and refractory infection being most common indication in right-sided endocarditis) is potentially life-saving and should never be delayed in an unstable patient. After treatment of this patient's IE, the VSD should be surgically closed.

Key points and global issues

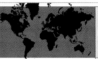

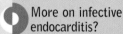

More on infective endocarditis?

See Chapter 18 of **Davidson's Principles & Practice** of **Medicine (21st edn)**

- Despite improvements in healthcare, the global incidence of IE has not decreased over the past decades. This apparent paradox is due to emerging risk factors such as intravenous drug use, an increasing incidence of degenerative valve disease in the elderly, an increasing use of prosthetic valves and occurrence of nosocomial infections. Furthermore, the overall incidence of complications related to IE has not changed significantly.

- The most common causative organism of IE in intravenous drug abusers is *Staphylococcus aureus*. It causes right-sided endocarditis with recurrent pulmonary emboli, manifesting as lung abscesses.

- The most common predisposing condition for IE in developing countries continues to be rheumatic heart disease, while in the Western world, degenerative valve disease, mitral valve prolapse, intravenous drug abuse and prosthetic valves top the list. The most common organism implicated in early endocarditis of a prosthetic valve is coagulase-negative staphylococci (*Staph. epidermidis*).

- Newly identified pathogens which are difficult to culture (e.g. *Bartonella* species) and multidrug-resistant organisms (*Staph. aureus*, *Enterococcus*) challenge conventional antimicrobial therapy. Newer serological and molecular techniques (which assist in blood culture-negative IE), novel antimicrobials and potential vaccines are emerging to meet this challenge.

- Antibiotic prophylaxis should be given to all patients with cardiac conditions, in whom the risk of IE is significant, to cover invasive procedures that may cause transient bacteraemia.

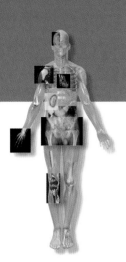

26

Rheumatic fever

PREM PAIS

Presenting problem

A 20-year-old carpenter's apprentice presents to his local hospital in India complaining of pain and swelling of his joints, together with fever, for the previous week. The pain and swelling first started in his knee joints. For the last 3 days, although the pain in the knees has eased, pain and swelling have appeared in his right elbow and left wrist. He has been unable to work since the onset of symptoms. A neighbouring physician prescribed diclofenac, which has given some temporary relief, and advised the young man to go to hospital. Together with the joint pain, he has been running a fever associated with sweating. He does not recall any preceding sore throat or fever. On questioning, he recalls that 8 years ago he had a similar episode of fever, pain and swelling of his knees, which was severe enough to keep him off school for a few weeks. He was not investigated at that time and, other than analgesics, took no medicines. He denies any history of shortness of breath or chest pain at the present or in the past.

What would your differential diagnosis include before examining the patient?

When a young man presents in India with arthritis involving a few large joints and fever, with a similar episode some years earlier, rheumatic fever (rheumatic arthritis) will be close to the top of the list of potential diagnoses. The absence of a history of preceding tonsillitis does not weaken this possibility; only about 40% of subjects will give this 'typical' history. If the previous episode was due to rheumatic fever, the patient could already have developed rheumatic valvular disease, as a proportion of patients with acute rheumatic fever subsequently develop rheumatic heart disease. If this is so, bacterial endocarditis, which at times causes arthritis, must also be considered, especially as it is a potentially life-threatening yet treatable condition. Also crippling yet treatable, is septic arthritis, but the sequential involvement of four joints makes this unlikely. Another condition to be considered is reactive arthritis. Here again, a preceding episode of diarrhoeal infection would be typical but is not essential. In reactive arthritis, there is usually involvement of the axial skeleton and often the joints of the fingers or toes; tendonitis, urethritis and uveitis may also occur. Finally, juvenile-onset spondyloarthropathy may present in young males with oligoarticular involvement of lower limb joints, and this is often associated with tendonitis.

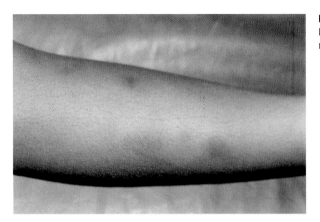

Figure 26.1 Classic lesions of erythema nodosum.

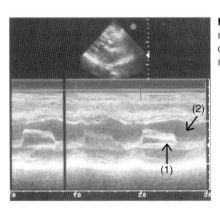

Figure 26.2 An M mode echo showing typical mitral stenosis (1) with paradoxical movement of the posterior leaflet and thickening of the mitral valve leaflets (2).

Examination

The patient weighs 60 kg and is febrile with a temperature of 38°C. His blood pressure is 110/76 mmHg and pulse rate 112 beats/min, with a regular rhythm and normal character. Both knee joints and the right elbow are swollen, red and tender and their movements are restricted because of pain. The left elbow is also tender, swollen and painful on movement. The young man has neither subconjunctival haemorrhages nor Roth's spots (seen on examination of the optic fund). There is no erythema marginatum, but lesions typical of erythema nodosum are found on the shins (Fig. 26.1). On examination of the precordium, the apical impulse is normal and there is no sternal lift. Auscultation at the cardiac apex reveals a loud first heart sound and a mid-diastolic rumbling murmur, with a pre-systolic accentuation and a soft systolic murmur. There is no accentuation of the pulmonary component of the second heart sound. There is no pericardial rub. The lungs are clear and neither liver nor spleen is palpable.

Has examination narrowed down your differential diagnosis?

The clinical findings suggest that this man has mitral stenosis, and this makes the present cluster of symptoms and signs most likely due to a recurrent episode of rheumatic fever. Erythema marginatum is a major criterion for the diagnosis of acute rheumatic fever but is seen in <5% of patients. Erythema nodosum is found much more often than erythema marginatum or rheumatic nodules, but is not specific for rheumatic fever. In the context of acute rheumatic fever it represents a reaction to recent streptococcal infection. There remains the possibility of infective endocarditis.

Investigations

Haemoglobin is 107 g/L (10.7 g/dL) and total white blood cell count is $14\,600 \times 10^9$/L (10^3/mm^3), with 84% neutrophils, 15% lymphocytes and 1% eosinophils. The erythrocyte sedimentation rate (ESR) is 90 mm/1st hour. The C-reactive protein (CRP) is increased at 87 mg/L and antistreptolysin O (ASO) antibody titre is positive (600 U), while rheumatoid factor is negative. Three blood cultures are negative and urinalysis is normal. A 12-lead ECG shows a sinus rhythm at 110/min and a PR interval of 0.22 s. A chest X-ray reveals cardiomegaly. A transthoracic echocardiogram shows thickened mitral valve cusps and an abnormal opening pattern of the mitral valve suggestive of mitral valvular stenosis (Fig. 26.2), with a mitral valve area of 1.6 cm^2. The left ventricle appears dilated but left ventricular systolic function is preserved; there is moderate mitral regurgitation but no vegetations are seen.

Does this narrow down your differential diagnosis?

The investigations suggest that the patient has rheumatic fever with carditis, superadded to pre-existing chronic valvular heart disease. Carditis is suggested because of the tachycardia, a possible new onset of mitral valve regurgitation and a dilated left ventricle on echocardiography. With regard to the diagnosis of rheumatic fever, this young man has two major Jones' criteria (Box 26.1), polyarthritis and carditis, and a number of minor criteria, i.e. fever, raised ESR and CRP, leucocytosis and 1st-degree heart block. He also has evidence of a preceding streptococcal infection – namely, a raised ASO antibody titre. The three negative blood cultures make infective endocarditis unlikely, although endocarditis caused by fastidious organisms cannot be excluded.

How will you treat this patient?

The patient should be treated as a case of rheumatic fever with carditis. If infective endocarditis is suspected, in most cases it would be best to await the results of blood culture before starting antibiotics. In sick patients, it is reasonable to begin antibiotic treatment for endocarditis once the blood cultures have been drawn and, if necessary, change the antibiotics after the blood culture results become available. This patient should be kept in bed and given 1.2 million units of benzyl penicillin intramuscularly. He should also be started on oral aspirin, three tablets of 325 mg each, 6-hourly – a total of 3.8 g daily (60 mg/kg). This should be continued until his ESR has fallen and then gradually tailed off. Given the high-dose

BOX 26.1

Jones' criteria for the diagnosis of rheumatic fever*

Major manifestations
- Carditis
- Polyarthritis
- Chorea
- Erythema marginatum
- Subcutaneous nodules

Minor manifestations
- Fever
- Arthralgia
- Previous rheumatic fever
- Raised ESR or CRP
- Leucocytosis
- 1st-degree atrioventricular block

Plus
- Supporting evidence of preceding streptococcal infection: recent scarlet fever, raised ASO or other streptococcal antibody titre, positive throat culture*

*Note: Evidence of recent streptococcal infection is particularly important if there is only one major manifestation.

aspirin therapy, it is usually prudent to prescribe a proton pump inhibitor too. Since the carditis is not symptomatic, he does not require treatment with diuretics or corticosteroids.

With this therapy, the patient improves rapidly. Within 10 days, his ESR comes down to 25 mm/h and the left ventricular dilatation on echo-screening almost completely regresses. He is discharged but advised not to return to his job, at least until his next review in 2 weeks. He is also advised to take 1.2 million units of benzathine penicillin i.m. once every 3–4 weeks, at least until he is 40 years old. The importance of this prophylaxis is explained to both the patient and his parents. Although oral antibiotics are often used as prophylaxis (phenoxy-methylpenicillin, sulfadiazine or erythromycin), it is easier to track the patient's compliance with intramuscular penicillin. In addition, he is warned to tell any doctor or dentist that he consults that he has valvular heart disease, so that pre-cautions could be taken to prevent 'infection in his heart'. He is also advised that, should he develop a fever persisting for over a week, it would be important for him to consult a doctor. At present, the mitral stenosis does not require any active intervention, but this may well be required in the years ahead. The young man is told about this and warned of the importance of coming for review at least once a year.

Key points and global issues

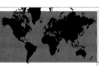

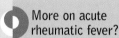

More on acute rheumatic fever?

See Chapter 18 of
Davidson's Principles
& **Practice** of
Medicine (21st edn)

• Although acute rheumatic fever (ARF) and its chronic sequela, rheumatic heart disease (RHD), have become rare in the most affluent populations, they continue to be a daily challenge to doctors who work in developing countries, where ARF is still the most common cause of acquired heart disease in childhood and adolescence.

• Poor living conditions with overcrowding and limited access to healthcare are responsible for the continuing high rate of this eminently preventable disease.

• Primary prevention of ARF (which involves providing antibiotic treatment for all symptomatic pharyngitis caused by group A *streptococcus*) has been unsuccessful because the majority of patients with ARF do not have a sore throat and therefore do not seek medical attention.

• Secondary prevention of ARF (which involves long-term administration of antibiotics to patients with a history of ARF or RHD, to prevent the recurrence of rheumatic fever) is the only proven cost-effective intervention available to date.

• An effective group A streptococcal vaccine (based on M-protein) is not yet on the horizon, and even if the obstacles of serotype coverage and safety were overcome, the cost of the vaccine would make it inaccessible to the populations that need it most.

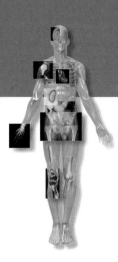

27

Acute breathlessness

M. K. DAGA

Presenting problem

A 55-year-old man presents with a 2-h history of right-sided chest pain, with worsening of his persistent breathlessness. The symptoms worsened rapidly while the patient was at work. He has been a smoker for the last 25–30 years. For the past 5–6 years, he has had a cough with expectoration during the winter months. His cough is worse on lying down. He has never been hospitalised for any other illness. He has no history of trauma to the chest and has not undergone any surgical intervention. However, he underwent therapy for pulmonary tuberculosis around 10 years ago.

What would your differential diagnosis include before examining the patient?

This is a middle-aged man with a history of chronic smoking and worsening of symptoms during winter months and that, of course, is suggestive of underlying chronic bronchitis. He has, however, experienced a rapid onset of chest pain associated with dyspnoea. The differential diagnosis is shown in Box 27.1. The absence of fever and a productive cough makes an acute infective exacerbation of chronic bronchitis and pneumonia less likely. There is no prior history of asthma and the pain is not typical of myocardial ischaemia. Acute left ventricular failure is possible, but there is no history of preceding peripheral oedema or nocturnal dyspnoea. A pulmonary embolus is a real diagnostic possibility and there need not be any obvious precipitating factor in the history. A pneumothorax should also be considered high on the list of possible diagnoses. Severe anxiety is very much a diagnosis of exclusion.

BOX 27.1
Causes of acute dyspnoea
• Pneumothorax
• Acute exacerbation of COPD
• Acute severe asthma
• Left ventricular failure
• Pneumonia
• Acute pulmonary embolism
• Severe anxiety

Examination

On examination, the patient is using his accessory muscles of respiration and has central cyanosis. His pulse rate is 116/min and his respiratory rate is 28 breaths/min. His blood pressure is 142/88 mmHg. His chest is barrel-shaped and the trachea is central. The chest wall movements on the right side are decreased and vocal fremitus is absent. The percussion note is hyper-resonant on both sides and the upper border of liver dullness is not found. Breath sounds are absent on the right side of the chest, while rhonchi and occasional crepitations are audible on the left side of the chest.

Has examination narrowed down your differential diagnosis?

Physical examination reveals signs of disease on both sides of the chest with evidence of an acute insult on the right side. Unilateral decreased chest wall movement can occur in several conditions and these include collapse of the lung, pleural effusion, a mass lesion or pneumothorax. The combination of a hyper-resonant percussion note with absent breath sounds is virtually diagnostic of pneumothorax. There is evidence of bronchospasm and hyperinflation on the left side, consistent with chronic obstructive airways disease. The presence of normal blood pressure and the midline location of the trachea provide reassurance that there is no tension pneumothorax.

Investigations

The chest X-ray shows a right-sided loculated pneumothorax with multiple emphysematous bullae (Fig. 27.1). On the left side, there are prominent bronchovascular markings with hyperinflated lung fields with a flattened left dome of the diaphragm. His arterial blood gas analysis, while breathing room air, reveals type I respiratory failure: PaO_2 7.4 kPa (56 mmHg), $PaCO_2$ 5.3 kPa (40 mmHg), oxygen saturation 80%; hydrogen ion 42 nmol/L (pH 7.38).

Has the diagnosis been clinched?

A simple chest X-ray confirms the clinical suspicion of pneumothorax. The chest X-ray is important, not only to confirm the diagnosis but also to give a clue as to any other underlying pulmonary or pleural disease. It also helps in planning the treatment of pneumothorax. There is rarely a need in such a case for any further investigations. However, care must be taken to distinguish between a large pre-existing emphysematous bulla and a pneumothorax. In such circumstances a computed tomography (CT) of the thorax is useful, as it provides additional information such as type of emphysema (smokers will have centriacinar emphysema;

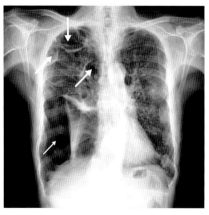

Figure 27.1 Chest X-ray showing a right side loculated pneumothorax (thin arrow) with multiple emphysematous bullae (thick arrows).

paraseptal emphysema can occur following tuberculosis and panacinar emphysema is a feature of α_1 antitrypsin deficiency), the presence of bullae and pulmonary artery hypertension.

How will you treat this patient?

Pneumothorax in the context of chronic airways disease can cause very marked respiratory compromise. The patient should be given supplemental oxygen preferably through a Venturi mask (starting at FiO_2 28% to maintain oxygen saturation at ~90%) and bronchodilators consisting of salbutamol (5 mg 6-hourly), ipratropium bromide (500 μg 6-hourly) and budesonide (500–1000 μg 12-hourly) through a nebuliser. As this patient has respiratory distress, an intercostal tube should be inserted and connected to an underwater seal bottle. This treatment will relieve his respiratory distress. A chest radiograph should be repeated to find out the status of re-expansion of the underlying lung. In addition to clinical examination, arterial blood gas analysis should also be repeated to ensure that there has been improvement in oxygenation and that there is no retention of carbon dioxide. The intercostal tube should be left in place until the leak seals and the underlying collapsed lung has completely expanded. Sometimes complications can occur following insertion of intercostal tube and include subcutaneous emphysema, re-expansion pulmonary oedema, bleeding and infection. He should be informed that recurrence of pneumothorax can occur in the future and that he may require chemical pleurodesis or surgery. Surgery is usually in the form of video-assisted thoracoscopic surgery (VATS), but clearly requires good pulmonary function. He should be advised about smoking cessation and optimal use of bronchodilators.

Key points and global issues

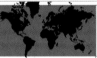

More on pneumothorax?

See Chapter 19 of **Davidson's Principles** & **Practice** of **Medicine (21st edn)**

- Pneumothorax can occur due to several lung diseases, however, globally, chronic obstructive pulmonary disease remains one of the important causes of secondary pneumothorax.

- Tuberculosis is also an important cause of pneumothorax in developing countries and may also present as hydropneumothorax or pyopneumothorax.

- *Pneumocystis jirovecii* is an important cause of pneumothorax in HIV/AIDS prevalent areas.

- Infection due to *Staphylococcus aureus* is frequently associated with pneumothorax.

- Mechanical ventilation, subclavian catheter placement and several other invasive procedures are important, but preventable, iatrogenic causes of pneumothorax.

- Early diagnosis and treatment of tension pneumothorax is crucial.

- Smoking cessation should be strongly encouraged.

28

Progressive breathlessness and cough

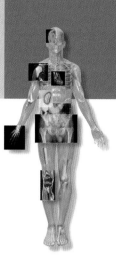

A. T. HILL

Presenting problem

A 62-year-old man is referred by his GP to a respiratory outpatient clinic, with a history of cough, sputum production and breathlessness. He has had a persistent cough for the past 12 years and produces a teaspoonful of mucopurulent phlegm on a daily basis. The breathlessness started 10 years previously and has progressively worsened, such that he is now breathless on climbing 12 stairs at a normal pace. He has no nocturnal chest symptoms and has received one course of antibiotics from his GP in the last year. His only past medical history is hypertension, which has been suboptimally controlled due to poor compliance with antihypertensive therapy. His current therapy is atenolol 50 mg once daily. He is a current smoker and has a 44-pack year history. He used to work in the demolition industry but took voluntary redundancy and retired at the age of 55.

What would your differential diagnosis include before examining the patient?

Cough and sputum production for more than 3 months of the year over 2 consecutive years meets the UK Medical Research Council definition of chronic bronchitis. The differential diagnosis should also include bronchiectasis, although patients with bronchiectasis normally have higher volumes of sputum production and suffer recurrent chest infections (this patient expectorates only a teaspoonful of mucopurulent phlegm a day and has had only one exacerbation in the past year).

The cause of the breathlessness is not clear at this stage. In view of the smoking history and the history of chronic bronchitis, he may be suffering from chronic obstructive pulmonary disease (COPD). Asthma should be considered, as the patient is on a β-blocker, but the lack of nocturnal symptoms and the development of progressive breathlessness over the last year is more in-keeping with COPD.

He was employed in the demolition industry and thus would have worked with asbestos. The differential diagnosis should include occupational lung disease – asbestos-related pleural thickening or asbestosis (interstitial pulmonary fibrosis due to asbestos).

In view of his non-compliance with the antihypertensive medication, hypertensive left ventricular failure should be excluded, although the lack of nocturnal breathlessness also goes against this diagnosis.

Examination

The patient is breathless on exertion but there is no cyanosis. He has obvious finger clubbing. Respiratory rate is 22 breaths/min, blood pressure is 160/90 mmHg, heart rate is regular at 96 beats/min and oxygen saturations are 94% breathing room air. His jugular venous pulse (JVP) is not elevated. Chest expansion and percussion are normal, but there are mid- to late fine inspiratory crackles on chest auscultation. Both heart sounds are normal and there is no peripheral oedema.

Initial investigations

Initial investigations are shown in Box 28.1.

Have examination and initial investigations narrowed down your differential diagnosis?

The clinical examination has been helpful in this circumstance. The findings are not typical of COPD. With COPD, one would have expected hyper-inflated lung fields, reduced chest expansion, hyper-resonance on percussion and reduced breath sounds. The initial investigations confirm that he has poorly-controlled hypertension, which has led to left ventricular hypertrophy identified on the electrocardiogram (ECG).

The examination findings of mid- to late inspiratory crackles and finger clubbing point to a diagnosis of pulmonary fibrosis. In view of this man's occupation, the possibility that the pulmonary fibrosis is due to heavy asbestos exposure, i.e. asbestosis, should be considered. Left ventricular failure could also cause the inspiratory crackles but would not be associated with finger clubbing. The typical chest X-ray findings in this type of case are often incorrectly interpreted as left ventricular failure.

Spirometry reveals a moderate to severe restrictive defect. This is the typical pattern

BOX 28.1	
Initial investigations	
ECG	Voltage criteria for left ventricular hypertrophy
Chest radiograph	Indistinct cardiac borders and bilateral reticulonodular shadowing suggestive of pulmonary fibrosis (Fig. 28.1)
Forced expiratory volume in 1 s (FEV$_1$)	1.3 L (46% of predicted)
Forced vital capacity (FVC)	1.6 L (42% of predicted)
FEV$_1$/FVC	81% (normal 73%)

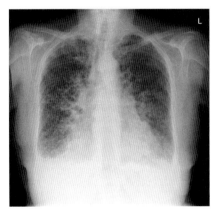

Figure 28.1 Chest X-ray showing indistinct cardiac borders and bilateral reticulonodular shadowing suggestive of pulmonary fibrosis.

seen in pulmonary fibrosis (in patients with COPD, an obstructive ventilatory defect would be expected).

Further investigations

An echocardiogram confirms left ventricular hypertrophy, with normal left ventricular function. More detailed lung function tests reveal that total lung capacity is reduced to 53% of predicted. Gas transfer for carbon monoxide is reduced to 50% of predicted. A high-resolution computed tomogram (CT) of the chest (mediastinal windows) reveals bilateral pleural plaques (Fig. 28.2); on the lung windows there is interlobular and intralobular septal thickening with honeycombing, particularly in the lower lobes and in a subpleural position (Fig. 28.3).

Does this narrow down your differential diagnosis?

To diagnose asbestosis, patients should have:

1. Significant asbestos exposure
2. Suitable lag time (usually 20+ years) between exposure and presentation of illness
3. Compared with patients with idiopathic pulmonary fibrosis (usual interstitial pneumonia), patients with asbestosis usually have a more indolent course with slower progression of breathlessness and slower radiographic progression of fibrosis
4. Mid- to late inspiratory crackles on examination
5. Finger clubbing (present in about 40% of cases)
6. A high-resolution CT of the chest showing pulmonary fibrosis predominantly in the lower lobes and in a subpleural distribution. There is usually interlobular and intralobular septal thickening, and in more advanced cases there is honeycombing. There may be subpleural lines and parenchymal bands. There may be accompanying bilateral pleural thickening and plaques
7. Lung function tests showing a restrictive defect; in more advanced cases a reduction in carbon monoxide gas transfer is seen
8. Bronchoalveolar lavage revealing asbestos bodies. This reflects a substantial lung burden with asbestos, but it only establishes the exposure, not the disease

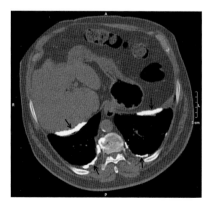

Figure 28.2 High-resolution CT of the chest (mediastinal windows). There are bilateral pleural plaques (arrows).

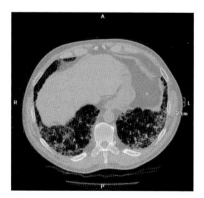

Figure 28.3 High-resolution CT of the chest (lung windows). There is interlobular and intralobular septal thickening with honeycombing, consistent with pulmonary fibrosis.

9. Final confirmation is by histological examination via thoracoscopic or open lung biopsy. This will help differentiate from other causes of pulmonary fibrosis. The Helsinki criteria for the histological diagnosis of asbestosis require at least two asbestos bodies per 5 μm thick tissue section measuring 1 cm^2. There remains controversy about the value of asbestos fibre counts and this is not routinely carried out.

This man is likely to have had significant asbestos exposure while working in the demolition industry, and meets the first six of the above criteria. There is no histological confirmation, but the overall clinical impression is that he has asbestosis.

How will you treat this patient?

Unfortunately, there is no treatment that will reverse the asbestosis. Smoking cessation is critical to reduce the risk of development of both lung cancer and mesothelioma. Supportive treatment is available. Oxygen therapy is helpful in advanced cases. Ambulatory oxygen can help patients leave the house and remain mobile. Long-term oxygen therapy is given when patients' PaO_2 is <7.3 kPa (55 mmHg). Diuretics are used once cor pulmonale with right ventricular failure develops. Both opiates and benzodiazepines may be useful in the terminal phase of the illness for palliation.

In the UK, asbestosis is an occupational lung disease and is compensatable. Claimants can receive a pension from the Department of Social Security but can also make a civil claim against their former employers. To pursue a civil claim, the claimants have to make a claim within 3 years of knowing the diagnosis.

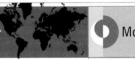

Key points and global issues

More on asbesto

- Internationally, asbestosis is an important occupational industrial disease. Prevention of asbestos-related disease should be a global priority.

See Chapter 19 of
Davidson's Principles
& **Practice** of
Medicine (21st edn)

- Chrysotile (a serpentine white asbestos that shears into smaller fibrils) is the most widely used form of asbestos. Straight asbestos fibres (amphiboles) include crocidolite (blue asbestos), amosite (brown asbestos) and tremolite. Russia and the Quebec Province in Canada are major producers of chrysotile, while South Africa produces crocidolite and amosite.

- All forms of asbestos are carcinogenic and can cause lung cancer, mesothelioma and other asbestos-related diseases. Although crocidolite appears to be more potent than others in inducing mesothelioma, all forms have an equal potential to cause bronchogenic carcinoma.

- A detailed occupational history enquiring about asbestos exposure should be sought in all individuals with respiratory disease. Such patients should be targeted for smoking cessation.

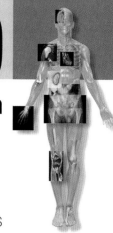

29

Pleuritic chest pain

J. A. INNES

Presenting problem

A 65-year-old man, who works for an international hotel group, is referred to the Accident and Emergency Department with a 2-week history of intermittent chest pains. He has a history of moderate chronic obstructive pulmonary disease (COPD) and also a 2-year history of prostate cancer, for which he receives androgen-suppressing treatment. Otherwise, he was well until 2 weeks prior to admission, when he developed sharp pain on inspiration below the right scapula. This made exercise, coughing and yawning painful. Two days later, he developed a mild cough productive of small amounts of yellow sputum. His symptoms settled within 5 days without specific treatment, but on the day of admission, a new sharp pain has developed posteriorly, at the base of the left lung. This time, the pain is more severe and even breathing at rest hurts.

What would your differential diagnosis include before examining the patient?

Pleuritic pain limiting breathing is usually due to infection, thromboembolism or inflammatory pleuritis. If unilateral, pneumothorax would be another possibility, but it is unlikely in this patient, who has bilateral pains separated in time. In any patient, but particularly in one with underlying COPD, pain which limits coughing will itself predispose towards infection by limiting airway clearance, so the history of yellow sputum does not really narrow the diagnostic possibilities. Inflammatory pleuritis occurs in connective tissue disease, especially systemic lupus erythematosus (SLE), but onset in a male of this age would be very unusual. Thus, the main possibilities are infection (bacterial or viral) causing pleural inflammation and thromboembolism. From the history, the patient may be predisposed to thromboembolism, both by his underlying prostatic malignancy and by his occupation (always remember to ask about recent long journeys). The most important feature of this history is the two sequential episodes of pleuritic pain separated in both time and site. This should raise a high index of suspicion with regard to thromboembolism.

Examination

The patient has a modestly elevated respiratory rate (20/min) and is reluctant to take deep breaths due to pain. His temperature is mildly elevated (38.1°C), but he has no pallor or cyanosis. Pulse is 90/min, there is sinus rhythm

and blood pressure is normal, as is the remainder of the cardiovascular examination. Examination of the chest reveals limited expansion on both sides due
to discomfort, and a soft pleural rub on inspiration posteriorly, at the left base.
There is no detectable abnormality in the abdomen.

 Initial investigations

Results of initial investigations are shown in Box 29.1.

Have examination and initial investigations narrowed your differential diagnosis?

In this common clinical situation, the examination has merely confirmed that the
pleura are inflamed at the left base, but it has not helped to distinguish the main
causes. Low-grade fever is typical in patients with pulmonary infarcts, as well
as in those with pneumonic infection. Small pulmonary emboli (PE) commonly
cause pleural pain without causing clinical features of right heart failure (raised
jugular venous pulse, right ventricular heave, loud P2); these usually occur only
with multiple or very large emboli (e.g. 'saddle emboli') obstructing a large
fraction of the pulmonary circulation. It is also common for clinical features of
deep venous thrombosis (DVT) to be absent in this situation. The diagnosis
remains ambiguous after initial investigations. Both pulmonary infarction and
infection can produce X-ray patches, modest elevation of the white cell count
and type 1 respiratory failure (hypoxia with normal CO_2). The elevated D-dimer
is also unhelpful, as this marker is raised by a number of conditions apart from
PE and indeed correlates with clinical outcome in pneumonia. Only a low value
(below 0.3 mg/L or 300 ng/mL) would have excluded thromboembolism.

Further investigations

The choice of further investigations is important here. Radionuclide ven-
tilation/perfusion scanning is likely to be unhelpful in this patient, because he
has a past history of COPD. This will typically cause multiple areas of matched
ventilation and perfusion abnormality obscuring any unmatched perfusion
defects. Computed tomogram (CT) pulmonary angiography (Fig. 29.1) is now
the investigation of choice in this area.

BOX 29.1	
Initial investigations	
Haemoglobin	137 g/L (13.7 g/dL)
WCC	12.1×10^9/L (10^3/mm³)
Oxygen saturation breathing room air	93%
Chest X-ray	Small patch of shadowing at the left base
D-dimer	1.45 mg/L (1450 ng/mL)
Arterial blood gas breathing air	
PO_2	8.5 kPa (64 mmHg)
PCO_2	4.5 kPa (34 mmHg)
H^+	39 nmol/L (pH 7.41)

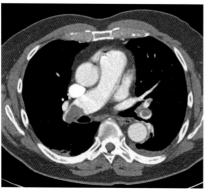

Figure 29.1 Image from the patient's CT pulmonary angiogram. Thrombus appears as dark filling defects in the right main pulmonary artery and also in the left lower lobe pulmonary artery, with a bright crescent of contrast surrounding it. There are also small areas of pleural reaction posteriorly on both sides corresponding to the sites of the patient's chest pains.

Does this narrow down your differential diagnosis?

The finding of thrombus, appearing as filling defects in otherwise contrast-filled lobar or segmental pulmonary arteries, is diagnostic of PE.

How will you treat this patient?

The main risk to the patient is of further major PE; therefore, as soon as there is a suspicion of thromboembolism from the history, the correct treatment is immediate formal anticoagulation using subcutaneous low molecular weight heparin (LMWH) pending further investigations. Oxygen should be given to relieve hypoxia, and analgesics should be given to ease pleural pain. There is evidence that continuing LMWH for at least 5 days while commencing oral anticoagulation leads to improved clearance of thrombus. If purulent sputum persists, it may be prudent to add antibiotics such as amoxicillin, as pulmonary infarcts easily become infected. In this patient, it would also be appropriate to reassess the prostatic carcinoma, in case it has spread to involve pelvic veins, precipitating his thromboembolism. More commonly, however, thrombosis with malignancy arises due to systemic activation of coagulation by the tumour.

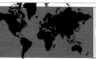

Key points and global issues

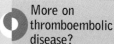

More on thromboembolic disease?

See Chapter 19 of
Davidson's Principles
& Practice of
Medicine (21st edn)

- PE and DVT are different manifestations of the same disease process, which is collectively known as venous thromboembolism (VTE).

- The diagnosis of PE is frequently missed and is difficult to confirm in resource-limited settings, due to non-availability of most of the diagnostic tools. Untreated PE is associated with a high mortality.

- When compared with unfractionated heparin (UFH), LMWH preparations are safe, efficacious and cost-effective for the treatment of acute VTE. However, at present, the evidence to support the use of LMWH in the management of massive PE is limited.

- Anticoagulant prophylaxis significantly reduces the risk for VTE in at-risk hospitalised medical patients.

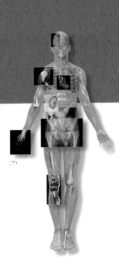

30
Haemoptysis

S. K. SHARMA

Presenting problem

A 45-year-old woman presents with a 3-month history of cough, expectoration and haemoptysis. She also complains of low-grade fever in the evenings. She has anorexia and has lost about 10 kg in weight during the last 2 months. She is a heavy cigarette smoker. Four years ago she received treatment for sputum smear-positive fibrocavitary pulmonary tuberculosis involving the left upper lobe. This involved directly observed thrice-weekly intermittent treatment with rifampicin, isoniazid, pyrazinamide and ethambutol for 2 months, and rifampicin and isoniazid for the subsequent 4 months.

What would your differential diagnosis include before examining the patient?

This patient had sputum smear-positive pulmonary tuberculosis 4 years ago and received a full course of antituberculosis treatment. She now presents again with a history of fever, toxaemic symptoms, haemoptysis, loss of appetite and weight loss. Bleeding from the cavity wall, rupture of Rasmussen's aneurysm (i.e. the dilatation of a small to medium-sized pulmonary artery in a tuberculosis cavity), direct erosion of capillaries/arteries by granulomatous inflammation, tuberculosis, endobronchiolitis, broncholith and cavernolith have all been postulated to be the mechanisms responsible for haemoptysis in patients with pulmonary tuberculosis. The causes of haemoptysis in a patient with a past history of tuberculosis are listed in Box 30.1.

Examination

Physical examination reveals mild pallor and crepitations in the infraclavicular and suprascapular areas on the left side. There is no evidence of peripheral lymphadenopathy. Physical examination is otherwise unremarkable.

Has examination narrowed down your differential diagnosis?

Physical examination points to a lesion in the left upper lobe. There is no other localisation clue. Physical examination can sometimes be unremarkable in patients with

BOX 30.1

Causes of haemoptysis in a patient with a past history of tuberculosis

- Reactivation tuberculosis
- Reinfection tuberculosis
- Post-tuberculosis bronchiectasis
- Aspergilloma
- Scar carcinoma

reactivation/reinfection tuberculosis, and several other conditions should be considered under the differential diagnosis. Further investigations are needed.

Further investigations

The patient is human immunodeficiency virus (HIV)-seronegative. Full blood count, serum biochemistry, urine examination and abdominal ultrasonography are normal. An oral glucose tolerance test rules out a diagnosis of diabetes mellitus. Sputum smear examination does not reveal acid-fast bacilli or malignant cells, and sputum culture does not grow mycobacteria. Sputum examination does, however, reveal fragments of fungal hyphae and sputum culture grows *Aspergillus fumigatus*. A chest X-ray reveals a left upper zone fibrocavitary lesion. Computed tomography (CT) of the chest (Fig. 30.1) reveals a cavity in the left upper lobe containing a radio-opaque shadow with a semicircular air crescent around it. The differential diagnosis for this radiographic presentation is shown in Box 30.2. When the CT is repeated with the patient in the prone position, the fungal ball is observed to have changed its position. An intradermal skin test with extracts of *Aspergillus fumigatus* is positive. Serum precipitins (double diffusion in gel method) and immunoglobulin G (IgG) against *Aspergillus fumigatus* are positive.

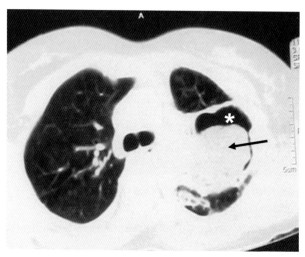

Figure 30.1 CT of the chest (lung window) showing a fungus ball (arrow) in a cavity in the left upper lobe. A semicircular, crescentic air shadow (asterisk) can also be seen around the radio-opaque fungus ball (air-crescent sign).

BOX 30.2

Differential diagnosis of a radio-opaque shadow in the lungs with a semicircular air crescent shadow ('air-crescent sign')

- Fungus ball
- Organised haematoma or pus inside a cavity
- Hydatid cyst
- Lung cancer

Does this narrow down the differential diagnosis?

Since she has been sputum smear-negative on two occasions, reactivation/reinfection pulmonary tuberculosis appears unlikely. The radiological evidence of the cavity in the left upper lobe, the positive skin test and the mycological and serological results strongly favour the diagnosis of aspergilloma in a tuberculosis cavity.

A fungus ball may be present for a long period without producing any clinical symptoms and may be incidentally detected. Most patients develop haemoptysis, which can sometimes be life-threatening, due to various causes such as mechanical friction, secretion of endotoxin with haemolytic properties, an anticoagulant factor derived from *Aspergillus*, local vasculitis and direct invasion of the blood vessels in the cavity by the fungal ball. Other clinical features include cough, weight loss, anorexia, fever and dyspnoea.

How will you treat this patient?

There is no consensus regarding the ideal treatment for aspergilloma. Systemic antifungal treatment is ineffective. Local instillation of antifungal agents using a bronchoscope has been used with varying results. Bronchial artery embolisation has been used for the management of recurrent haemoptysis in some patients. Some authorities have advocated surgery because of the potential for haemoptysis, which can sometimes be massive. Surgery is indicated if the haemoptysis is repetitive, severe or life-threatening. Asymptomatic patients and those with mild infrequent haemoptysis should be carefully monitored.

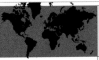

Key points and global issues

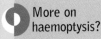

More on haemoptysis?

See Chapter 19 of
Davidson's Principles
& Practice of
Medicine (21st edn)

- Fungus balls are particularly common in areas of endemic tuberculosis, e.g. India, sub-Saharan Africa.

- HIV infection has contributed to an increasing prevalence of tuberculosis.

- In Western countries, fungal balls have been described in cystic fibrosis, sarcoidosis, bronchiectasis, asbestosis, histoplasmosis and bronchial cysts.

- The 'air-crescent sign' can be identified by plain film chest tomography, as well as by CT.

31

A solitary radiographic pulmonary lesion

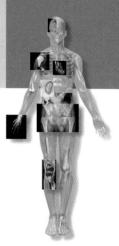

S. K. SHARMA

Presenting problem

A 55-year-old asymptomatic man is referred to the chest clinic because a solitary lesion has been detected in the left lower hemithorax on a chest X-ray taken as part of preoperative evaluation for hernia surgery about 2 months previously. He is a heavy cigarette smoker who is healthy, but for left-sided indirect inguinal hernia. Otherwise, his general health has been good in the past and he is not taking any form of medication. There is no history of contact with animals or international travel.

What would your differential diagnosis include before examining the patient?

The evaluation of a solitary pulmonary radiographic lesion in an asymptomatic patient is a common diagnostic dilemma. The goal in evaluating such a lesion is to distinguish a benign from a potentially malignant lesion. Considering the age of this patient and his smoking habit, malignant conditions like bronchogenic carcinoma and solitary metastasis would top the list of possibilities (Box 31.1), but benign conditions such as tuberculosis, fungal infections, hydatid disease and Wegener's granulomatosis, among others, must be ruled out.

Examination

The patient is apyrexial, and there is no evidence of Horner's syndrome, cutaneous lesions or peripheral lymphadenopathy. No abnormal masses are noted on palpation of the abdomen and examination of the respiratory system is normal. In short, the physical examination is unremarkable.

Has examination narrowed down your differential diagnosis?

The physical examination is not infrequently unremarkable in patients with a solitary pulmonary radiographic lesion. Narrowing down of the differential diagnosis requires more investigations.

Further investigations

Full blood count, serum biochemistry, urine examination and abdominal ultrasonography are normal. Sputum smear does not reveal acid-fast bacilli or malignant cells, and sputum culture does not grow mycobacteria or fungi. This man is human immunodeficiency virus (HIV)-seronegative. A tuberculin skin test (5 tuberculin units), complement fixation and enzyme-linked immunosorbent assay (ELISA) tests for hydatid disease, a serological panel for coccidioidomycosis, antineutrophil cytoplasmic antibodies (ANCA) and rheumatoid factor (RF) are all negative. A repeat chest X-ray (Fig. 31.1) confirms a solitary

BOX 31.1

Common aetiological causes of a solitary radiographic pulmonary lesion

Malignant causes
- Bronchogenic carcinoma
- Lymphoma
- Carcinoid tumour
- Metastasis

Benign causes
- Congenital
  Bronchogenic cyst
  Bronchial atresia
- Infections
  Granulomatous infections, e.g. mycobacterial (tuberculosis), fungal (coccidioidomycosis)
  Lung abscess
  Round pneumonia
  Septic embolisation
  Nocardiosis
  Parasitic, e.g. hydatid disease, *Dirofilaria* (dog heart worm)
  Infected bulla
- Connective tissue disorders
  Wegener's granulomatosis
  Rheumatoid arthritis (necrobiotic nodule)
- Vascular
  Arteriovenous malformation
  Pulmonary infarction
  Pulmonary artery aneurysm
  Pulmonary venous varix
  Haematoma
- Airway diseases
  Mucocoele
- Neoplasms
  Hamartoma
  Inflammatory pseudotumour
- Unknown aetiology

pulmonary radiographic lesion in the left lower zone. There is no evidence of calcification.

Does this narrow down the differential diagnosis?

The patient has been asymptomatic and apyrexial throughout and there is no evidence of immunosuppression. Therefore, a lung abscess, pneumonia or septic embolism is unlikely. The negative serological panel for fungal infections, together with no history of travel to areas where fungal infections such as coccidioidomycosis are endemic, argues against possible fungal causes. The absence of eye- and kidney-related symptoms and arthralgias, normal urinalysis and negative ANCA and RF tests rule out Wegener's granulomatosis and rheumatoid arthritis as possible causes. As the patient is a heavy smoker and the available investigations are inconclusive, a further diagnostic evaluation is required.

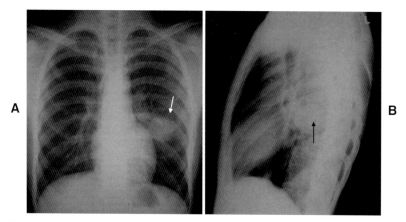

Figure 31.1 Chest radiograph showing a solitary pulmonary radiographic lesion (arrows) in the left lower zone. (A) Postero-anterior view. (B) Lateral view.

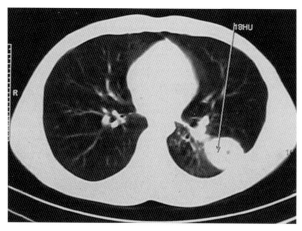

Figure 31.2 Contrast-enhanced spiral CT of the chest showing an enhancing (18 HU) solitary pulmonary lesion. There is no evidence of mediastinal lymphadenopathy.

Definitive investigations

Fibreoptic bronchoscopy is unremarkable. The bronchoscopic aspirate does not reveal acid-fast bacilli or malignant cells.

Contrast-enhanced computed tomography (CT) of the chest (Fig. 31.2) verifies a solitary, smooth, round lesion in the lung, with no evidence of calcification. The lesion shows an attenuation value of 18 Hounsfield units (HU) after the administration of intravenous contrast. There is no evidence of mediastinal lymphadenopathy. The attenuation value of 18 HU argues against cystic lesions such as hydatid cyst or lung abscess and suggests a high probability of a malignant lesion (normal lung has attenuation values between −400 and −600; cystic lesions are close to zero.) The CT findings in patients with benign and malignant solitary pulmonary nodules are contrasted in Box 31.2. In a patient with a solitary radiographic pulmonary lesion, round margins, the presence of

BOX 31.2

CT findings in solitary benign and malignant lesions

Variable	Benign more likely	Malignant more likely
Size	<3 cm	>3 cm
	80% of benign nodules are <2 cm in size	42% of malignant nodules are <2 cm in size
Growth (defined as ≥26% increase in diameter)	Doubling time <1 month or >18 months	Doubling time 1–18 months
Margins	Smooth, well-defined	Spiculated, tabulated margins
Satellite lesions	Frequent	Rare
Calcification	Frequently present	Rare
Presence of fat	50% hamartomas will have fat detectable on thin section CT	Seldom seen
Cavitation	Frequent in tuberculosis, Wegener's granulomatosis, pulmonary infarction and lung abscess	Rare, although squamous cell carcinoma can cavitate
Air bronchograms or bubbly low attenuation	May be rarely seen in organising pneumonia, sarcoidosis, pulmonary infarcts	Frequently seen in adenocarcinoma, especially localised bronchoalveolar carcinoma

central, laminated, diffuse or 'popcorn' calcification, the presence of fat within the lesion, homogeneous attenuation, the presence of satellite nodules and a CT density value of <15 HU all favour a benign aetiology. In the present patient, the lesion has a smooth round margin without spiculation. However, about 20% of malignant lesions can have a round margin. Positron emission tomography (which has high sensitivity and specificity in evaluating lung lesions) is not available at the centre where the patient is being evaluated, as is the case in most developing countries.

A CT-guided percutaneous needle biopsy reveals a well-differentiated squamous cell carcinoma. Abdominal ultrasonography, CT of the brain and a radionuclide bone scan do not reveal any evidence of metastatic disease. In view of the patient's age and smoking history, preoperative pulmonary function tests are carried out and found to be normal. Cardiac status evaluation, including an electrocardiogram and echocardiography, are normal.

How will you treat this patient?

Unfortunately, the majority of patients with bronchogenic carcinoma of squamous cell histology are inoperable by the time the diagnosis is made. This patient is lucky in that his solitary radiographic pulmonary lesion has been identified incidentally and confirmed to be a primary bronchogenic carcinoma. There is no evidence of involvement of central mediastinal structures or tumour spread to distant sites. Thus, the patient has stage I disease (N0, M0, tumour confined within visceral pleura). He does not have any significant comorbid condition and his cardiac status and respiratory reserve are adequate to allow a surgical resection. Although the overall prognosis in bronchogenic carcinoma is very poor, with around 80% of patients dying within 1 year of diagnosis, patients with a well-differentiated squamous cell carcinoma which has not metastasised are amenable to surgical treatment and have the best prognosis. This patient should be advised to have surgical resection of the tumour, as this carries the best hope of long-term survival; the 5-year survival rate in stage I disease is over 75%. Many patients with squamous cell carcinoma have undetectable microscopic metastases at diagnosis. After surgery, this patient should also receive adjuvant chemotherapy with carboplatin- or cisplatin-based regimens.

Key points and global issues

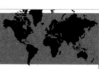

More on solitary radiographic pulmonary lesions?

See Chapter 19 of **Davidson's Principles & Practice** of **Medicine (21st edn)**

- Tobacco smoking is the most important cause of lung cancer. In contrast to developed countries where a decreasing trend is being observed, smoking, especially bidi smoking, is on the rise in developing countries. Thus, the burden of lung cancer is expected to increase in the developing world in the years to come.

- Even in developed countries like the USA and UK, smoking prevalence and deaths from lung cancer continue to increase in women, and more women now die of lung cancer than breast cancer.

- In spite of the advent of CT imaging, the widespread availability of fibreoptic bronchoscopy and facilities for histopathological and cytopathological diagnosis, even in developed countries patients with lung cancer too often present late in the disease, when it is inoperable and only palliative treatment is possible. These facilities are not widely available in developing countries; given that tobacco smoking is increasing there, lung cancer, detected at a stage where nothing other than palliative care will be possible, is likely to emerge as a major public health problem.

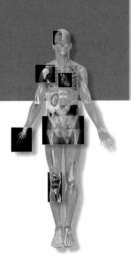

32

Pleural effusion

S. K. SHARMA

Presenting problem

A 25-year-old man presents with a 5-day history of right-sided chest pain and describes it as a 'catch in the breath'. It gets worse with deep breathing and coughing. During this period, he has developed a fever, which is more pronounced in the evening. He also complains of a dry cough. Over the past 2 days, he has developed breathlessness, which has worsened rapidly. He does not complain of a rash, oral ulcers, photosensitivity or joint pains. He is an otherwise healthy bank clerk who has not suffered from any other illness. He does not smoke or drink alcohol and is not taking any medication.

What would your differential diagnosis include before examination?

When an otherwise healthy young male presents with right-sided pleuritic chest pain and fever, the diagnostic possibilities include pleurisy, pneumonia, venous thromboembolism (VTE) with pulmonary infarction and pneumothorax. In a patient with pneumonia, the illness starts with fever and the pleuritic chest pain develops later on due to involvement of the overlying costal parietal pleura. Sudden onset of pain and breathlessness are features of pneumothorax. In VTE with pulmonary infarction, the patient presents with haemoptysis, breathlessness and pleuritic chest pain; fever is usually not present and usually there is an appropriate clinical setting for venous thrombosis. When a patient presents with pleuritic chest pain followed by fever and progressive breathlessness, the possibility of acute pleurisy going on to pleural effusion is the most likely diagnosis.

Examination

Physical examination reveals mild pallor. His pulse is regular at 110 beats/min and his blood pressure is 120/82 mmHg. Respiratory rate is 26/min. There is no evidence of a rash, oral ulcers, arthritis or peripheral lymphadenopathy. Signs of chronic liver disease are absent. The trachea is shifted to the left side and the apical impulse is shifted laterally. The right side of the chest moves less with respiration. Tactile vocal fremitus is reduced. On percussion, a stony dull note is elicited on the right side and this dullness does not shift with change in posture. Breath sounds and vocal resonance are almost absent on the right side. There is no succussion splash. Abdominal, cardiovascular and neurological examinations are normal. The rest of the physical examination is unremarkable.

Has the examination narrowed down your differential diagnosis?

Physical examination points to a right-sided pleural effusion.

Further investigation

He is human immunodeficiency virus (HIV) seronegative. A full blood count, serum biochemistry and urine examination are normal. Random blood glucose is not elevated. A sputum specimen is not available for testing. A tuberculin skin test (5 TU) is positive (14×20 mm) after 48 h. Serological tests for antinuclear and rheumatoid factors are negative. A chest radiograph (Fig. 32.1A) reveals a dense uniform opacity in the lower and lateral parts of the right hemithorax, shading off above and medially into the translucent lung, suggestive of a right-sided pleural effusion. Echocardiography and ultrasonography of the abdomen are normal. Contrast-enhanced tomography of the chest (Fig. 32.1B) suggests the presence of a right-sided pleural effusion. There are no

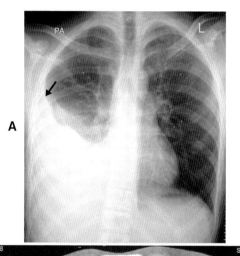

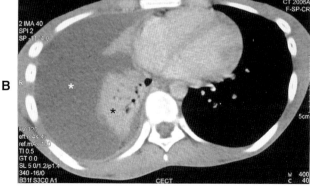

Figure 32.1 (A) Chest radiograph (postero-anterior view) showing right-sided pleural effusion (arrow). (B) Contrast enhanced computed tomogram of the chest showing pleural effusion. The white asterisk indicates fluid and the black asterisk indicates the collapsed lung.

loculations; the diaphragm and subdiaphragmatic space are normal. An appropriate site for thoracocentesis is localised on ultrasonography of the chest and marked.

After securing written informed consent, under local anaesthesia, a diagnostic thoracocentesis is first performed and 50 mL of a serous amber-coloured pleural fluid is aspirated. Then, needle biopsy of the pleura is obtained and a further 600 mL of pleural fluid is drained. The pleural fluid is subjected to cell count, biochemical analysis, cytopathology, Gram stain, Ziehl–Neelsen stain, bacterial and mycobacterial culture. The pleural fluid serum protein ratio is >0.5; pleural fluid serum lactate dehydrogenase (LDH) ratio is >0.6, suggesting that it is an exudative pleural effusion. Furthermore, the pleural fluid is lymphocyte rich, adenosine deaminase (ADA) level in the pleural fluid is 86 U/L (cut-off value >35 U/L is suggestive of tuberculosis) and the fluid is negative for acid-fast bacilli (AFB) and malignant cells. The pleural biopsy reveals caseating epithelioid granulomas. Pleural fluid culture grows *M. tuberculosis* 6 weeks later.

Does this narrow down the differential diagnosis?

The differential diagnosis for an exudative pleural effusion is shown in Box 32.1. The patient is an otherwise healthy man who developed pleurisy with a pleural effusion which is exudative, lymphocyte rich and negative for AFB and malignant cells. He is tuberculin skin test positive; the pleural fluid grew *M. tuberculosis* and the pleural biopsy revealed granulomatous inflammation. The diagnosis in this young person is tuberculosis pleural effusion.

How will you treat this patient?

The patient should be started on antituberculosis treatment (2-month intensive phase with isoniazid, rifampicin, pyrazinamide and ethambutol, followed by a 4-month continuation phase with isoniazid and rifampicin). The drugs can be administered either daily or thrice weekly under direct observation as advocated by the National TB Control Programmes of the respective country.

Since there is strong evidence suggestive of tuberculosis in the form of a positive tuberculin skin test, a needle biopsy of the pleura indicating granulomatous inflammation, pleural fluid growing *M. tuberculosis*, and the patient does not have any other contraindication for corticosteroid use, prednisolone 20 mg daily by mouth can be administered for 4–6 weeks to prevent pleural thickening. Chest radiographs should be repeated during follow-up at the end of 2 and 6 months. Close follow-up is essential as some patients become defaulters. During follow-up visits patients should be evaluated clinically, radiologically and biochemically. Liver function tests should be done if symptoms suggest hepatotoxicity and serum uric acid checked if generalized body aches occur. It is mandatory to rule out acute viral hepatitis in endemic areas in patients who are diagnosed with hepatotoxicity due to antituberculosis treatment. Once diagnosed with hepatotoxicity, isoniazid, rifampicin and pyrazinamide should be

---

BOX 32.1

Common causes of an exudative pleural effusion

- Tuberculosis
- Pneumonia
- Malignant disease
- Bronchogenic carcinoma and other causes of pleural metastases such as breast cancer
- Lymphoma
- Pulmonary infarction
- Subdiaphragmatic causes, e.g. amoebic liver abscess, pancreatitis
- Connective tissue disorders, e.g. systemic lupus erythematosus

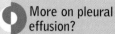

immediately stopped until liver function tests return to normal values. Ethambutol, an aminoglycoside and a quinolone should be administered during this period. While on antituberculosis treatment gastrointestinal related adverse events are quite common and these usually respond to symptomatic treatment.

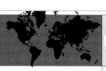

Key points and global issues

More on pleural effusion?

See Chapter 19 of
**Davidson's Principles
& Practice** of
Medicine (21st edn)

• Pleural effusion is the second most common site of extrapulmonary tuberculosis (the first being lymph node tuberculosis) and is a common cause of pleural effusion in areas endemic for tuberculosis. With the advent of a global pandemic of HIV infection and acquired immunodeficiency syndrome (AIDS), tuberculosis is once again emerging as an important cause of pleural effusion.

• In areas where tuberculosis is highly endemic, a positive tuberculin skin test in an adult patient only indicates evidence of infection but does not necessarily suggest active disease. Furthermore, tuberculin anergy is common in patients with HIV infection and AIDS. Therefore, tuberculin skin test results should be cautiously interpreted in patients with a tuberculosis pleural effusion in such areas. Interferon-γ release assays (IGRAs) are available but do not differentiate between latent TB infection and active TB disease.

• In resource-poor countries, facilities for pleural fluid cell count, protein and sugar estimation are commonly available. Though pleural fluid Ziehl–Neelsen staining and Gram staining are available, their yield is low. An elevated ADA level in the pleural fluid may aid in the diagnosis. Pleural fluid culture usually takes more than 3 months. Molecular methods such as polymerase chain reaction, although costly for developing countries, can provide early diagnosis; however, false-positivity of the tests in endemic areas needs to be kept in mind.

• Patients with an exudative pleural effusion that is rich in lymphocytes often receive empirical antituberculosis treatment under programme conditions as facilities for further detailed diagnostic testing are often not available. They are often referred to teaching hospitals attached to medical schools for further diagnostic work-up if they do not improve.

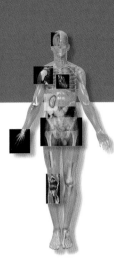

33

Day-time sleepiness

P. T. REID

Presenting problem

During the assessment of a 40-year-old man with hypertension, systematic enquiry reveals a history of excessive day-time sleepiness and poor concentration. He has no other symptoms. However, his wife reports that he snores loudly and that, on occasion, she has noticed he appears to stop breathing and she shakes him to make sure he is alive. He has smoked 20 cigarettes/day for 30 years, drinks 30 units of alcohol per week and is overweight. His high blood pressure is treated with lisinopril and bendroflumethiazide. His work involves periods on night shift and he is concerned that he has fallen asleep behind the wheel of the car when sitting at traffic lights. He lives at home with his wife; they have two young children aged 6 months and 3 years.

What would your differential diagnosis include before examining this patient?

Enquiry into the sleep history is good practice during any assessment. This man may be experiencing fragmentation of normal sleep through shift work or is having poor-quality sleep while he raises his young family. However, one of the most important and treatable causes of excessive day-time sleepiness is obstructive sleep apnoea hypopnoea syndrome (OSAHS) and this should be at the forefront of any clinician's mind. Other causes of excessive day-time tiredness include depression, hypothyroidism, certain drugs such as β-blockers or selective serotonin re-uptake inhibitors, and excessive use of sedatives or stimulants. Periodic limb movement disorder, narcolepsy and idiopathic hypersomnolence should also be considered.

Examination and initial investigations

The patient is 1.63 m tall, weighs 110 kg and has marked central obesity. His mandible and tongue appear normal and inspection of the upper airway reveals no evidence of nasal or pharyngeal obstruction. He is in sinus rhythm and his blood pressure is 180/110 mmHg. No abnormal findings are noted on examination of the respiratory, cardiovascular or neurological systems.

Simple spirometry reveals a mild obstructive ventilatory defect with no significant reversibility (Box 33.1) and the Epworth Sleepiness Scale (ESS) is 17/24. Thyroid function tests are normal.

BOX 33.1

Spirometry results

	Baseline	Predicted*
FEV$_1$	2.3 L	3.36 L (2.85–3.87 L)
VC	3.9 L	4.01 L (3.4–4.62 L)
FEV$_1$/VC	0.59	0.8
20 min following 2.5 mg salbutamol		
FEV$_1$	2.34 L	
VC	3.95 L	

*Median (range) predicted values for a 40-year-old man who is 1.63 m tall. FEV$_1$, forced expiratory volume in 1 second; VC, vital capacity.

Have examination and initial investigations narrowed down your differential diagnosis?

The most likely diagnosis remains OSAHS. In this condition, the upper airway collapses intermittently and repeatedly during sleep. Partial obstruction results in snoring; complete collapse requires an increased respiratory effort to overcome the obstruction, resulting in a transient wakening of the patient. This pattern occurs repeatedly throughout the night, resulting in poor-quality sleep, excessive day-time sleepiness and poor concentration. The condition is more common in men, particularly if they are obese (this patient has a body mass index of 41.4) and have a collar size >17 inches (42.5 cm). Abnormalities in the anatomy of the upper airway may increase the likelihood of obstruction, such as an abnormally small mandible, macroglossia, large tonsils or uvula. Examination should also consider whether there are any features of hypothyroidism, acromegaly or Marfan's syndrome.

The ESS is a validated questionnaire for assessing the likelihood of falling asleep in a variety of situations. The maximum score is 24. All patients, and their partners, should complete an Epworth questionnaire; an ESS >10 suggests significant day-time sleepiness and should prompt referral to a sleep service.

Further investigations

The patient undergoes a formal sleep study. Figure 33.1 details the polysomnography (PSG) and shows multiple apnoeic and hypopnoeic events (apnoea being a 10-second breath hold, and hypopnoea being a 10-second event where there is continued breathing, but ventilation is reduced by at least 50% from the previous baseline during sleep). The apnoea/hypopnoea index (AHI) is 63.4. The oximetry trace shows multiple episodes of desaturation, with the lowest oxygen saturation being 57%. There is no evidence of periodic leg movements. A diagnosis of obstructive sleep apnoea (OSA) is made when the AHI score is >5 events/h, while the diagnosis of OSAHS requires the additional presence of day-time sleepiness.

Does this narrow down your differential diagnosis?

Sleep studies confirm the diagnostic suspicion and provide an indication of the severity. The study demonstrates that this patient has OSAHS and the AHI of 63.4 indicates severe disease. PSG is expensive and more limited sleep studies (e.g. a measure of airflow, thoraco-abdominal movement, oximetry and heart

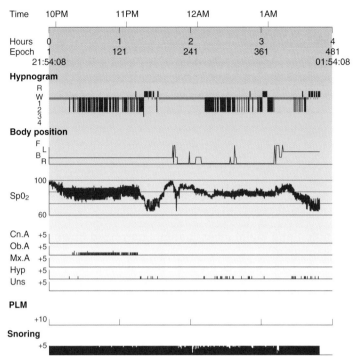

Figure 33.1 The use of polysomnography (PSG) allows the simultaneous recording of breathing and sleep pattern over a period of time (in this example, over 4 h). Typical recordings include an electroencephalogram (not shown here), a measure of respiratory airflow, thoraco-abdominal movement (allowing identification of hypopnoeas and apnoeas) and oxygen saturation (allowing the identification of significant desaturation events). Some centres also record body position (front, back, left and right) and the occurrence of snoring. In this case, the patient experiences multiple apnoeic and hypopnoeic events; the apnoea/hypopnoea index (AHI) is 63.4 (Box 33.2). The oximetry trace shows multiple episodes of desaturation, with the lowest SaO_2 being 57% (Box 33.3). There is no evidence of periodic leg movements (PLM).

BOX 33.2

Respiratory events (REM and non-REM sleep)

Parameter	REM	Non-REM	Sleep
Obstructive apnoeas	0	46	71
Hypopnoeas	9	23	42
AHI (h)	–	–	63.4

AHI, apnoea/hypopnoea index; REM, rapid eye movement.

BOX 33.3

SaO_2 summary

SaO_2 awake average	96%
Lowest SaO_2	67%
Average SaO_2 desaturation	9%
Number of desaturations $\geq 4\%$	75

rate) are often sufficient for first-line investigation. Oximetry alone is rarely adequate.

How will you treat this patient?

The AHI provides an indication of the severity of OSAHS and current evidence suggests that patients with an AHI ≥15 or a 4% oxygen saturation dip rate at the level of >10/h benefit from treatment. This man should be advised to lose weight (although this is rarely successful) and avoid alcohol, which exacerbates the condition. He should be referred for establishment of continuous positive airways pressure (CPAP), which functions as a pneumatic splint preventing upper airway collapse during sleep. Treatment with CPAP has been shown to improve day-time sleepiness, cognitive function, vigilance, mood and quality of life. The main problem with CPAP therapy is adherence and it is important to review the patient with this in mind. Use for <2 h per night suggests long-term compliance is likely to be poor. Intra-oral devices are often considered for patients with mild OSAHS and those patients unable to tolerate CPAP. Surgery may be considered in carefully selected patients.

Patients with OSAHS and excessive day-time sleepiness are at increased risk of road traffic accidents. In the UK, the law requires that all patients with OSAHS should inform the Driver Vehicle and Licensing Authority (DVLA) of the diagnosis. Driving is permitted, provided the patient demonstrates satisfactory control of symptoms. Hypertension appears to be independently associated with OSAHS and treatment with CPAP has also been shown to assist in lowering BP, thereby potentially helping to lower the risk of cardiovascular events or stroke.

Key points and global issues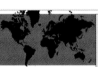

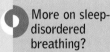
More on sleep-disordered breathing?

See Chapter 19 of
Davidson's Principles
& **Practice** of
Medicine (21st edn)

- OSAHS is an emerging public health problem worldwide because of its significant association with obesity, hypertension, insulin resistance and increased cardiovascular morbidity.

- In general, the disease often remains undiagnosed because of a low level of awareness among primary physicians.

- Prevalence of the disease in the Western population is approximately 4% in males and 2% in females.

- Truncal obesity, increased neck circumference (43 cm in males and 40 cm in females), male gender, increasing age (up to 65 years), hypothyroidism, acromegaly and, in the Chinese population, craniofacial features that compromise the upper airway are important risk factors.

- A clinical diagnosis of OSA may be made on the basis of a characteristic history (snoring and day-time sleepiness) and physical examination (anthropometry and neck circumference), but overnight PSG is the gold standard investigation to confirm the diagnosis. Access to PSG may be limited in resource-poor countries.

- Nasal CPAP is the usual first-line treatment but is costly.

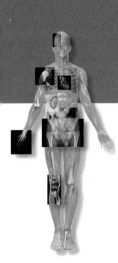

34

Chronic wheeze

P. KUNA

Presenting problem

A 29-year-old male baker is referred to the Pulmonary and Allergic Diseases outpatient department with a history of bouts of breathlessness, recurrent respiratory infections and effort intolerance, due to breathlessness and chest tightness, occurring typically 10–15 min after completion of exercise. The first episode of shortness of breath occurred 8 years previously and since that time, it has become a frequent complaint. Respiratory symptoms wake him almost every night, impairing his life considerably. He has worked in the same bakery for the last 10 years and recently has noticed that contact with flour triggers breathlessness and wheezing, accompanied by watery rhinorrhea and bouts of sneezing. The patient reports occasional temporary improvement during summertime and feels that his condition is steadily deteriorating, with no apparent cause. He is otherwise well, does not take any medications, except for short cycles of oral antibiotics periodically for bronchitis and occasional oxymetazoline for relief of nasal symptoms. He used to smoke (20 cigarettes a day for 5 years) but gave this up 3 years previously.

What would your differential diagnosis include before examining the patient?

Breathlessness is a common complaint due to cardiac and pulmonary conditions, with a peak incidence in the 5th and 6th decades of life. Given this patient's relatively young age, cardiac disorders that should be considered would include mainly congenital conditions, valvular abnormalities and arrhythmias. However, a pulmonary cause seems more likely. Interstitial lung disease is a possibility, but the paroxysmal nature of his symptoms indicates a functional disorder rather than structural pathology. Undoubtedly, bronchial asthma and chronic obstructive pulmonary disease should be at the top of the differential diagnosis list.

Examination

Routine physical examination is essentially unremarkable – the patient is a normally built young man with no apparent abnormalities, a regular pulse rate of 70/min, and supine blood pressure of 116/80 mmHg on his left arm and 110/80 mmHg on his right arm. The heart sounds are clear and regular, there are no murmurs. Auscultation of the lungs is normal. There is no lower extremity oedema.

Has examination narrowed down your differential diagnosis?

Physical examination is frequently normal in patients with a history of paroxysmal breathlessness and so may not narrow down the differential diagnosis. Although normal chest auscultation and similar blood pressure value on both arms do not rule out congenital heart defects or valvular abnormalities completely, they do make such diagnoses seem less likely.

Investigations

Routine haematology, biochemistry and liver function tests are normal. An echocardiogram reveals normal appearance and function of the valves and heart muscle with ejection fraction of 70%. A standard 12-lead ECG shows sinus rhythm confirmed on 24-h ambulatory ECG monitoring (sinus rhythm at rest and on exertion with no pathologies whatsoever). A chest radiograph is normal.

Basic spirometry demonstrates a forced expiratory volume in 1 second (FEV_1) of 2.90 L/min (70% of predicted value), forced vital capacity (FVC) of 5.02 L/min (103% of predicted value) and FEV_1/FVC of 59.86% (Fig. 34.1). At 15 min after inhalation of salbutamol (albuterol), the spirometric values are as follows: FEV_1 3.78 L/min (30% increase from baseline), FVC 5.26 L/min (4% increase from baseline) and FEV_1/FVC of 71, 87%.

Skin prick tests with an extended panel of allergens are performed, the patient develops a positive wheal and flare response to grass pollens, cat's dander, rye, wheat, rye flour and wheat flour.

Does this narrow down your differential diagnosis?

Airflow limitation found on basic spirometry indicates the presence of obstructive pulmonary disease, either asthma or COPD. A reversibility test with an inhaled short-acting β-agonist is a simple tool used to differentiate between those

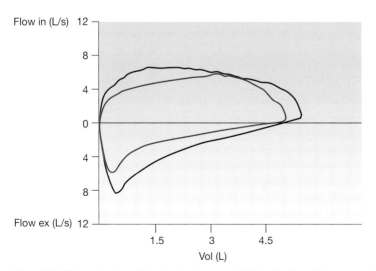

Figure 34.1 Change in spirometric values during a reversibility test – the red lines represent the baseline readings and the black lines are the results after the nebulised salbutamol.

two conditions – an increase of 12% and 200 mL in spirometric values is a cut-off point for a positive result according to The Global Initiative for Asthma (GINA) guidelines. The positive reversibility test, in conjunction with a consistent clinical history and positive skin prick test results, confirms allergic asthma diagnosis.

Further investigations

Specific IgE antibodies against the allergens of rye flour, wheat flour, barley flour and rice flour are detected in this patient's peripheral blood.

An inhalation challenge with different types of flour leads to a significant decrease in FEV_1 and PEF values at time points specific for early and delayed allergic reaction. Changes in spirometry are accompanied by rhinitis symptoms (sneezing and rhinorrhea). In view of patient's medical history (onset of symptoms approximately 1 year after the beginning of exposure at work, contact with allergens at work triggers exacerbations, temporary improvements during vacations), the above tests confirm the diagnosis of occupational asthma and rhinitis.

How will you treat this patient?

Occupational asthma can be reversible if it is diagnosed early and properly treated. Although long-term exposure to allergens at work worsens the condition, many patients refuse to even consider changing to a different job. Treatment of occupational asthma does not differ from treatment of other types of asthma – the patient should be prescribed inhaled glucocorticoids for daily use and a short-acting, inhaled β-agonist as a rescue medication in case of dyspnoea. Exposure to flour should be rigorously avoided. The patient should be re-evaluated after 3 months. If there is improvement, a step-down approach to therapy should be implemented to keep him on the lowest doses of inhaled glucocorticoids securing adequate disease control. The patient should also be prescribed an oral glucocorticoid, with a written management plan explaining how to take this drug, in case of a severe exacerbation.

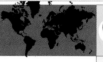

Key points and global issues

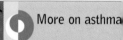

More on asthma

- Occupational asthma is now the most common occupational respiratory disorder – it accounts for 5% of all adult-onset asthma.

  See Chapter 19 of
  Davidson's Principles
  & **Practice** of
  Medicine (21st edn)

- Occupational asthma should be considered in all adults with asthma of working age, particularly if symptoms subside during time away from work, e.g. weekends, holidays.

35

Hyponatraemia

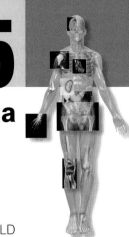

M. J. FIELD

Presenting problem

A consultation is requested on the neurosurgery ward for a 71-year-old man who has become confused and aggressive on the ward. He was admitted 14 days previously following a motor vehicle accident in which he received numerous injuries to the head and trunk. An intracerebral haematoma in the left parietal lobe was identified on computed tomography (CT) (Fig. 35.1) and evacuated 8 days following his admission. In the immediate postoperative period, he was ventilated in the intensive care unit and, following discharge from there, he developed a right lower lobe pneumonia, which was treated with intravenous antibiotics. His behaviour has been deteriorating for several days by the time of consultation, and routine biochemistry has shown that the plasma sodium has fallen from 136 mmol/L (mEq/L) on the day of admission to 117 mmol/L (mEq/L).

What would your differential diagnosis include before examining the patient?

Hyponatraemia generally indicates a relative excess of water in relation to sodium in the extracellular fluid. It can develop in a context where the total body sodium content is low, normal or high. In the present clinical situation, it is possible that a disturbance of total body sodium (and hence extracellular fluid volume) has occurred during his period of hospital treatment, but it is even more likely that he has developed water retention without a major underlying disturbance of sodium balance. It is important to check that he has not been given an excess of sodium-free intravenous fluids, such as 5% glucose, which would aggravate any tendency to water retention. Both cerebral injury and lung pathology have the potential to stimulate the release of antidiuretic hormone (vasopressin) from the hypothalamus–posterior pituitary axis. Therefore, the syndrome of inappropriate secretion of antidiuretic hormone (SIADH) seems the most likely working diagnosis.

Examination

On examination, the patient is disoriented and somewhat aggressive to those around him. There is a dressing over his craniotomy wound. On examination of the cardiovascular system, the blood pressure is normal lying and sitting, and there is no evidence of tissue dehydration (hypovolaemia), or of peripheral oedema suggestive of sodium retention. Examination of the lung

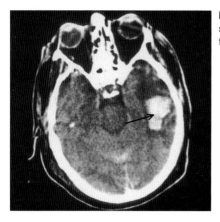

Figure 35.1 Cerebral CT scan of the patient, showing an intracerebral haematoma (arrow) in the left parietal lobe.

fields reveals some reduction of air entry and crepitations at the right base, consistent with resolving pneumonia. There are no focal neurological signs, although complete examination is difficult because of his confused state. The intravenous fluid charts show that no sodium-free fluids have been administered since his admission to hospital.

Has examination narrowed down your differential diagnosis?

The hyponatraemia appears to have developed here in the context of normovolaemia; in the absence of a large administered load of free water, the most likely diagnosis remains SIADH. If the hyponatraemia had developed more insidiously and over a longer time period, hypothyroidism and impaired adrenocortical function would need to be considered. A number of drugs can cause SIADH (e.g. carbamazepine, phenothiazines and clofibrate), but none had been used in this patient.

Further investigations

Repeat plasma biochemistry analysis is shown in Box 35.1. A single urine specimen is taken at the same time as the above blood specimen and shows: urine sodium 53 mmol/L (mEq/L), urine osmolality 603 mmol/kg. Plasma ADH concentration is 3.2 pmol/L (3.5 pg/mL).

Does this narrow down your differential diagnosis?

The low plasma osmolality confirms that the measured hyponatraemia is real, rather than being an artefact, and it suggests that the patient's disturbed mental function is likely to reflect a degree of cerebral oedema. (The head injury itself and the chest infection may also be contributing to his confusion.) The finding of a high urine osmolality, associated with a high urine sodium concentration, is consistent with SIADH rather than a hypovolaemic cause of water retention or an oedema-forming hypervolaemic state, both of which are typically associated with renal sodium retention and low urine sodium concentrations. The ADH concentration is elevated above the near-zero levels that would be expected in the face of the low plasma osmolality. In the present context, this is consistent with SIADH, as there is neither an osmotic nor a circulatory (non-osmotic) stimulus to its release.

How will you treat this patient?

The mainstay of treatment for SIADH is fluid restriction. Carefully supervised restriction of fluid intake to 600 mL/day is the appropriate first step in management of this patient's water retention disorder, and gradual elevation in his plasma sodium and the level of mental function can be expected. Given the significant cerebral pathology and surgical intervention, as well as the resolving pneumonia, SIADH may persist for some time, and sometimes an adjunctive measure to assist free water clearance can be used. Depending on local experience, this may take the form of oral demeclocycline (600–900 mg/day), or alternatively oral urea therapy (30–45 g/day) can be instituted under careful supervision. Intravenous infusion of hypertonic (3%) saline should be reserved for situations where hyponatraemia is severe, has developed very abruptly, and is associated with marked neurological complications such as seizures. Overly rapid correction of hyponatraemia, which has developed over 2 days or more, brings the risk of inducing severe neurological injury due to osmotic demyelination of cerebral neurons.

Key points and global issues

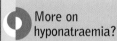

More on hyponatraemia?

See Chapter 16 of **Davidson's Principles & Practice** of **Medicine (21st edn)**

- Important factors to take into account in assessing the hyponatraemic patient are the clinical volume status, and the apparent rate of development of the disorder.

- Clinical hypovolaemia and a low urine sodium concentration suggest that the hyponatraemia is depletional (associated with a sodium deficit), while clinical euvolaemia and a high urine sodium concentration are consistent with dilutional hyponatraemia, as in SIADH. (Note, however, that in dilutional hyponatraemia due to excess water intake alone, the urine osmolality and urine sodium concentration are both low.)

- Hypovolaemic causes of hyponatraemia are encountered in areas where gastroenteritis is common and where water rather than electrolyte-containing rehydration solutions are used.

- Assay of plasma ADH is quite unnecessary to make the diagnosis of SIADH, given the appropriate clinical context and consistent plasma and urine biochemistry results.

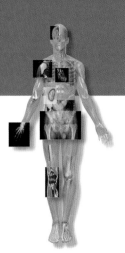

36

Hypokalaemia

M. J. FIELD

Presenting problem

A 26-year-old man is found incidentally to have a plasma potassium of 2.4 mmol/L (mEq/L) following an elective hernia repair. He has an apparently healthy diet, is taking no prescribed or illicit drugs, and specifically denies using purgatives or diuretics. He says he has experienced occasional tingling in his fingertips and a few episodes of spasm in the hands over the previous 10 years. The initial blood test results are shown in Box 36.1.

What would your differential diagnosis include before examining the patient?

The association of hypokalaemia with a high plasma bicarbonate is a common one. It is possible that the high bicarbonate is associated with a primary metabolic alkalosis and is contributing to the hypokalaemia by causing shift of potassium into cells. However, in this case, the very low potassium concentration suggests that there is some factor causing excessive potassium loss from the body, although this might also be associated with loss of acid.

Both gastrointestinal and renal causes for such potassium loss should be considered. In the case of gastrointestinal losses, the association with alkalosis would particularly suggest vomiting, but there is no report of this here (although the possibility of surreptitious self-induced vomiting has to be kept in mind, especially if there were a psychosocial setting suggestive of anorexia nervosa). Renal losses of potassium are a more likely underlying cause in this patient. A useful distinction is between renal potassium loss caused by primary mineralocorticoid excess, which is associated with renal sodium retention and hypertension, and other causes which are associated with normal or low volume states and in which blood pressure is normal or low.

The neuromuscular symptoms are suggestive of episodes of low ionised calcium concentration in the extracellular fluid, probably due to alkalosis causing increased binding of calcium to plasma albumin.

Examination

The patient is a normally built young man in apparent good health. There is no obvious evidence of frank hypovolaemia, and the blood pressure is 115/75 mmHg

BOX 36.1	
Initial investigations	
Sodium	148 mmol/L (mEq/L)
Potassium	2.4 mmol/L (mEq/L)
Chloride	98 mmol/L (mEq/L)
Bicarbonate	34 mmol/L (mEq/L)
Urea	6.5 mmol/L (18.21 mg/dL)
Creatinine	140 μmol/L (1.58 mg/dL)
Calcium	2.21 mmol/L (8.86 mg/dL)
Magnesium	0.78 mmol/L (1.9 mg/dL)
Albumin	41 g/L (4.1 g/dL)

lying and 110/80 mmHg standing. Neurological examination is normal, and tests for muscular irritability associated with hypocalcaemia (Chvostek's and Trousseau's signs) are negative.

Has examination narrowed down your differential diagnosis?

The absence of hypertension argues against primary mineralocorticoid excess. A renal tubular disorder associated with potassium wasting, and possibly also acid wasting, is now more likely, although covert diuretic use still needs to be excluded.

Further investigations

A set of arterial blood gases is useful to define more precisely the disorder of acid–base balance. This shows H^+ 31 nmol/L (pH 7.51), PO_2 11.9 kPa (89 mmHg), PCO_2 6.9 kPa (52 mmHg), base excess +5 mmol/L (mEq/L). Plasma renin activity is 25 ng/mL per hour (normal range 4–8), and plasma aldosterone is 480 pmol/L (17.3 ng/dL) (normal range 100–500 pmol/L (3.6–18 ng/dL)). A 24-h urine collection is also performed and the results are shown in Box 36.2.

A urine drug screen is negative for diuretics and all other drugs.

BOX 36.2	
24-h urine results	
Volume	3.2 L
Osmolality	350 mmol/kg
Sodium	44 mmol/L (mEq/L)
Potassium	38 mmol/L (mEq/L)
Chloride	29 mmol/L (mEq/L)

Does this narrow down your differential diagnosis?

The blood gases confirm that the hypokalaemic state is associated with a significant metabolic alkalosis, with some compensatory hypoventilation. The plasma renin and aldosterone results indicate secondary hyperaldosteronism, consistent with an acute or chronic hypovolaemic stimulus, i.e. the aldosterone concentration is in the high normal range and is associated with an increased plasma renin activity.

The urine results show that the patient is polyuric and has a relatively dilute urine, especially taken in the context of a high-range plasma sodium (and thus a high plasma osmolality). This is consistent with a partial defect of the urinary concentrating mechanism (i.e. partial nephrogenic diabetes insipidus). The appearance of significant quantities of sodium and chloride in the urine, in the face of this patient's low blood pressure and activated renin system, suggests that there is a primary renal tubular leak of sodium chloride, while the high urine potassium level in the setting of hypokalaemia suggests that there is a simultaneous tubular leak of potassium. The high urine chloride effectively excludes surreptitious vomiting, as this is associated with marked renal chloride conservation. The negative drug screen excludes surreptitious diuretic abuse.

While the plasma magnesium is in the low normal range, this suggests some parallel loss of magnesium as part of the primary problem, rather than profound magnesium depletion itself being the cause of the hypokalaemia.

All of these results are consistent with Bartter's syndrome. This condition mimics loop diuretic therapy in virtually every way, in that there is an inherited defect of the carrier mechanism mediating reabsorption of sodium, potassium and chloride in the thick ascending limb of the loop of Henle. The consequences are:

1. Sodium wasting leading to hypovolaemia and activation of the renin–angiotensin–aldosterone system
2. Potassium wasting, both from the loop of Henle itself and also because of enhanced potassium secretion in the late distal/cortical collecting duct segment, due to high sodium delivery and high aldosterone levels
3. An impaired urinary concentration mechanism (nephrogenic diabetes insipidus). This is partly caused by the failure to build up a medullary concentration gradient, due to faulty loop of Henle action. In addition,

there is resistance to the action of antidiuretic hormone (ADH) associated with the hypokalaemia and also increased medullary prostaglandin synthesis (which is also stimulated by hypokalaemia).

The metabolic alkalosis is due to increased urinary excretion of acid, provoked in part by aldosterone-stimulated distal acid secretion. The low-range plasma magnesium is a direct result of the impaired thick ascending limb reabsorptive mechanisms.

How will you treat this patient?

While the underlying tubular transport defect in this condition cannot be reversed, much can be done to alleviate the high rates of urinary loss of potassium and acid, which bring about many of the most troublesome consequences of this disorder. Therapy usually involves three elements:

1. Oral supplements of potassium chloride (e.g. slow-release KCl) are generally required, although even in high doses, they are not adequate by themselves to correct the hypokalaemia, due to continuation of tubular mechanisms driving high potassium excretion rates. Typically, 6–12 slow-release KCl tablets are needed per day.
2. Much can be gained by interfering with aldosterone action in the late distal/cortical collecting duct segment. This can be achieved using either spironolactone (50–100 mg/day) or amiloride (10–20 mg/day), both of which serve to inhibit the secretion of potassium and acid in exchange for reabsorbed sodium in this tubular segment.
3. In some cases, it can be beneficial to prescribe an inhibitor of prostaglandin synthesis, such as a non-steroidal anti-inflammatory drug (NSAID, e.g. indometacin), since increased renal prostaglandin synthesis amplifies urinary losses of sodium and potassium, while inhibiting ADH action. However, once potassium balance is restored by the above two measures, continued prostaglandin inhibition may not be necessary.

Key points and global issues

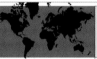

More on hypokalaemia?

See Chapter 16 of
Davidson's Principles & Practice of
Medicine (21st edn)

- The initial approach to hypokalaemia must consider causes of potassium redistribution into cells, then move to assess whether losses are through the gastrointestinal tract or the kidney.
- In many parts of the developing world, hypokalaemia will be most commonly associated with malnutrition and/or gastroenteritis. In such cases, especially where diarrhoea is the predominant symptom, the hypokalaemia will typically be associated with metabolic acidosis.
- Chronic diuretic therapy in patients with chronic valvular heart disease secondary to rheumatic heart disease is frequently associated with hypokalaemia in the developing world. Where digoxin is also administered to control the heart rate, careful monitoring for hypokalaemia is required, as serious arrhythmias can occur when diuretics and digoxin are administered concomitantly. Potassium supplementation should be provided on a regular basis to these patients.
- Diuretic and laxative abuse should always be considered in the differential diagnosis of hypokalaemia.
- Hypokalaemia may increase the difficulty in weaning patients from mechanical ventilation.

37

Metabolic acidosis

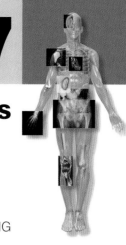

A. CUMMING

Presenting problem

A 34-year-old man presents to the Emergency Department complaining of acute left loin pain. This developed suddenly 2 h earlier, and is very severe but fluctuating in intensity. He has vomited twice. Prior to this, he has been well, but gives a history of bilateral back/loin discomfort over many years, ascribed to osteoarthritis of the spine.

He mentions an episode of right renal colic at the age of 19. He suffered bilateral wrist fractures in an occupational accident 1 year earlier. He has worked most of his life overseas as an ecologist, and has recently returned to the UK. There is no other relevant past history or family history and he is on no regular medications.

What would your differential diagnosis include before examining the patient?

Given his previous history, renal colic must be very high on the differential diagnosis list. Pyelonephritis should also be considered, but there is no history of systemic upset. Other causes of acute abdominal pain, e.g. pancreatitis, gastritis and diverticular disease, should not be excluded just yet.

Examination

He is extremely tender in the left loin, but there is no evidence of tenderness or peritonism over the anterior abdomen. He is afebrile and examination is otherwise unremarkable.

Has examination narrowed down your differential diagnosis?

Everything seems to be pointing towards the left kidney and in the absence of a fever, the history and examination are highly suggestive of left-sided renal colic, most likely due to a calculus. Renal papillary necrosis is unlikely in the absence of a history of diabetes. There are many possible underlying causes of renal stone formation including hypercalcaemia, ileal disease (increases oxalate absorption), renal tubular acidosis, medullary sponge kidney, familial hypercalciuria.

Initial investigations

Urinalysis shows +blood and no other abnormalities. Blood test results are shown in Box 37.1.

An urgent ultrasound examination shows bilateral renal calcification, typical of nephrocalcinosis (Fig. 37.1), and also a calculus lodged at the left vesico-ureteric junction.

Initial investigations

Venous blood

Urea	8.4 mmol/L (23.5 mg/dL)
Sodium	136 mmol/L (mEq/L)
Potassium	3.1 mmol/L (mEq/L)
Bicarbonate	10 mmol/L (mEq/L)
Creatinine	108 μmol/L (1.22 mg/dL)
eGFR	63 mL/min
Calcium	2.03 mmol/L (8.14 mg/dL)
Phosphate	0.68 mmol/L (2.11 mg/dL)
Alkaline phosphatase	245 units/mL
Haemoglobin	144 g/L (14.4 g/dL)
White cell count	11.3×10^9/L (10^3/mm^3)

Arterial blood

Hydrogen ion	50 nmol/L (7.3 pH)
$PaCO_2$	3.3 kPa (24.8 mmHg)
Bicarbonate	11 mmol/L (mEq/L)
PaO_2	11.4 kPa 85.5 (mmHg)

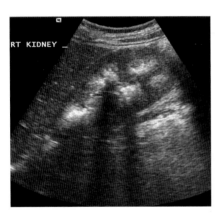

RT KIDNEY

Figure 37.1 This renal ultrasound examination demonstrates diffuse intrarenal calcification of the right kidney, affecting the medulla most severely and with some sparing of the renal cortex. The left kidney showed similar appearances.

Have the initial investigations narrowed down your differential diagnosis?

The major presenting clinical problems are left renal colic due to left ureteric calculus and diffuse bilateral nephrocalcinosis.

The biochemistry demonstrates a number of abnormalities. There is a metabolic acidosis, with a partial degree of respiratory compensation, but a very low plasma bicarbonate concentration (Fig. 37.2).

Taken together with the hypokalaemia, these features strongly suggest a diagnosis of renal tubular acidosis. In metabolic acidosis due to other causes (e.g. renal failure, diabetic ketoacidosis, lactic acidosis), potassium shifts out of cells and the plasma potassium rises.

In the absence of glycosuria or (tubular) proteinuria, and of any of the common causes of Type 2 (proximal) RTA, the most likely diagnosis is Type 1 (distal) RTA. Hypokalaemia and nephrocalcinosis are typical of this condition. There is no evidence of any of the common causes of secondary Type 1 RTA (such as

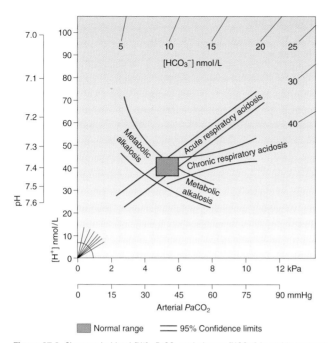

Figure 37.2 Changes in blood [H⁺], $PaCO_2$ and plasma [HCO_3^-] in stable compensated acid–base disorders. The rectangle indicates limits of normal reference ranges for [H⁺] and $PaCO_2$. The bands represent 95% confidence limits of single disturbances in human blood *in vivo*. When the point obtained by plotting [H⁺] against $PaCO_2$ does not fall within one of the labelled bands, compensation is incomplete or a mixed disorder is present.

autoimmune and hyperglobulinaemic states, drugs such as amphotericin, obstructive uropathy and sickle cell disease), and in the absence of a relevant family history, this is most likely a sporadic, idiopathic case.

The primary defect is an inability to secrete hydrogen ions in the distal tubule. This causes metabolic acidosis. In particular, because of intracellular acidosis in the proximal nephron, proximal sodium reabsorption is impaired. This leads to relative contraction of the extracellular fluid compartment, hypovolaemia and secondary hyperaldosteronism. Excessive sodium is delivered to the distal nephron, and under the influence of the increased aldosterone levels, this promotes increased exchange of sodium for potassium distally, leading to hypokalaemia. In this case, in the context of reduced fluid intake and vomiting on admission, the ECF contraction, together with partial obstruction of the left ureter, was sufficient to increase the urea and creatinine and lower the GFR.

Similarly, intracellular acidosis in the proximal nephron inhibits calcium reabsorption, leading to hypercalciuria and renal stone formation. Plasma calcium levels are reduced, causing secondary hyperparathyroidism, which is associated with increased urinary phosphate losses and hypophosphataemia. Intracellular acidosis inhibits the renal conversion of 25-hydoxyvitamin D3 to the active 1,25-dihydroxyvitamin D3. Together these abnormalities contribute to metabolic bone disease (rickets in children, osteomalacia in adults). The raised alkaline phosphatase is a marker of this condition, which will likely have contributed to his previous fractures. His long-term back discomfort could reflect the renal stone disease and/or osteomalacia.

Further investigations

Measurement of the urinary pH gives a value of 6.7 which, in the context of metabolic acidosis and acidaemia, indicates a failure of urinary acidification. In the presence of metabolic acidosis, a urine pH of >5.5 is pathognomonic of RTA. Further, more detailed tests of urinary acidification such as administration of an ammonium chloride load are not necessary in this case, but may be necessary where the abnormalities are less clear-cut.

Skeletal survey shows typical features of osteomalacia. Plasma parathyroid hormone level is moderately raised at 13.5 pmol/L (135 pg/mL).

Plasma chloride is 119 mmol/L (mEq/L). This indicates a normal anion gap, typical of renal tubular acidosis.

$([Na^+]+[K^+])-([Cl^-]+[HCO_3^-])=10$ mmol/L (mEq/L)

(normal $=8$–12 mmol/L (mEq/L))

Urinary estimations of amino acids and urate are normal, excluding a diagnosis of Fanconi syndrome (often associated with Type 2 proximal RTA). Urinary excretion rates of sodium, potassium, calcium and phosphate are all elevated.

Detailed genetic studies in kindreds (not carried out in this case) most often show mutations of Band 3 (the basolateral HCO_3 transporter of the intercalated cell in the distal nephron) or of the apical proton pump vH^+-ATPase.

How will you treat this patient?

Two hours after admission, the patient spontaneously passed a stone per urethra. Subsequent analysis of the calculus showed it to be composed primarily of calcium and phosphate.

After completion of the relevant investigations, life-long treatment with alkali should be initiated, in the form of oral sodium bicarbonate 1.5 mmol/kg body weight daily. This is titrated to achieve a normal plasma bicarbonate level. As the acidosis corrects, the secondary abnormalities of hypokalaemia, hypercalciuria and secondary hyperparathyroidism will progressively improve. Long-term potassium supplementation is usually unnecessary, and skeletal radiology after 1 year of treatment should demonstrate resolution of the osteomalacic features. Regular renal imaging should be performed to ensure that there is no further progression of the nephrocalcinosis.

Key points and global issues

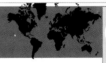

More on metabolic acidosis and kidney stones?

- Long-term alkali therapy is beneficial in preventing or controlling the secondary features of renal tubular acidosis and should be initiated as early as possible.

See Chapters 16 and 17 of **Davidson's Principles & Practice** of **Medicine (21st edn)**

- Diagnosis in this case may have been delayed because of his work in remote and rural settings overseas, with irregular access to healthcare services and routine biochemical and radiological screening.

- There are clusters of hereditary renal tubular acidosis in various geographical locations, e.g. Thailand, Malaysia, Papua New Guinea, Turkey, Saudi Arabia, North Africa and USA. In many cases, specific gene mutations have been identified.

- Hot climates may exacerbate the ECF contraction typical of Type 1 RTA, leading to worsening of secondary aldosteronism and hypokalaemia, and predisposing to intrarenal calcium/phosphate stone formation.

38

Hypomagnesaemia

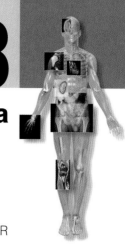

A. N. TURNER

Presenting problem

A 28-year-old male pharmacy worker is admitted to hospital complaining of muscular cramps over several weeks, worsening over the last few days, during which time he has developed progressively more severe weakness so that he now cannot stand. He has no significant past medical history, is a non-smoker who describes moderate alcohol intake, and is not on any medication. Initial investigations show potassium 2.4 mmol/L (mEq/L) and the patient is given intravenous potassium, which raises it to 3.0 mmol/L (mEq/L); his symptoms continue, however. Further tests show that plasma calcium is normal, but magnesium concentration is low at 0.45 mmol/L (1.1 mg/dL) (Box 38.1).

What would your differential diagnosis include before examining the patient?

Hypomagnesaemia rarely occurs as an isolated biochemical abnormality, and hypokalaemia is the most commonly associated abnormality, as in this patient; the symptoms may be attributable to both. Deficient magnesium intake and major shifts in magnesium balance, as may occur in 'hungry bones' syndrome, are exceptionally rare. Thus, hypomagnesaemia is invariably a consequence of magnesium loss and the initial diagnostic question is whether the losses are occurring through the gastrointestinal tract or the kidneys. In the absence of any history, renal loss is more likely, although patients may sometimes be reluctant to admit to gastrointestinal disease. Alcohol abuse is a common cause of

BOX 38.1	
Further investigations	
Sodium	136 mmol/L (136 mEq/L)
Potassium	2.4 mmol/L (2.4 mEq/L)
Bicarbonate	33 mmol/L (33 mEq/L)
Urea	4.2 mmol/L (25 mg/dL)
Creatinine	90 μmol/L (1 mg/dL)
Calcium	2.35 mmol/L (9.4 mg/dL)
Phosphate	0.8 mmol/L (2.48 mg/dL)
Magnesium	0.45 mmol/L (1.1 mg/dL) (0.75–1.05)

hypomagnesaemia – it has a magnesiuric effect promoting renal loss, overall diet may be poor resulting in low oral intake of magnesium and there may be chronic alcohol-related diarrhoea promoting gastrointestinal loss of magnesium. The patient is slightly alkalotic (raised bicarbonate) and has a normal phosphate, which rules out renal tubular acidosis and generalised proximal tubular disorders.

Examination

Routine examination is essentially normal, apart from global weakness. Pulse is 72/min and supine blood pressure is 110/64 mmHg. There are no signs of malnutrition, liver disease, thyroid disease or any other disorder. Prolonged inflation of the blood pressure cuff leads to spasm of the muscles of the forearm (Trousseau's sign).

Has examination narrowed down your differential diagnosis?

The absence of signs of liver disease or undernutrition makes gastrointestinal loss still less likely as an explanation. Although Trousseau's sign is typically associated with hypocalcaemia, it may also occur in hypomagnesaemia and does not help with the differential diagnosis.

Further investigations

A 24-h urine collection was performed and the following electrolyte results were obtained: potassium 90 mmol (mEq)/24 h (normal range ~40–100 mmol (mEq)/24 h); chloride 242 mmol (mEq)/24 h (normal range ~110–250 mmol (mEq)/24 h); magnesium 4 mmol (19.4 mg)/24 h (normal range ~3.3–4.9 mmol (8.0–11.8 mg)/24 h).

Has the diagnosis been clinched?

On-going urinary magnesium loss at a time of hypomagnesaemia confirms that the primary problem is renal. If there was an acute cause of renal hypomagnesaemia, the urine magnesium would clearly be elevated, but in chronic disorders a steady-state is achieved with urine (and GI) losses matching daily intake. The normal 24-h urinary chloride helps to exclude concealed vomiting as a cause of magnesium losses. Of the list of conditions that can cause renal hypomagnesaemia, the normal phosphate and lack of acidosis (phosphate loss and acidosis are common in tubular disorders) rule out several possibilities. The most likely cause is Gitelman's syndrome, in which there is a mutation in the sodium chloride co-transporter in the distal tubule. This is the target of thiazide diuretics, and patients with Gitelman's syndrome have many characteristics of patients overtreated with diuretics, showing modest sodium wasting and hypokalaemia. It is not clear why hypomagnesaemia is such a prominent feature of Gitelman's syndrome (more severe than in patients on diuretics), but it is diagnostically helpful. Bartter's syndrome is an analogous condition in which the abnormality is in the loop of Henle, similar to the target of loop diuretics. Sodium losses are usually much more severe, leading to presentation in childhood. Hypomagnesaemia is not a prominent feature, but hypercalciuria is common.

The patient's job in a pharmacy raises the important question of whether the abnormalities could be due to undeclared exposure to diuretics. This is very difficult to exclude altogether, although the degree of hypomagnesaemia makes this less likely. Diuretic exposure may have worsened the abnormality in a patient with another underlying cause. Diuretic abuse is associated with disorders of body image such as anorexia nervosa and bulimia. There are some rarer causes of renal magnesium wasting, and confirmation of Gitelman's requires genetic testing.

How will you treat this patient?

Initially, treatment involves replacement of potassium and magnesium intravenously. Magnesium is not easy to supplement orally, as magnesium salts cause diarrhoea. Supplementation of potassium is easier and large amounts may be required. Potassium-sparing diuretics (spironolactone, amiloride) may be useful for the hypokalaemia and help to conserve magnesium too. However, they may further lower blood pressure. Although it may be difficult to identify precipitating causes for some attacks, gastrointestinal upset is a common cause and alcoholic binges may increase magnesium excretion, so the patient should be warned to temper his alcohol intake.

Key points and global issues

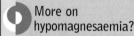 More on hypomagnesaemia?

- After sodium, potassium and calcium, magnesium is the fourth most abundant cation in the human body. It is the second most abundant intracellular cation.

  See Chapter 16 of **Davidson's Principles** & **Practice** of **Medicine (21st edn)**

- Magnesium deficiency is frequent in hospitalised patients (about 65% in intensive care units and 12% in general wards). Diabetes mellitus and alcohol consumption are commonly associated with magnesium deficiency.

- Symptoms of magnesium deficiency are non-specific and the deficiency frequently coexists with other abnormalities such as hypokalaemia, hypocalcaemia and metabolic alkalosis.

- Monitoring for magnesium deficiency is important in emergency rooms and intensive care units in critically ill patients. Access to facilities for laboratory monitoring of magnesium may be limited in the developing world.

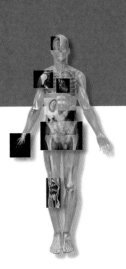

39

Haematuria

S. JAIN

Presenting problem

A 20-year-old man presents to the outpatient department with a 3-day history of facial puffiness and passing red-coloured urine. There is no associated loin or abdominal pain. He had a sore throat and fever 10 days ago. He has no previous history of note and does not take any regular medication.

What would your differential diagnosis include before examining the patient?

The red urine in this young patient suggests haematuria, indicating bleeding in the urinary tract, anywhere from the glomerulus to the urethra. Haematuria can present in various ways. It can be intermittent or persistent; painful or painless; microscopic or macroscopic. It must be emphasised, however, that not one of these variations in itself is enough to diagnose the cause of bleeding. All patients with haematuria will eventually require investigations. It must also be remembered that a very small amount of blood (as little as 1 mL) can change the colour of 1 L of urine.

Red urine is not always due to haematuria; it may be caused by haemoglobinuria, myoglobinuria, porphyria, the ingestion of beetroot and certain drugs such as Furadantin and Pyridium. Urine dipsticks can detect 1–2 red blood cells (RBCs) per high-power field but can also give false-positive results. Discoloured urine, not due to haematuria, and a false-positive dipstick result can be distinguished from haematuria by the absence of RBCs on urine microscopy. Isolated haematuria (absence of proteinuria with no other cells or cellular casts on microscopy) indicates bleeding from the urinary tract, and common causes include stones, tumours, tuberculosis and prostatitis.

Haematuria in an adult is of either glomerular or extraglomerular origin. The glomerular causes of haematuria include post-streptococcal glomerulonephritis (PSGN), IgA nephropathy and Henoch–Schönlein purpura, mesangioproliferative glomerulonephritis and Alport's syndrome (hereditary nephritis with haematuria, sensorineural deafness and ocular abnormalities). Gross haematuria with blood clots is most unlikely to have a glomerular cause and suggests a post-renal source in the urinary collecting system. Extraglomerular causes of haematuria include renal stones, renal tumours, cysts, renal infarction, bladder tumours, acute urinary tract infection, chronic infections such as tuberculosis and schistosomiasis, and the use of anticoagulants.

In this case, some of the causes of haematuria can be ruled out immediately. Acute urinary tract infection typically presents with fever, shaking chills and rigors, dysuria, pyuria, haematuria and increased frequency of micturition. Acute cystitis and urethritis in women can produce gross haematuria. Renal stones usually produce painful

BOX 39.1

Initial investigations

Haemoglobin	145 g/L (14.5 g/dL)
Serum sodium	140 mmol/L (mEq/L)
Serum potassium	4.6 mmol/L (mEq/L)
Urea	14.2 mmol/L (40 mg/dL)
Serum creatinine	266 μmol/L (1.8 mg/dL)
Urine examination	
Albumin	++
Microscopy	50–60 RBCs per high-power field, with occasional RBC casts

haematuria, whereas tuberculosis classically presents with painless haematuria along with fever. About 90% of renal stones can be demonstrated confidently on plain X-ray of the abdomen. Urogenital tumours should be suspected in older patients presenting with isolated painless haematuria.

The facial puffiness in this patient is most likely to be due to a decline in glomerular filtration (due to inflammation of glomeruli), with subsequent fluid and salt retention.

Examination

This man has facial puffiness, most prominent below the eyes, and pitting oedema of both lower legs. His blood pressure is 150/96 mmHg. The remainder of the physical examination is normal. The results of initial investigations are detailed in Box 39.1.

Have examination and initial investigations narrowed down your differential diagnosis?

The most important test in the evaluation of haematuria is urinalysis. The presence of RBC casts in this patient's urine is characteristic of glomerular pathology. Although this finding is specific, the absence of RBC casts does not exclude glomerular disease. An associated proteinuria of >500 mg/day also favours a glomerular cause for the haematuria. RBC morphology can help to differentiate a glomerular from a non-glomerular origin of haematuria. Glomerular haematuria is characterised by the presence of dysmorphic (altered shape) RBCs, while they are round or oval in non-glomerular haematuria when examined by phase-contrast microscopy. The raised blood urea and serum creatinine in this patient suggest renal insufficiency.

The presence of hypertension, oedema, haematuria and renal insufficiency suggests an acute nephritic syndrome; this is the clinical correlate of acute glomerular inflammation, characterised by gross haematuria (red or 'smoky' urine) and 'nephritic urinary sediment' (dysmorphic RBCs, RBC casts, leucocytes and subnephrotic proteinuria (<3 g/day) on urinalysis). Important causes of acute nephritic syndrome include PSGN, membranoproliferative glomerulonephritis, rapidly progressive glomerulonephritis (RPGN) and vasculitis. The absence of skin nodules, ulcers and nasal or ear discharge argues against a diagnosis of vasculitis in this patient. The history of a recent upper respiratory tract or skin infection clearly favours a diagnosis of PSGN or IgA nephropathy. Characteristically, the latent period between the preceding infection and the onset of nephritis is shorter in IgA nephropathy (24–48 h) compared with acute post-infectious glomerulonephritis (about 10 days). IgA nephropathy derives its name from the IgA deposits in the mesangium that are detected by immunofluorescence. Several episodes of occult or overt exacerbations of nephropathy following pharyngeal infections culminate in end-stage renal disease (ESRD). As renal and serological abnormalities in IgA nephropathy (a renal-limited form of glomerulonephritis) and Henoch–Schönlein purpura (a systemic disease) are similar, both conditions are considered in the spectrum of a single disease.

Further investigations

Throat culture for streptococci is negative. The anti-streptolysin O (ASO) titre is high and the serum complement (C3) level is low. Tests for anti-neutrophilic cytoplasmic antibody (ANCA), anti-nuclear and anti-glomerular

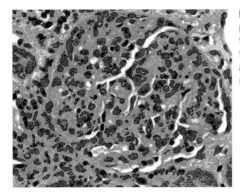

Figure 39.1 Renal histopathology of post-streptococcal glomerulonephritis. Note the diffuse hypercellularity of glomeruli due to endocapillary proliferation of mesangial and endothelial cells and to an influx of neutrophils.

basement membrane (GBM) antibodies, and circulating cryoglobulins are negative. Hepatitis B and C serologies and human immunodeficiency virus (HIV) enzyme-linked immunosorbent assay (ELISA) are negative. A percutaneous renal biopsy is performed and this shows an acute diffuse proliferative glomerulonephritis. There is diffuse hypercellularity of glomeruli due to endocapillary proliferation of mesangial and endothelial cells and to an influx of neutrophils (Fig. 39.1).

Does this narrow down your differential diagnosis?

Yes. The presence of a raised ASO titre and low complement (C3) and the renal biopsy findings confirm PSGN, i.e. glomerulonephritis following a throat infection with a nephritogenic strain of a group A β-haemolytic streptococcus. The complement levels usually return to normal within 8 weeks. If the serum C3 levels were to be persistently depressed, one should think of membranoproliferative glomerulonephritis, occult sepsis, systemic lupus erythematosus or endocarditis as the cause of this patient's glomerulonephritis.

How will you treat this patient?

Treatment should be largely supportive. He needs bed-rest and the administration of a loop diuretic (furosemide) and antihypertensive drugs (calcium channel blocker). Potassium-sparing diuretics should be avoided, as they might produce hyperkalaemia. A low-salt diet with fluid restriction should be recommended. Penicillin therapy is usually given for 10 days. The majority of patients with PSGN usually undergo spontaneous remission within 7–10 days of the onset of the disease. However, a few adult patients with PSGN may have persistent proteinuria and deranged renal functions on long-term follow-up.

Key points and global issues

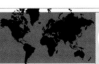

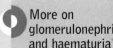

More on glomerulonephritis and haematuria

See Chapter 17 of **Davidson's Principles & Practice** of **Medicine (21st edn)**

- Acute PSGN is becoming rare in developed countries.
- In developing countries, PSGN is a common cause of acute nephritic syndrome, especially among children. The prognosis is excellent and spontaneous recovery occurs in most cases.
- IgA nephropathy is also common in southern Europe and Asia. It is more common in blacks than in whites.

40

Nephrotic syndrome

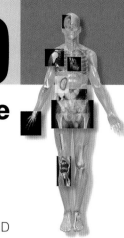

J. GODDARD

Presenting problem

A 43-year-old man presents to the Accident and Emergency Department with left pleuritic chest pain and minor haemoptysis. He gives a 3-month history of increasing bilateral leg swelling that is now up to his thighs. He has gained 10 kg in weight over this time. His wife has noticed that his eyes are puffy. He has previously been well, except for what he describes as arthritis. He has not sought medical advice about this.

What would your differential diagnosis include before examining the patient?

In addition to the usual differential diagnoses for the respiratory symptoms, with pulmonary embolism and pneumonia at the top of the list, the oedema raises the possibility of an underlying systemic problem. Increased hydrostatic pressure will cause dependent oedema. The patient could have bilateral leg deep venous thromboses (DVTs), but this would be unlikely to be associated with increasing swelling up to the thighs. It is possible that this patient has had multiple thromboembolic events with consequent raised right heart pressure and right heart failure causing peripheral oedema. Oedema may also be a consequence of liver disease and malnutrition, both of which could be associated with infection. However, both infection and thromboembolism are recognised complications of nephrotic syndrome, which typically presents as increasing oedema.

Examination and initial investigations

Blood pressure is 160/105 mmHg. The patient has pitting oedema to the mid-thighs. Heart sounds are normal and the jugular venous pulse (JVP) is elevated at +7 cm. On abdominal examination, there is no organomegaly or ascites. Chest auscultation reveals a pleural rub heard over the left lateral chest. Oxygen saturation is 98% on air.

The chest X-ray is normal but the electrocardiogram (ECG) shows a sinus tachycardia. A computed tomography pulmonary angiogram (CTPA) demonstrates a left subsegmental pulmonary embolism but no other abnormality. Doppler ultrasound demonstrates a DVT in the right calf. The left leg venous system appears normal. Initial blood tests are shown in Box 40.1. Urinalysis shows 4+ proteinuria, but no haematuria.

Have examination and initial investigations narrowed down your differential diagnosis?

The cause for the pleuritic chest pain is revealed as a pulmonary embolism secondary to a right leg DVT. The normal chest X-ray and otherwise normal CTPA (aside from the pulmonary embolism) go against chronic lung disease and secondary right heart failure (cor pulmonale) as a cause for his bilateral leg oedema. The depressed serum albumin could suggest either liver disease or malnutrition. However, the strongly positive urinalysis for protein suggests nephrotic syndrome is the underlying cause of the low serum albumin. The peripheral oedema is a consequence of low oncotic pressure and avid sodium retention.

Further investigations

The 24-h urine protein excretion is 9.6 g. Serum cholesterol is 12.5 mmol/L (483 mg/dL).

Has the diagnosis been clinched?

The abnormally high urinary protein excretion, associated with the low serum albumin, confirms nephrotic syndrome. Low oncotic pressure stimulates the liver to increase lipoprotein synthesis, resulting in hypercholesterolaemia.

Over 50% of cases of nephrotic syndrome are due to primary renal disease. The three major non-inflammatory glomerular conditions are minimal change nephropathy, focal and segmental glomerulosclerosis (FSGS) and membranous nephropathy. If a primary renal cause for this man's nephrotic syndrome is suspected, it may be appropriate to treat with empirical steroids, as these would be used initially for both minimal change nephropathy and FSGS.

While these renal conditions are usually idiopathic, this patient should be screened for conditions known to be associated with them, or other causes of nephrotic syndrome, e.g. the use of non-steroidal anti-inflammatory drugs (NSAIDs), Hodgkin's lymphoma and other haematological malignancies have been implicated in minimal change disease. Membranous nephropathy can also be associated with NSAIDs, which this patient might have bought at a pharmacy and taken for his arthritis. It is also one form of renal involvement in systemic lupus erythematosus (which could also link to this patient's arthritis). Additionally, malignancy, hepatitis B, syphilis and rarely hepatitis C may underlie this condition. Primary FSGS is, by definition, idiopathic (Fig. 40.1). It may be familial. Secondary FSGS, which is the consequence of glomerular hypertrophy or scarring due to another condition, causes proteinuria but rarely nephrotic syndrome. Inflammatory or proliferative glomerulonephritides will usually also be associated with haematuria, so are less likely in this case. A monoclonal band on serum or urine electrophoresis might point towards AL amyloidosis as a cause for this patient's nephrotic syndrome and should be excluded. Chronic inflammatory conditions that may cause AA amyloid should be considered. Proteinuria as a consequence of diabetic nephropathy can be severe enough to cause nephrotic syndrome, but diabetes has usually been present for at least 10 years for involvement to progress to this stage.

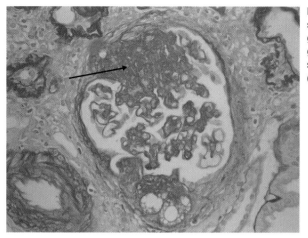

Figure 40.1 Focal and segmental glomerulosclerosis. The glomerulus in the centre shows a segmental scar (arrow).

How will you treat this patient?

Ideally, he should have a renal biopsy to establish the cause for his nephrotic syndrome, as some conditions, e.g. minimal change and primary FSGS, are treated with immunosuppression. However, he also needs anticoagulation for his thromboembolic disease; a renal biopsy must either be performed under tightly controlled conditions with intravenous heparin, which can be rapidly discontinued if post-biopsy bleeding occurs, or be postponed. His blood pressure will also need to be lowered before biopsy to reduce the risk of bleeding.

With regard to his volume overload, loop diuretics will increase natriuresis and help reduce oedema. Daily measurement of weight will help establish whether this measure is successful. The patient should also be advised about taking a low-salt diet. He may need a combination of loop diuretics and a thiazide, but care must be taken not to achieve over-diuresis, as intravascular volume depletion may cause worsening of renal function. Angiotensin-converting enzyme (ACE) inhibitors may also be used to reduce proteinuria with regular careful monitoring of renal function and, again, care to avoid volume depletion. His hypercholesterolaemia should also be treated with a statin, but should resolve as his proteinuria reduces. His risk of thrombotic complications will continue as long as the nephrotic syndrome persists, and he should be anticoagulated accordingly. If his nephrotic syndrome persists for a long period, then pneumococcal and meningococcal vaccination should be considered.

Key points and global issues

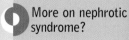

More on nephrotic syndrome?

See Chapter 17 of
Davidson's Principles
& Practice of
Medicine (21st edn)

- Nephrotic syndrome is the consequence of urinary protein loss due to an intrinsic renal lesion and is characterised by overt proteinuria (usually >3.5 g/24 h), hypoalbuminaemia (<30 g/L) and oedema, due to a combination of low oncotic pressure and avid sodium retention.

- It is a procoagulant state due to urinary losses of inhibitors of coagulation and an increase in liver synthesis of procoagulant factors.

- It is frequently associated with infective complications due to urinary losses of γ-globulins.

- Hypercholesterolaemia is common, with a consequent higher rate of atherosclerosis if the underlying condition is chronic.
- Human immunodeficiency virus (HIV) can cause a 'collapsing' variant of FSGS that presents with nephrotic syndrome.
- Tuberculosis is a common cause of AA amyloidosis, which can present with nephrotic syndrome.

41

Acute kidney injury

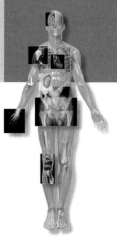

M. KING

Presenting problem

A 72-year-old man is referred to an Emergency Department with a 2-week history of loss of appetite and left loin pain. He was prescribed co-amoxiclav (course completed) for a presumed urinary tract infection, but if anything, he now feels more unwell with lethargy and severe generalised weakness. He has a background history of chronic kidney disease, type 2 diabetes mellitus and hypertension. Present medications include ramipril, metformin, bendroflumethiazide, bisoprolol, aspirin and simvastatin. His creatinine concentration usually sits around 150 μmol/L (1.69 mg/dL), with an estimated glomerular filtration rate of 38 mL/min per kg, but prior to referral, his GP had checked his renal function and had found it had deteriorated significantly.

He admits to some loose stools after starting the antibiotic. He also has chronic back pain that is unchanged in character. His loin pain has now resolved and he describes no other urinary symptoms. A 12-lead electro-cardiogram (ECG) is performed by one of the nurses and shows peaked T waves, diminished R waves, widened QRS complexes and loss of p waves (Fig. 41.1).

What would your differential diagnosis include before examining the patient?

The ECG suggests hyperkalaemia. The diagnosis should be confirmed immediately by checking his blood urea and electrolytes, but the results should not delay treatment. Urgent treatment, by administering 10 mL of 10% calcium gluconate intravenously over 10 min, is directed towards stabilisation of the myocardium and prevention of cardiac arrhythmias. Other treatment might include insulin in a dextrose infusion (10 units insulin in 125 mL 20% glucose), 5 mg nebulised salbutamol and a 1.26% sodium bicarbonate infusion.

Severe hyperkalaemia is seen almost exclusively in the setting of acute kidney injury. Other rarer causes include rhabdomyolysis, Addison's disease, tumour lysis syndrome and renal tubular acidosis.

Examination and initial investigations

On examination, pulse is 105/min, regular, blood pressure 104/75 mmHg, respiratory rate is 25/min and temperature is 37.2°C. Jugular venous pressure is normal at 2 cm. The rest of the examination is normal.

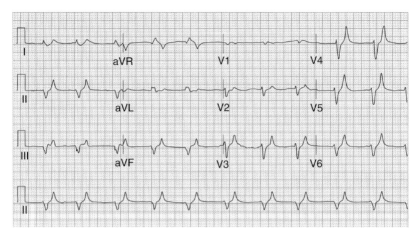

Figure 41.1 A 12-lead ECG showing features consistent with acute hyperkalaemia.

Blood urea is significantly elevated at 37.6 mmol/L (105.3 mg/dL) with a serum creatinine of 487 μmol/L (5.5 mg/dL). Serum sodium is 131 mmol/L (mEq/L) and potassium is elevated at 7.8 mmol/L (mEq/L). Venous bicarbonate is 18 mmol/L (mEq/L). Random blood glucose is 9.7 mmol/L (174.6 mg/dL). There is a mild anaemia with a haemoglobin of 103 g/L (10.3 g/dL) and MCV of 84 fL. The patient is catheterised and urinalysis shows a trace of blood and a trace of protein.

Have examination and initial investigations narrowed down your differential diagnosis?

The diagnosis is acute kidney injury (AKI). Although the potential causes are numerous, the commonest cause of AKI, particularly in the acute hospital setting, is acute tubular necrosis (ATN). ATN results from effective renal ischaemia and the predominant insults are, therefore, ones of hypotension, hypoxia and/or intravascular volume depletion. A list of some other potential insults is provided in Box 41.1. AKI is frequently multifactorial in aetiology.

Background renal disease makes this patient more susceptible to the development of AKI. The history of anorexia, diarrhoea and diuretic use may suggest a period of intravascular depletion ('dehydration'). Antibiotics are a common cause of allergic interstitial nephritis. Linking a new drug with the onset of AKI may be crucial in reaching this diagnosis but a causative association is not always obviously apparent. The history of loin pain could suggest a urological/obstructive aetiology. This can be excluded by a renal ultrasound scan looking for hydronephrosis. Although ACE inhibitors are indicated for many patients with stable chronic kidney disease, they can contribute to the development of AKI when patients are unwell. Anaemia and back pain are frequent medical problems. However, both are potential features of multiple myeloma. A myeloma screen is often considered a routine test in cases of renal failure. A history of pain may imply the use of analgesia. Use of non-steroidal anti-inflammatory drugs should be specifically asked about. Bland urinalysis makes an intra-renal disease such as a glomerulonephritis most unlikely. In summary, the patient is at risk of developing AKI during any intercurrent illness and he has a number of 'renal insults' identified in his history. His bland urinalysis would be against an intrinsic

BOX 41.1

Common 'renal insults' in the hospital setting

Insult/condition	Mechanism
Non-steroidal anti-inflammatory drugs (NSAIDs)	Loss of 'autoregulation' of renal blood flow/interstitial nephritis
Angiotensin-converting enzyme inhibitors	Loss of 'autoregulation' of renal blood flow
Aminoglycosides (e.g. gentamicin)	Tubular toxicity
Amphotericin	Tubular toxicity
CT SCAN (iodine-based radio-contrast)	Contrast induced nephropathy
Opiate based medication	Excessive dosage may cause hypotension and renal hypoperfusion
Hypotension (sepsis, drugs, excessive GI loss and blood loss)	Renal hypoperfusion and acute tubular necrosis
New drugs (especially loop diuretics and antibiotics)	Allergic interstitial nephritis
Vascular intervention	Angiography may cause cholesterol emboli
Vascular surgery/abdominal aortic aneurysm repair	Renal artery clamping leading to ATN
Pre-existing renal disease	Lower level of renal reserve and increased susceptibility to further damage

glomerular renal disease and a diagnosis of pre-renal failure developing into ATN is most likely.

How will you treat this patient?

The clinical features of tachycardia and relatively low blood pressure suggest that intravascular volume may be suboptimal. Fluid resuscitation with careful monitoring of fluid status and urine output would be the initial line of management. Ramipril and bendroflumethiazide should be discontinued. Metformin should also be discontinued due to the theoretical risk of lactic acidosis. Because of the severity of the hyperkalaemia, the patient should be managed in a high dependency area with continuous cardiac monitoring. A renal tract ultrasound is indicated to exclude obstruction. If urine output is poor and/or hyperkalaemia is refractory to treatment the patient may require renal replacement treatment/dialysis.

Key points and global issues

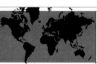

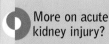
More on acute kidney injury?

See Chapter 17 of
Davidson's Principles
& **Practice** of
Medicine (21st edn)

- Acute kidney injury has many potential causes, but most frequent is ATN.

- ATN is commonly multifactorial in origin and often frequent 'renal insults' can be identified from a patient's history.
  The diagnosis is often assumed if insults can be identified and if renal and post-renal causes can be excluded by the presence of a bland urinalysis and a normal renal tract ultrasound, respectively.

- ATN is usually self-limiting if intravascular volume is optimised and further renal insults avoided, but in severe cases, renal replacement therapy may be required.

- Although renal biopsy may be considered a definitive test in the diagnosis of ATN, it carries a significant associated risk of haemorrhage and is not necessary in most cases.

- Although ATN tends to be the commonest cause of AKI worldwide, there are significant geographical differences in the underlying insult(s). In particular diarrhoea and obstetric related problems are common causes of AKI in younger patients in developing countries.

- The nature of poisons causing AKI also shows a wide degree of regional variation.

42

Chronic renal failure

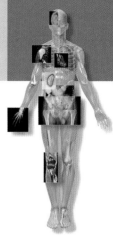

V. SAKHUJA

Presenting problem

A 22-year-old man presents with a history of diarrhoea for 2 days. He has been treated with intravenous fluids at a peripheral clinic. Although the diarrhoea has settled, there has been a decrease in his urine output and he has become breathless. Consequently, he has been transferred to a referral hospital. For the last 6 months, the patient has noticed puffiness of his face in the mornings, and tiredness, but has not sought medical attention. He denies nocturia. At the age of 7 years, he developed swelling of his feet and face, and reported to his parents that he was passing blood in his urine. He remembers that he had a kidney biopsy but cannot recall any further details.

What would your differential diagnosis include before examining the patient?

Oliguria and breathlessness, in the setting of likely dehydration following diarrhoea, are suggestive of acute renal failure with fluid overload. However, this would be unusual in a young adult, unless the diarrhoea has caused severe dehydration. Tiredness is a non-specific symptom and could be due to a host of conditions. However, coupled with a history of facial puffiness in the mornings, it should suggest pre-existing chronic renal failure (CRF). The fact that this man had a probable nephritic illness in childhood, warranting kidney biopsy, should further strengthen the suspicion that he has chronic rather than acute renal failure.

Examination

The patient is pale, tachypnoeic and unable to lie down. Puffiness of the face is evident and he has bilateral pitting pedal oedema. He is hypertensive, with a blood pressure of 180/100 mmHg and a pulse rate of 110/min. Auscultation of the lungs reveals bilateral coarse crepitations. The heart sounds are normal and there are no murmurs or pericardial rub. The results of initial investigations are provided in Box 42.1.

Have examination and initial investigations narrowed down your differential diagnosis?

Based on the clinical findings of crepitations in the lungs in an orthopnoeic patient, a diagnosis of pulmonary oedema is appropriate. Excessive intravenous fluid therapy in a setting of oliguric renal failure can precipitate a fluid overload

Initial investigations

Haemoglobin	80 g/L (8.0 g/dL)
Blood urea	39.6 mmol/L (240 mg/dL)
Serum creatinine	720 μmol/L (8.2 mg/dL)
Serum sodium	135 mmol/L (mEq/L)
Serum potassium	7.8 mmol/L (mEq/L)
Serum calcium	2.1 mmol/L (8.4 mg/dL)
Serum phosphate	2.8 mmol/L (8.7 mg/dL)
Serum albumin	32 g/L (3.2 g/dL)
Urine examination	
Albumin	++ (by dipstick)
Microscopy	1–2 granular casts per high-power field, no erythrocytes or pus cells seen
Chest X-ray	Typical bat-wing appearance of pulmonary oedema
Ultrasound	Right kidney length 8.0 cm, left kidney 8.2 cm, kidney outlines smooth

state. However, probable anaemia and hypertension are two important clinical findings in this patient that once again point towards underlying CRF. A diagnosis of CRF is usually suspected in the setting of a constellation of signs and symptoms including oedema, hypertension, anaemia and the uraemic syndrome. Pulmonary oedema can be the result of a cardiac pathology too, but the setting of oliguria after diarrhoea, history of early morning facial puffiness and essentially normal cardiac auscultation makes this unlikely.

The blood results clearly indicate that this man has renal failure. Bilaterally shrunken kidneys on ultrasound establish that there is at least a chronic element to this. Hyperkalaemia is another life-threatening complication of CRF in this patient and warrants urgent intervention.

Establishing an underlying diagnosis may have important implications for this man when considering renal transplantation in the future. Diabetes mellitus and glomerular disease are the most common causes of chronic kidney disease. He has no history of the former, but the history of a nephritic illness in childhood indicates that the most likely aetiology of his CRF is chronic glomerulonephritis. A history of polyuria and nocturia, in the absence of significant hypertension or oedema, might have suggested chronic interstitial nephritis. However, these differences become blurred in end-stage renal disease. The renal ultrasound has excluded polycystic kidney disease. Other rarer causes of CRF to be considered would include renovascular disease and systemic inflammatory diseases, such as systemic lupus erythematosus and vasculitis.

Further investigations

The patient's previous biopsy slides are reviewed and reveal membranoproliferative glomerulonephritis (Fig. 42.1). Hepatitis (B and C) and human immunodeficiency virus (HIV) serology are negative. Serial blood cultures are also negative.

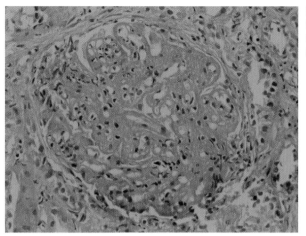

Figure 42.1 Renal biopsy showing membranoproliferative glomerulonephritis.

How will you treat this patient?

He needs immediate dialysis in view of fluid overload and hyperkalaemia. A trial of high-dose intravenous furosemide and conservative measures for hyperkalaemia (injection of calcium gluconate, glucose–insulin infusion and potassium-binding resins) may be used to buy time. Box 42.2 lists the indications for dialysis in CRF.

If the acute insult of diarrhoea and consequent dehydration is significant, this young man's renal function may improve partially and there may be no further need for dialysis. In such a non-dialysis-dependent patient with CRF, there are many facets to therapy. Anaemia can be improved by recombinant human erythropoietin and parenteral iron therapy. Hyperphosphataemia and hypo-

> **BOX 42.2**
>
> **Indications for dialysis in chronic renal failure**
>
> - Clinical symptoms and signs of uraemic syndrome
> - Fluid overload
> - Hyperkalaemia
> - Uraemic pericarditis
> - Severe metabolic acidosis

calcaemia, as seen in this patient, can be corrected by the use of phosphate binders and 1-α-hydroxylated analogues of vitamin D. This will also prevent, or at least control, renal osteodystrophy. However, these drugs should be judiciously used, with frequent monitoring of calcium, phosphate and parathyroid hormone levels, for fear of precipitating hypercalcaemia. It is possible to retard progression of CRF by tight control of blood pressure (target <130/85 mmHg; and <125/75 mmHg if proteinuria >1 g/day) and by reducing proteinuria, both of which can be achieved by using angiotensin-converting enzyme (ACE) inhibitors or angiotensin receptor blockers. Restriction of dietary sodium and diuretics will help in control of oedema.

Membranoproliferative (or mesangiocapillary) glomerulonephritis can be associated with chronic infections such as hepatitis B and bacterial endocarditis, but often no underlying cause is found. Immunosuppressive therapy is of no proven benefit. Our patient is likely to progress to end-stage renal disease over a period of time and will eventually require long-term renal replacement therapy. The options at that stage would be renal transplant, maintenance haemodialysis or continuous ambulatory peritoneal dialysis. Given his young age, 5-year survival on haemodialysis would be in excess of 80%, but this treatment is associated with a poor quality of life. His best option for long-term survival and quality of life would be a renal transplant.

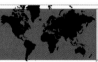

Key points and global issues

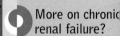

More on chronic renal failure?

See Chapter 17 of **Davidson's Principles** & **Practice** of **Medicine (21st edn)**

- In any patient who presents with unexplained renal failure, it is important to distinguish between chronic renal failure, acute renal failure and an acute insult superimposed on pre-existing chronic renal failure.

- The most common cause of CRF in the Western world is diabetic nephropathy. In the developing world, chronic glomerulonephritis has been the most frequently found cause, but the incidence of diabetic nephropathy is rapidly increasing.

- Long-term renal replacement therapy is very expensive and financial constraints often preclude such treatment in the majority of patients in resource-poor countries.

- Cadaveric renal transplant programmes are well established in the Western world. In the developing world, transplants from live relatives are much more common than cadaveric transplants.

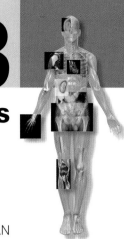

43

Thyrotoxicosis

A. G. FRAUMAN

Presenting problem

A 53-year-old contract supervisor presents to his local GP with a 3–4-month history of tremor with intermittent anxiety and sweating. He has also lost some 10 kg weight over this time period. He had intermittent diarrhoea 2 months earlier. There is no neck swelling or pain and no palpitations. He has no visual disturbance. He has a past history of hypertension and is a non-smoker. He drinks 3–4 light beers per week. He has had no recent domestic or financial stresses and has a family history of a mother who died at the age of 83 of breast cancer whom, he recalls, had also had a thyroidectomy. He is on enalapril for hypertension.

What would your differential diagnosis include before examining the patient?

Many of the symptoms here clearly point to a diagnosis of thyrotoxicosis and, in that regard, the history of thyroid disease in a 1st-degree relative may be of relevance. Many of the symptoms would also fit with an anxiety state and, given that he has hypertension, the possibility of phaeochromocytoma should also just be kept at the back of one's mind.

Examination

Clinically he appears well. He has a fine tremor and some palmar sweatiness. Pulse is 100/min and regular; his blood pressure is 130/60 mmHg. Cardiovascular, respiratory and abdominal examinations are unremarkable. He has a small diffuse goitre, but no bruit. Other than a 'staring' appearance, he has no signs of ophthalmoplegia.

Has examination narrowed down your differential diagnosis?

Goitres are common in the general population and most affected individuals will have normal thyroid function. In this context, however, with a typical history and some eye signs, thyrotoxicosis must be a racing certainty!

Investigations

Full blood count, electrolytes, liver function and random glucose are normal. ECG shows a sinus tachycardia. Thyroid function tests are abnormal: free T4 50.5 pmol/L (3926 pg/dL), total T3 4.6 nmol/L (299 ng/dL),

TSH <0.05 mU/L. Repeat thyroid function tests are conducted and these confirm thyrotoxicosis.

Has the diagnosis been clinched?

Hyperthyroidism is confirmed! The major differential diagnosis is now that of toxic multinodular goitre or Graves' disease. Less commonly seen are thyrotoxicosis due to exogenous thyroxine administration, thyroiditis or toxic adenoma. To establish a more definitive assessment of the aetiology, isotopic scanning (^{99m}technetium pertechnetate) is valuable in this context as treatment plans will differ according to aetiologies (Fig. 43.1). Thus, if a toxic multinodular goitre is present, antithyroid treatment to achieve euthyroidism, followed by radioactive iodine would be appropriate. If Graves' disease is present a prolonged (approximately 12–18 month) course of antithyroid treatment would be indicated as this has a significant permanent remission rate (see below).

Further investigations

TSH receptor antibody titres are measured and are positive. Thyroid isotopic scanning is performed (figure) and this reveals a diffuse increase in uptake, consistent with Graves' disease.

How will you treat this patient?

This patient should initially be started on antithyroid medication such as carbimazole or propylthiouracil, e.g. 5–40 mg/day or 50–400 mg/day, respectively. In a patient such as this, with moderately severe hyperthyroidism biochemically, larger doses are started initially and titrated downwardly (initially monthly), according to the patient's clinical and biochemical response. All patients should be warned of the development of an unexpected sore throat or a rash. The former may reflect the rare but potentially fatal risk of agranulocytosis, which occurs in <1% of all patients. If this were to occur, it will usually happen within the first few months of treatment and an urgent blood count must be done. β-Blockers can be used, e.g. propranolol (80–160 mg/day) if the patient has significant adrenergic symptoms. Repeat TSH receptor antibody level measurement towards the end of the treatment course may be helpful to predict the likelihood of

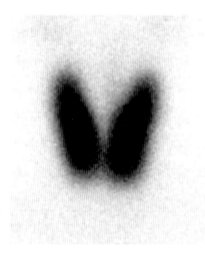

Figure 43.1 ^{99m}Technetium pertechnetate scan with diffusely increased thyroid uptake.

remission (if the TSH receptor antibody level normalises) or relapse (if the TSH receptor antibody level remains elevated). There is an approximately 50% chance of remission after a 12–18-month treatment course with antithyroid medications in Graves' disease and if the hyperthyroidism relapses after treatment cessation, a repeat course of antithyroid medications for a further 12–18 months could still have comparable remission rates. Alternatively, radioactive iodine or thyroidectomy may be considered if further relapse occurs or hyperthyroidism is difficult to control. Although this patient had minor eye signs at presentation, development of more active eye signs such as conjunctivitis, chemosis, proptosis or ophthalmoplegia may ensue and prednisolone therapy may be appropriate.

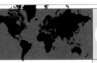

Key points and global issues

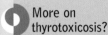

More on thyrotoxicosis?

See Chapter 20 of
Davidson's Principles
& **Practice** of
Medicine (21st edn)

- Graves' disease is a common cause of hyperthyroidism and although more prevalent in women compared with men, the diagnosis should always be entertained in a male presenting with unexplained anxiety and sweating.

- The differential diagnosis from an anxiety state is important and the possibility of hyperthyroidism is not uncommonly overlooked in the context of a patient who has a history of background anxiety.

- Hyperthyroidism is easily diagnosed when thought of and is generally easily managed with antithyroid drugs, radioactive iodine or thyroidectomy.

- TSH receptor antibody levels (TRAb) in patients with Graves' disease can be useful for prognostic purposes.

- Graves' eye disease (or Graves' ophthalmopathy), although not present initially in all patients, may develop during the course of Graves' disease (including after achievement of euthyroidism) and needs to be monitored carefully. Smoking is a major risk factor. Ophthalmology input may be necessary for more rapid or problematic cases of Graves' ophthalmopathy.

- Graves' disease may uncommonly present with hypokalaemic periodic paralysis in Asian populations.

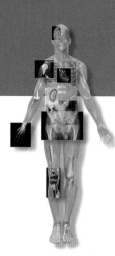

44

Solitary thyroid nodule

I. SHERIF

Presenting problem

A 46-year-old woman presents with a 3-month history of a lump in the front of her neck. The lump is painless and moves up and down when she eats or drinks. She had no difficulty in swallowing or breathing, but admits that, since she discovered it, she has been more anxious and sometimes notices tremor of the hands. Her weight has been steady, her appetite good and her bowels and periods remain regular. The lump has not changed in size since she first became aware of it.

What would your differential diagnosis include before examining the patient?

Thyroid enlargement is one of the commonest presentations in thyroid disease. The enlargement can be due to diffuse or multinodular goitre or a solitary nodule. The history does not help, except when there is acute pain suggesting haemorrhage into a cyst or (de Quervain's) thyroiditis. In the latter, one would expect there to be some systemic upset and the whole thyroid would be painful, whereas haemorrhage into a cyst would lead to more localized swelling. Symptoms of anxiety are common in patients with any lump here because of fear of malignancy. Most thyroid nodules are non-functioning and should produce no symptoms of hyperthyroidism. It is almost impossible to tell whether a nodule is benign or malignant from the history alone, although a rapid increase in size is of concern.

Examination and initial investigations

The woman looks well and does not have tachycardia. Her hands are warm, but not sweaty, and she has no tremor. There is a swelling in the anterior neck that moves with swallowing and the overlying skin looks normal. Palpation confirms the presence of 1.5 cm nodule in the right lobe of the thyroid which is firm and mobile with no adjacent lymph node enlargement. The rest of the thyroid is not palpable.

Full blood count, erythrocyte sedimentation rate and thyroid function tests are normal (Box 44.1).

Have examination and initial investigations narrowed down your differential diagnosis?

Yes, the examination and blood tests confirm that we are dealing with a non-functioning solitary thyroid nodule. Toxic nodules (either solitary or in the

BOX 44.1

Initial investigations

Full blood count	Normal
ESR	30 mm/1st hour
U&E, glucose	Normal
	fT4 – 11.2 pmol/L (0.87 ng/dL)
Thyroid function	T3 – 1.2 nmol/L (78.1 ng/dL)
	TSH – 1.2 mU/L (µU/mL)

context of a multinodular goitre) would result in a suppressed TSH. Similarly, the normal thyroid function tests and ESR exclude a subacute thyroiditis. We do not know if the nodule is solid or cystic, benign or malignant.

Further investigations
An ultrasound of the thyroid confirms the presence of a solitary nodule in the right lobe of the thyroid (Fig. 44.1). This nodule has a cystic central area, but is predominantly solid. No microcalcification is seen and there is no associated cervical lymphadenopathy. A fine-needle aspiration is performed. Cytology is reported as suspicious of a follicular neoplasm.

Does this narrow down your diagnosis?
Thyroid ultrasonography is commonly performed and will confirm that a nodule is in the thyroid; it gives an accurate measure of size and determines if there is a cystic component. Ultrasound cannot, however, definitely distinguish a benign lesion from a malignant one. There are some features which may raise suspicion of malignancy, such as microcalcification, irregular margins and central vascularity, but these are not absolutely specific. Similarly, isotope scanning is not particularly helpful – 'hot' nodules are rarely malignant, but can be; most solitary nodules in euthyroid patients are 'cold' and most of these are benign, but a small proportion will be malignant.

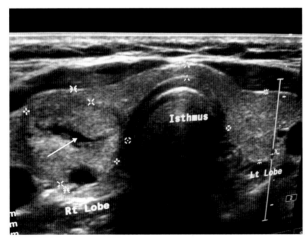

Figure 44.1 Ultrasound of thyroid showing nodule in right lobe; the nodule is predominantly solid, but the central area (arrow) is cystic.

Fine-needle aspiration is now the investigation of choice and this may be done with or without ultrasound guidance, providing the nodule is palpable. Cytology may be non-diagnostic, non-neoplastic, diagnostic of malignancy (papillary, medullary, anaplastic or lymphomatous) or, as in this case, follicular. Most of the time, patients with follicular cytology will turn out to have a follicular adenoma, but occasionally it may be due to a follicular carcinoma. These two neoplasms cannot be distinguished by cytology.

How will you treat this patient?

Thyroid lobectomy is usually recommended for patients with follicular cytology. The pathologists can then look at the whole specimen and work out if the follicular lesion is an adenoma or a carcinoma. Follicular neoplasms are usually surrounded by a capsule – capsular and/or vascular invasion are clearly features of carcinomas. High risk features include size of the tumour (>4 cm), age of the patient (>45 years) and evidence of vascular invasion. For high risk patients, completion thyroidectomy and ablative treatment with radioactive iodine (3700 MBq; 100 mCi) is recommended. TSH is a growth factor for thyroid cells, including malignant cells, and so all patients with follicular carcinomas should receive a dose of levothyroxine that is sufficient to suppress TSH concentration.

Serum thyroglobulin (Tg) level is a very useful tumour marker in this situation. Tg should be undetectable following thyroid ablation and TSH suppression, and a detectable or increasing TG (in the absence of TG antibodies) suggests recurrence of the disease or metastasis. Overall though, prognosis in differentiated thyroid cancer is generally very good and even patients with metastatic disease may live for many years. Metastases can be treated with high doses of radioactive iodine and, occasionally, external beam radiotherapy. Chemotherapy is of no benefit, but early trials of tyrosine kinase inhibitors show promise in those with iodine-refractory metastatic disease.

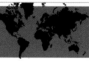

Key points and global issues

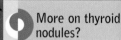

More on thyroid nodules?

- Differentiated thyroid carcinoma is a curable disease provided certain basic principles are followed.
- Fine-needle aspiration cytology is easy, reliable and can be done in any hospital with a histopathology service.

See Chapter 20 of **Davidson's Principles** & **Practice** of **Medicine (21st edn)**

- L-thyroxine is one of the cheapest drugs, but problems with bioavailability of different generic preparations may affect the optimal TSH suppression needed.

45

Secondary amenorrhoea

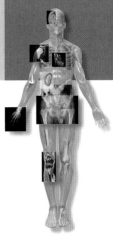

G. A. WITTERT

Presenting problem

A 30-year-old nulliparous woman presents with a 6-month history of amenorrhoea since discontinuing the combined oral contraceptive pill. Menarche occurred at the age of 13 and she rapidly established a regular bleeding pattern with no menstrual abnormality. At the age of 18, she commenced a combined oral contraceptive, which she discontinued because she wished to start a family.

There is no history of weight cycling or unusual eating patterns. She is a triathlete and trains daily. She has no unusual stress, but her mood has been somewhat labile and she has not been sleeping well. She has not had any gynaecological procedures at any time. Over the last few months, there has been a noticeable reduction in libido, and increasing discomfort during intercourse. She has not had any hot flushes and has not noticed the presence of breast milk. She has no headache or visual disturbance. There are no other symptoms of any sort – in particular, no symptoms of any other hormonal deficiency or excess. She is not taking medication of any kind.

What would your differential diagnosis include before examining the patient?

The scenario, in particular the loss of libido and discomfort during intercourse, suggests oestrogen deficiency, either due to loss of gonadotrophin production or ovarian failure. Galactorrhoea, when present, suggests excess prolactin production as the cause of failure of gonadotrophin production; this will need to be looked for on examination. Depression, weight loss, eating disorders and excessive exercise, particularly if accompanied by caloric restriction, may also cause failure of gonadotrophin secretion. The physical activity undertaken by this patient may be an issue. A careful assessment of nutritional status is required. Loss of gonadotrophin production may be caused by a pituitary or hypothalamic tumour or infiltrative disorder (sarcoidosis, haemochromatosis), but there are no features in the history to suggest either. Autoimmune ovarian failure should be considered. Oestrogen deficiency symptoms would not be typical of pregnancy; nevertheless this should be excluded, since it is possible to conceive before the first period occurs after discontinuing the pill.

Examination

The patient's weight is normal (BMI: 21). The skin is normal and there are no signs of acne, hirsutism or dysmorphic features. There is no evidence of pregnancy. Bilateral expressible galactorrhoea is present, along with atrophic vaginitis. There are no clinical features of any hormone excess (e.g. growth hormone, cortisol) or deficiency (e.g. thyroxine). There are no abnormalities of vision or visual fields.

Has examination narrowed down your differential diagnosis?

The presence of galactorrhoea in the setting of oestrogen deficiency symptoms suggests the presence of hyperprolactinaemia. A number of medications (e.g. antiemetics, antipsychotics) can increase prolactin, but she is not taking any of these. A prolactin-secreting microadenoma, or stalk compression from a larger pituitary tumour, or interference of dopamine production as a result of a

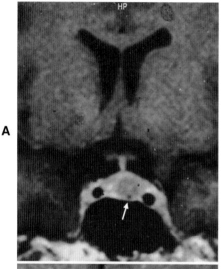
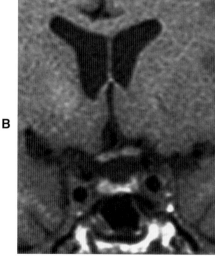

Figure 45.1 Secondary amenorrhoea. (A) An MRI obtained post-gadolinium. The section is a coronal view through the pituitary gland. The optic chiasm and pituitary stalk can be seen as enhancing structures. The internal carotid in each cavernous sinus appears black. A 0.9 cm unenhancing lesion, typical of microadenoma, is visible in the pituitary gland (arrow). (B) For comparison, a normal pituitary MRI is also presented.

hypothalamic tumour or infiltrative disorder, are possible causes. The absence of compressive symptoms or evidence of any other hormone excess or deficiency makes an isolated prolactin-secreting microadenoma the most likely cause.

Investigations

The following hormone results are obtained: follicle-stimulating hormone <1 U/L (<0.1 µg/L), luteinising hormone <1 U/L (< 0.1 µg/L), prolactin 140 µg/L (ng/mL) (normal range 0–25 µg/L (ng/mL) or equivalent), thyroid-stimulating hormone (TSH) 1 mU/L, free T_4 13 pmol/L (1000 pg/dL).

A magnetic resonance image (MRI) of the pituitary is obtained. A coronal section through the pituitary, obtained after the administration of gadolinium (Fig. 45.1) shows a 0.9 cm unenhancing tumour, typical of a microadenoma.

Does this narrow down your differential diagnosis?

The patient has a prolactin-secreting microadenoma with otherwise normal pituitary function.

How will you treat this patient?

A long-acting dopamine receptor 2 agonist (D2RA), such as cabergoline, will normalise prolactin levels, shrink the tumour and restore normal menstrual function and fertility with minimal side-effects. Short-acting D2RAs, e.g. bromocriptine, cause significant side-effects (nausea, vomiting, nasal stuffiness and postural hypotension) and the dose needs to be titrated up slowly. Although there is no evidence of harm, D2RAs should be discontinued once pregnancy occurs and need only be reinstated if clinically significant tumour growth occurs (headaches and visual disturbance). In some cases, the problem resolves after delivery.

Where appropriate expertise is available, selective microadenomectomy via a trans-sphenoidal approach can be offered.

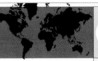

Key points and global issues

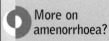

More on
amenorrhoea?

See Chapter 20 of
Davidson's Principles
& **Practice** of
Medicine (21st edn)

- Amenorrhoea after discontinuing the combined oral contraceptive pill is not due to the use of the pill *per se*, regardless of how long it has been used. A cause should also be vigorously sought.

- Secondary amenorrhoea, regardless of cause, results in a decrease in bone mineral density and predisposes to significant osteoporosis later in life. Such patients should be specifically targeted for screening and prevention strategies.

- Obesity is now as common as, or perhaps more so than, under-nutrition as a global problem. Particularly when severe and associated with insulin resistance or obstructive sleep apnoea, it may result in secondary amenorrhoea as part of the spectrum of polycystic ovarian syndrome.

- Tuberculosis, as well as being a rare cause of pituitary failure, can cause endometrial adhesions which obliterate the endometrial cavity and result in amenorrhoea.

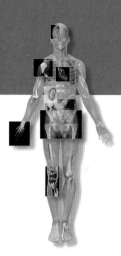

46

Hypercalcaemia

M. W. J. STRACHAN

Presenting problem

A 75-year-old woman is referred to an endocrine clinic with a 4-month history of malaise and increased thirst. Five years ago she had an episode of severe pain in her left loin which settled after a few hours and for which she did not seek medical attention. The lady thinks that she has lost a few inches in height over the last few years and a recent X-ray of her thoracic spine showed several wedge fractures. She does not take any regular medication. Prior to referral, her GP checked some routine blood tests and these identified an elevated serum calcium concentration (Box 46.1).

What would your differential diagnosis include before examining the patient?

The two most common causes of hypercalcaemia are hyperparathyroidism and malignancy. The vertebral fractures are not particularly discriminatory, given the high prevalence of osteoporosis in women of this age; they could be coincidental, or a consequence of hyperparathyroidism or even neoplastic disease (e.g. myeloma). The history suggests that the patient may have had a renal calculus in the past and this would be more in-keeping with hyperparathyroidism. Thyrotoxicosis and glucocorticoid insufficiency can cause hypercalcaemia, but it is invariably mild and asymptomatic.

The woman is not taking lithium or any vitamin D preparations, but vitamin D excess can be caused by sarcoidosis and other granulomatous disorders, and this should certainly be considered if the more common causes are excluded.

Examination

The patient looks a little dry and has a stooped posture. No masses are felt in the breasts or the abdomen.

Has examination narrowed down your differential diagnosis?

As is often the case in endocrinology, if there is no easy spot diagnosis (e.g. a patient with an acromegaloid or Cushingoid appearance), then detailed

BOX 46.1
Initial investigations
• Urea 18.3 mmol/L (51.26 mg/dL)
• Creatinine 105 μmol/L (1.19 mg/dL)
• Sodium 144 mmol/L (mEq/L)
• Potassium 3.4 mmol/L (mEq/L)
• Calcium 2.89 mmol/L (11.56 mg/dL)
• Phosphate 0.63 mmol/L (1.95 mg/dL)
• Albumin 35 g/L (3.5 g/dL)

examination is often unrewarding. There is, though, a general rule of thumb with hypercalcaemia that if the patient is well enough to come to an outpatient clinic, then the likely cause is hyperparathyroidism. However, if the patient requires admission to hospital, then in all probability, there is underlying neoplastic disease. (All rules of thumb, of course, are there to be broken!) If a patient is not already known to have cancer or this is not evident from the initial history, examination and investigations, then the key discriminatory test is measurement of serum parathyroid hormone (PTH).

Further investigations

The serum PTH concentration is 12.6 pmol/L (126 pg/mL) and 24-h urine calcium is 9.4 mmol/24 h (376 mg/24 h).

Does this narrow down your differential diagnosis?

The PTH concentration is high and so the diagnosis is almost certainly primary hyperparathyroidism – 'almost certainly' because a rare trap for the unwary is familial hypocalciuric hypercalcaemia. This inherited disorder can cause elevated serum calcium and PTH concentrations, but can usually be diagnosed by the finding of a low 24-h urinary calcium concentration and the identification of borderline hypercalcaemia in close relatives.

If the PTH had been low, then malignant hypercalcaemia would have been most likely and further investigations, such as protein electrophoresis, urine Bence Jones protein and a CT of the chest and abdomen, would have been indicated.

How will you treat this patient?

Primary hyperparathyroidism is invariably caused by a solitary parathyroid adenoma and so the definitive therapy is parathyroidectomy. Standard indications for surgery are shown in Box 46.2, but selection of patients is not always straightforward. This woman, providing she is fit enough for a general anaesthetic, should have

> **BOX 46.2**
>
> **Indications for surgery in primary hyperpara-thyroidism**
>
> - Complications of hyperparathyroidism, e.g. renal stones, renal impairment (with no other identifiable cause) and osteoporosis
> - Symptoms of hyperparathyroidism
> - Age <50 years
> - Serum calcium >2.85 mmol/L (11.4 mg/dL)

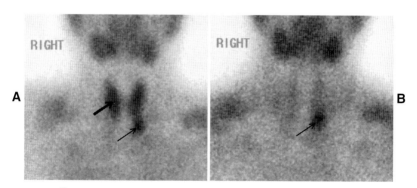

Figure 46.1 ^{99m}Technetium-sestamibi scan. (A) Initial uptake into the thyroid (thick arrow) and left inferior parathyroid gland (thin arrow). (B) After 3 h – there is only uptake in the abnormal parathyroid.

surgery because of her relatively high serum calcium, thin bones and high urine calcium excretion. If an ultrasound scan of the kidneys showed evidence of nephrocalcinosis or nephrolithiasis, then the case for surgery would be even stronger.

In some centres, preoperative localisation of a parathyroid adenoma with ^{99m}technetium-sestamibi scanning (Fig. 46.1) and contemporaneous ultrasound allows targeted resection using minimally invasive techniques. Postoperative hypocalcaemia is not uncommon during the first 2 weeks while residual suppressed parathyroid tissue recovers.

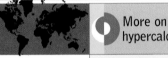

Key points and global issues

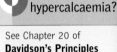

More on hypercalcaemia?

- ^{99m}Technetium-sestamibi scanning is not essential, as an experienced surgeon will locate a parathyroid adenoma by careful neck exploration in over 90% of patients.

See Chapter 20 of
Davidson's Principles
& **Practice** of
Medicine (21st edn)

- Granulomatous disorders, including tuberculosis, fungal infections and berylliosis, can cause hypercalcaemia secondary to vitamin D excess.

- Rarely, human immunodeficiency virus (HIV)-associated *Pneumocystis jirovecii* infection can be associated with severe hypercalcaemia.

47

Hypocalcaemia

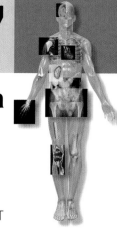

G. A. WITTERT

Presenting problem

A 54-year-old man presents with a 3-month history of increasing muscle cramps in the lower back, legs, feet and hands. More recently, he has noticed some tingling and burning in the fingers and around the mouth. Four months ago he had a thyroidectomy for a large multinodular goitre. He takes thyroxine and a thiazide diuretic for mild hypertension. He has a sedentary job, works long hours and spends little if any time out of doors. Initial blood tests reveal a low plasma calcium (Box 47.1).

What would your differential diagnosis include before examining the patient?

The patient has symptoms and biochemistry consistent with hypocalcaemia. If the plasma calcium level falls very rapidly, or if the proportion of ionised calcium decreases acutely when the plasma calcium level is already low, laryngospasm, bronchospasm, tetany or seizures may occur.

The most common causes are hypoparathyroidism due to iatrogenic or autoimmune destruction of the parathyroid glands, deficiency or abnormal metabolism of vitamin D, magnesium deficiency and chronic renal failure.

In this patient, the parathyroid glands may have been removed or their blood supply damaged during the previous thyroid surgery. Other factors which need

BOX 47.1	
Initial investigations	
Total calcium	1.8 mmol/L (7.2 mg/dL)
Ionised calcium	0.9 mmol/L (3.6 mg/dL)
Phosphate	0.6 mmol/L (1.86 mg/dL)
Albumin	39 g/L (3.9 mg/dL)
Sodium	137 mmol/L (mEq/L)
Potassium	3.0 mmol/L (mEq/L)
Creatinine	120 μmol/L (1.36 mg/dL)
Urea	7.0 mmol/L (19.6 mg/dL)
TSH	2.5 mU/L

to be considered include the possibility of vitamin D deficiency due to lack of exposure to sunlight and magnesium deficiency due to the thiazide diuretic. Severe magnesium deficiency results in impaired secretion of parathyroid hormone and resistance to its action. Magnesium deficiency is not infrequent in response to thiazides and, unlike hypokalaemia, is often overlooked.

Hypocalcaemic states are best categorised according to the level of para-thyroid hormone (PTH). Ordinarily, PTH secretion is exquisitely sensitive to changes in ionised calcium. In hypoparathyroid states, the level of PTH is inap-propriately low for the level of calcium. Elevated PTH levels (secondary hyper-parathyroidism) suggest normal PTH responsiveness to the low plasma calcium.

Examination

This man is well nourished and there is no evidence of gastrointestinal disease. The scar from the previous thyroid surgery is evident and no thyroid remnant is palpable. There is no vitiligo, mucocutaneous candidiasis or skin lesions of any sort. Twitching of the circumoral muscles occurs in response to tapping the facial nerve just anterior to the ear (Chvostek's sign). Carpal spasm is elicited by inflation of the blood pressure cuff to 20 mmHg above the systolic blood pressure for 3 min (Trousseau's sign; Fig. 47.1). There is no obvious ocular calcification, proximal muscle weakness or disorders of movement.

Has examination narrowed down your differential diagnosis?

The examination, together with investigations so far, suggest that the low calcium, which is causing significant neuromuscular irritability, is responsible for this patient's symptoms and that malabsorption, liver or renal disease are unlikely to be factors in the abnormalities of calcium or vitamin D homeostasis. In the absence of evidence of any autoimmune or other system disease process, it seems that any abnormality of PTH, if present, is likely to be due to be the result of the previous thyroid surgery.

Further investigations

Further tests reveal magnesium 0.65 mmol/L (1.58 mg/dL), 25 hydroxy-vitamin D 45 nmol/L (18 ng/mL) and PTH 1 pmol/L (10 pg/mL).

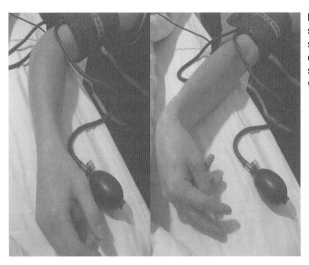

Figure 47.1 Trousseau's sign. Inflation of the sphygmomanometer cuff causes carpal muscle spasm in an individual with hypocalcaemia.

Does this narrow down your differential diagnosis?

The low PTH level suggests that the primary problem is hypoparathyroidism, most likely as a consequence of damage to the parathyroid glands or their blood supply during surgery. Although the magnesium level is low and may be contributing to the problem, it is usually only when it is very low (0.4 mmol/L (0.97 mg/dL) or less) that it is likely to be the primary cause of hypoparathyroidism. The renal handling of potassium and magnesium is similar, and the low potassium and magnesium are both related to the thiazide diuretic, which induces renal loss of both electrolytes. On the other hand, thiazides decrease renal calcium loss. The low vitamin D is the result of inadequate sun exposure and, while not the primary cause of the problem, will compromise not only the patient's ability to maintain plasma calcium, but also skeletal, muscular and metabolic integrity, and may even increase his cancer risk.

How will you treat this patient?

Commence an oral calcium supplement equivalent to 1–2 g of elemental calcium per day. The thiazide diuretic should be replaced with an angiotensin-converting enzyme (ACE) inhibitor or angiotensin 2 receptor antagonist, and potassium and magnesium should be replaced orally. Sunlight exposure of unprotected skin should be encouraged where feasible for 10 min/day in summer and 20 min/day in winter. If this is not feasible or if the vitamin D level remains low, an oral supplement should be given. If the plasma calcium remains low, oral 1,25-dihydroxyvitamin D (0.25–1.0 μg) is added. The plasma calcium level should be maintained in the lower part of the normal range.

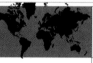

Key points and global issues

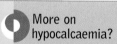

More on
hypocalcaemia?

See Chapter 20 of
Davidson's Principles
& **Practice** of
Medicine (21st edn)

- The biologically active vitamin D metabolite, 1,25(OH)$_2$D, is not exclusively produced in the kidney, but is also synthesised in many other tissues such as the prostate, colon, skin and osteoblasts. There is a relationship between vitamin D deficiency and various types of cancer, bone diseases, autoimmune diseases, hypertension and cardiovascular disease.

- Approximately 90% of all requisite vitamin D has to be formed in the skin through the action of the sun. Strict sun protection causes vitamin D deficiency, which is being recognised to be prevalent even in the sunniest countries. The problem can be a particular issue in pregnant women, the institutionalised elderly with dark skin, and other groups where sun exposure does not occur.

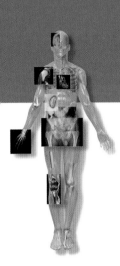

48

Cushing's syndrome

W. F. MOLLENTZE

Presenting problem

A 25-year-old woman presents to an endocrine clinic with a 4-year history of amenorrhoea, progressive weight gain (10 kg during the past year), fatigue and difficulty in climbing stairs and rising from a deep chair. The lady mentions that her body shape has changed with an increase in waist circumference. Her face has become rounder and hairy and she also noticed that she bruises easily. She finds it difficult to concentrate, experiences headaches and feels depressed and tearful of late. She denies ever having taken any form of glucocorticoid treatment. Her GP has found that her blood pressure was increased on several occasions.

What would your differential diagnosis include before examining the patient?

At least three conditions need to be considered in the differential diagnosis at this stage: polycystic ovarian syndrome (PCOS), primary hypothyroidism and Cushing's syndrome. Although obesity, especially central obesity, is present in most patients with PCOS, it is not recognised as a diagnostic feature of the syndrome. Oligo- or amenorrhoea and hirsutism, however, are both defining features of PCOS but myopathy is not part of this syndrome. Patients with primary hypothyroidism, especially of gradual onset, may complain of weight gain, fatigue and menstrual irregularity. While menorrhagia is the classic menstrual abnormality in female patients with primary hypothyroidism, oligo- and amenorrhoea can also occur. Proximal muscle weakness is an unusual but important feature of primary hypothyroidism. The combination of easy bruising, proximal muscle weakness and hypertension in any obese patient is, however, highly suggestive of Cushing's syndrome.

Examination

The patient weighs 63 kg and her height is 1.56 m (BMI: 25.89). She has an obvious Cushingoid and plethoric appearance (Fig. 48.1) with prominent broad purple striae (Fig. 48.2) over the abdomen and breasts. Ankle oedema is present, as well as mild hirsutism on the upper lip and cheeks. Her supine blood pressure is 170/120 mmHg. The lady is unable to rise from a squatting position (Fig. 48.3). The patient's GP performed some initial investigations before referring the patient (Box 48.1).

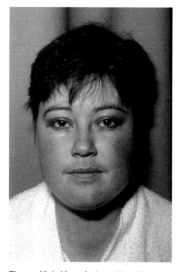

Figure 48.1 Moon facies with mild hirsutism.

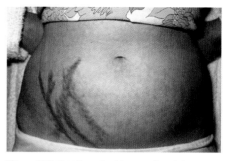

Figure 48.2 Broad purple striae over the abdomen.

Figure 48.3 The patient is unable to rise from a squatting position, indicating proximal muscle weakness.

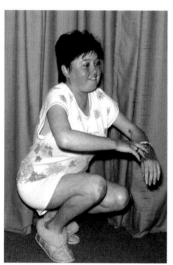

BOX 48.1	
Initial investigations	
Serum sodium	146 mmol/L (mEq/L)
Serum potassium	2.1 mmol/L (mEq/L)
24-h urinary free cortisol	3850 nmol (1395 μg) (normal range 30–300 nmol (10–100 μg))
09.00 hours s-cortisol	1151 nmol/L (41.72 μg/dL) (normal range 220–660 nmol/L (8–24 μg/dL))
23.00 hours s-cortisol	1127 nmol/L (40.85 μg/dL) (normal range 50–410 nmol/L (2–15 μg/dL))

s, serum.

Have examination and initial investigations narrowed down your differential diagnosis?

The clinical manifestations in this patient, combined with hypokalaemia, increased 24-h urinary free cortisol secretion and loss of circadian rhythm, are almost diagnostic of Cushing's syndrome. Two more conditions which have overlapping clinical and biochemical features with Cushing's syndrome should now also be considered before embarking on more expensive investigations. Pseudo-Cushing's syndrome caused by alcohol excess may mimic some of the features of Cushing's syndrome, such as central obesity, proximal muscle weakness and overproduction of cortisol. A thorough history, including collateral information, may be useful in this regard. Liver enzymes are frankly abnormal in these patients. Major depressive illness may also be associated with increased 24-h urinary free cortisol excretion, but proximal muscle weakness, purple striae and severe hypokalaemia argue in favour of an organic illness.

Further investigations

The standard low-dose dexamethasone suppression test, consisting of dexamethasone 0.5 mg every 6 h taken orally for 48 h, is now required to confirm the presence of Cushing's syndrome. This is immediately followed by the standard high-dose dexamethasone suppression test, consisting of 2 mg dexamethasone every 6 h, to establish the cause of Cushing's syndrome. The reason for performing these two investigations consecutively is, first, that the results of the adrenocorticotrophic hormone (ACTH) assays become available only after some time and, second, for convenience, since the patient is best admitted to hospital to ensure adherence to the test protocol. The results of these tests are shown in Box 48.2.

BOX 48.2

Results of the dexamethasone suppression tests

Standard low-dose test

Day 1	09.00 h	s-cortisol	1200 nmol/L (43.49 pg/dL) (before the first dose of dexamethasone)
Day 1	09.00 h	p-ACTH*	6.61 pmol/L (30 pg/mL)
Day 2	09.00 h	s-cortisol	1215 nmol/L (44.04 pg/dL)
Day 2		24-h urinary free cortisol	3740 nmol (1356 pg)

High-dose 48-h test

Day 3	09.00 h	s-cortisol	1129 nmol/L (40.93 pg/dL) (before the first high dose of dexamethasone)
Day 3	09.00 h	p-ACTH*	7.27 pmol/L (33 pg/mL)
Day 4	09.00 h	s-cortisol	1107 nmol/L (40.12 pg/dL)
Day 4		24-h urinary free cortisol	3853 nmol (1397 pg)
Day 5	09.00 h	s-cortisol	1058 nmol/L (38.34 pg/dL) (after completion of high-dose dexamethasone test)
Day 5	09.00 h	p-ACTH*	6.17 pmol/L (28 pg/mL)

*Normal range 0–15.63 pmol/L (0–71 pg/mL). s, serum; p, plasma.

Does this narrow down your differential diagnosis?

The patient's 09.00 h s-cortisol concentration on day 3, as well as the 24-h urinary free cortisol during day 2, fails to suppress after 48 h of low-dose dexamethasone, confirming the presence of Cushing's syndrome. The 'detectable' baseline p-ACTH concentration of 6.61 pmol/L (30 pg/mL) on day 1 in the presence of excess cortisol may point towards a pituitary or ectopic source of this patient's Cushing's syndrome. After 48 h of high-dose dexamethasone the 09.00 h ACTH concentration, as well as the 09.00 h s-cortisol and 24-h urinary free cortisol concentrations, fail to suppress. These findings argue against a pituitary tumour. An X-ray of the chest is requested and shows no evidence of a possible source of ectopic ACTH production. A computed tomogram (CT) of the abdomen demonstrates a 2.5 cm tumor in the left adrenal gland. A magnetic resonance image (MRI) of the brain shows some cerebral atrophy and the pituitary gland appears normal. The fact that ACTH was detectable in this patient at baseline, as well as after the high dose dexamethasone suppression test, is unusual for a cortisol-producing adrenal tumour, as normally the ACTH levels would be undetectable.

How will you treat this patient?

The patient should be referred for a left adrenalectomy after correcting the hypokalaemia with intravenous potassium chloride and controlling the elevated blood pressure with an angiotensin-converting enzyme (ACE) inhibitor. Preoperatively, excess cortisol concentrations can be reduced by treatment with metyrapone. Since the cortex of the contralateral adrenal gland may be atrophic in spite of the measurable amounts of ACTH, the adrenalectomy must be conducted under full glucocorticoid cover including intravenous hydrocortisone, followed by full replacement doses of oral hydrocortisone as soon as the patient is allowed to eat. Full recovery of the hypothalamic–pituitary–adrenal axis is expected within 2–12 months, during which period the replacement dose of hydrocortisone can be tapered gradually.

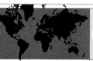

Key points and global issues

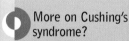
More on Cushing's syndrome?

See Chapter 20 of **Davidson's Principles** & **Practice** of **Medicine (21st edn)**

- Corticotrophin-releasing hormone (CRH) is not freely available in developing countries and even the availability of dexamethasone is under threat in some.

- Although Cushing's syndrome may be fairly obvious clinically, the definitive biochemical diagnosis, including establishing the exact aetiology and often the anatomical localisation of the underlying disorder, may prove to be extremely challenging.

- Most, if not all, patients with suspected Cushing's syndrome should preferably be referred to a centre with experience in the management of such patients.

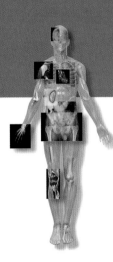

49

Adrenal insufficiency

W. F. MOLLENTZE

Presenting problem

A 27-year-old woman is referred by her GP to an endocrine clinic with gradual onset of fatigue, anorexia, weight loss and hyperpigmentation dating back to her second and last pregnancy 5 years ago. She also complains of amenorrhoea of 4 months' duration, intermittent diarrhoea and orthostatic dizziness.

What would your differential diagnosis include before examining the patient?

Fatigue is a frequent complaint in an endocrine clinic. Hypothyroidism is unlikely since the patient lost weight and she also complains of amenorrhoea and not menorrhagia. Rheumatoid arthritis and multiple sclerosis are examples of autoimmune conditions associated with fatigue and could easily be excluded on further enquiry. Chronic fatigue syndrome may follow after a viral infection such as infectious mononucleosis, influenza or hepatitis. Anorexia nervosa should also be considered in the differential diagnosis of weight loss and amenorrhoea. The absence of similar complaints during adolescence would argue against this condition. None of the above conditions is, however, characterised by hyperpigmentation. Primary adrenocortical failure, pellagra and malabsorption (Box 49.1) may also present with hyperpigmentation, weight loss and diarrhoea.

Examination

This young woman's height is 1.69 m and she weighs 52 kg (BMI: 18.2). Generalised hyperpigmentation is present but is more pronounced on the sun-exposed areas (Fig. 49.1). Her hair is dark, and dark freckles are also present over the anterior chest wall. Pressure areas, such as the elbows, the skin over spinous processes and underneath the brassiere straps, are also darker than surrounding skin. The patient's pulse rate is 88/min and blood pressure is 100/70 mmHg lying down and 60/40 mmHg in the erect position. Vitiligo is absent and no abnormal

---

BOX 49.1

Causes of diffuse hyperpigmentation

Endocrinopathies
- Addison's disease
- Nelson's syndrome
- Ectopic ACTH secretion

Metabolic
- Porphyria cutanea tarda
- Haemochromatosis
- Vitamin B_{12} and folate deficiency
- Pellagra
- Malabsorption

Autoimmune
- Hepatic cirrhosis
- Systemic sclerosis

Drug-induced
- Amiodarone
- Busulfan
- Chloroquine
- Minocycline
- Phenothiazines
- Psoralens

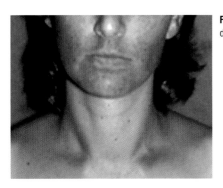

Figure 49.1 Hyperpigmentation in Addison's disease.

BOX 49.2	
Initial investigations	
Sodium	131 mmol/L (mEq/L)
Potassium	5.4 mmol/L (mEq/L)
Urea	7.1 mmol/L (19.9 mg/dL)
Creatinine	106 pmol/L (1.20 mg/dL)
Glucose	3.7 mmol/L (66.65 mg/dL)

pigmentation is present on the oral mucous membranes. Initial blood test results are shown in Box 49.2.

Have examination and initial investigations narrowed down your differential diagnosis?

Although the hyperpigmentation in this patient is highly suggestive of primary adrenocortical failure (Addison's disease), it is by no means diagnostic. The absence of vitiligo does not exclude Addison's disease since it is seen in only 10–20% of patients with the autoimmune variety. The orthostatic decrease in blood pressure and the raised plasma urea and creatinine are suggestive of primary adrenal insufficiency, but may also be due to hypovolaemia secondary to chronic diarrhoea and malabsorption. Hyponatraemia and hyperkalaemia in the presence of hypovolaemia, however, argue strongly in favour of primary adrenal insufficiency.

Further investigations

The patient's morning (08.00 hours) plasma cortisol concentration is 47.1 nmol/L (1.71 µg/dL) and the corresponding plasma corticotrophin (ACTH) concentration is 53.5 pmol/L (243 pg/mL). This woman's thyroid function test results are normal but her thyroid microsomal antibody titre is positive to a titre of 1:6400. A computed tomogram (CT) of the adrenal glands reveals atrophy of both glands, and the serum ferritin concentration is within the normal range.

Does this narrow down your differential diagnosis?

The clinical picture and the finding of low serum cortisol and elevated ACTH concentrations all but clinch the diagnosis of primary adrenocortical failure. In less clear-cut cases, a short Synacthen test should be performed, as the identification of a low stimulated cortisol concentration is a more robust marker of glucocorticoid deficiency than a random or early morning cortisol. In this case, this might be considered superfluous.

Common causes of chronic primary adrenocortical failure include autoimmune adrenalitis (Addison's disease) and infections such as tuberculosis and human immunodeficiency virus-acquired immunodeficiency syndrome (HIV/AIDS). Measurement of antibodies directed against the adrenal cortex is helpful to diagnose autoimmune adrenalitis, but unfortunately this assay is not widely available. The presence of thyroid microsomal antibodies in this patient argues in favour of an underlying autoimmune process. The absence of calcification or evidence of metastatic disease in the adrenal glands rules out tuberculosis and underlying malignancy respectively as aetiological factors.

How will you treat this patient?

Both glucocorticoid and mineralocorticoid replacement therapy should be provided. Hydrocortisone (cortisol) 15 mg orally on waking and 5 mg orally at approximately 18.00 hours constitute the glucocorticoid regimen of choice. This dosage regimen is usually sufficient but may need to be increased to 20 mg and 10 mg, respectively, in some patients. Unfortunately, measurement of 'trough and peak' cortisol concentrations is not very helpful for determining the optimum dosage of hydrocortisone. Furthermore, the pharmacokinetics of hydrocortisone makes it very hard to mimic circadian cortisol secretion. Therefore, some patients may still experience daily episodes of lassitude and fatigue in spite of an adequate total daily dose of hydrocortisone. In some individuals it may be prudent to advise a small dose after lunch and to postpone the evening dose till bedtime. Cortisol is a powerful appetite stimulant and excessive weight gain usually indicates overtreatment. Hyperpigmentation should improve within several weeks to a few months. Persistent hyperpigmentation indicates insufficient chronic suppression of ACTH secretion.

Fludrocortisone (9α-fluorohydrocortisone) is the mineralocorticoid of choice and can be initiated with 0.05 mg orally on waking. The objective of fludrocortisone treatment is to prevent further sodium loss, to restore intravascular volume and to prevent hyperkalaemia. Adequacy of fludrocortisone replacement can be monitored by routinely measuring blood pressure in the supine as well as the upright position, in addition to the serum sodium and potassium concentrations. Over-treatment with fludrocortisone should be suspected when the blood pressure becomes elevated and oedema and hypokalaemia develop.

Patient education is of the utmost importance in the long-term successful management of primary adrenal insufficiency. Patients should be advised to increase their salt intake during summer in regions known for hot, dry summers. The dose of hydrocortisone must be doubled during periods of emotional and physical stress, e.g. febrile periods, and the GP should be notified if this exceeds 3 days. Parenteral hydrocortisone and intravenous saline must be administered during episodes of vomiting. Patients should also be carefully followed for the development of other autoimmune endocrinopathies such as hypothyroidism and premature ovarian failure.

In known patients, as well as in previously undiagnosed ones, an acute adrenal crisis should be suspected if they present in shock, especially when this is accompanied by anorexia, nausea, vomiting, weakness and abdominal pain with deep tenderness on palpation. Intravenous saline should be infused as required to

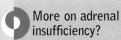
normalise haemodynamic indices and care must be taken not to correct hypo-natraemia too rapidly. Hypoglycaemia may be a rare presentation of acute adrenal insufficiency in adults.

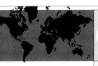

Key points and global issues

More on adrenal insufficiency?

See Chapter 20 of
Davidson's Principles
& Practice of
Medicine (21st edn)

- As the incidence of HIV/AIDS increases, especially in developing countries, overt adrenal insufficiency may become more prevalent due to a necrotising adrenalitis secondary to cytomegalovirus infection or tuberculous involvement; Kaposi's sarcoma may also metastasise to the adrenal glands.

- Synacthen (ACTH1–24) is not available in some developing countries.

- Assays for antibodies directed at the adrenal cortex are also not widely available in developing countries.

- Patients with chronic adrenal insufficiency must be advised to increase their salt intake during summer in countries with hot dry summers.

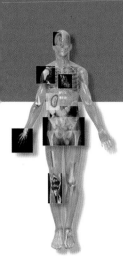

50

Spontaneous hypoglycaemia

M. W. J. STRACHAN

Presenting problem

A 78-year-old Caucasian woman is admitted to hospital in a coma (Glasgow Coma Score (GCS, 5). She was found collapsed at home by her husband, who reports that his wife has been experiencing increasingly frequent dizzy spells over the previous 4 months. These episodes typically occur first thing in the morning, before breakfast, or later in the day, particularly if she has been working in her large garden. These spells are often relieved by a cup of sweet tea and a biscuit. She is an otherwise fit woman and her only medication is low-dose aspirin and simvastatin.

On the patient's arrival in the Emergency Department, the triage nurse performs a capillary blood glucose test, and a level of 1.3 mmol/L (23.4 mg/dL) is recorded on the meter. Venous blood samples are taken and the patient is given 50 mL of 50% dextrose intravenously. Within 5 min, her GCS has risen to 15. The laboratory glucose is subsequently reported at 1.6 mmol/L (28.8 mg/dL).

What would your differential diagnosis include before examining the patient?

The differential diagnosis of acute hypoglycaemia is very extensive. In the first instance, of course, it is crucial to confirm that you are dealing with a hypoglycaemic disorder and, for that, all constituents of Whipple's triad should be met (Box 50.1). In addition, laboratory confirmation of the low blood glucose concentration is essential, because bedside meters are not sufficiently accurate in the hypoglycaemia range. Clearly, though, your patient should not have treatment deferred while awaiting the pronouncement from the laboratory, and intravenous dextrose (or intramuscular glucagon) should be administered when venous blood samples have been taken.

> ### BOX 50.1
> **Whipple's triad**
>
> - The patient must have symptoms of hypoglycaemia.
> - The patient must have biochemical evidence of hypoglycaemia.
> - The symptoms must resolve when the hypoglycaemia is corrected.

Often, the cause of acute hypoglycaemia is obvious. The husband does not report that his wife has diabetes mellitus and he looks affronted when excess alcohol consumption is suggested! Pituitary and adrenocortical insufficiency rarely cause acute hypoglycaemia in adults, but can in children. Disorders of carbohydrate metabolism would also have presented in early life and acute liver failure, sepsis and kidney failure are much less likely, given the prolonged history. This implies a more insidious process, such as endogenous insulin excess (insulinoma) or a non-islet cell tumour causing hypoglycaemia. Drug-related causes should always be considered in an individual with hypoglycaemia. Aspirin can cause hypoglycaemia, but only in very high doses. If the patient's husband has diabetes (or a close family member or friend), then the possibility of factitious or felonious hypoglycaemia should not be discounted.

Examination

The woman is apyrexial and cardiovascularly stable, with good peripheral perfusion. Her skin is normal and she is well nourished, if indeed slightly overweight. A left-sided hemiparesis is noted on arrival in the department, but this quickly resolves on correction of the hypoglycaemia. No abnormal masses are noted on palpation of the abdomen.

Has examination narrowed down your differential diagnosis?

Transient neurological phenomena are not uncommon in elderly patients and it is important to exclude hypoglycaemia in anyone with acute neurological symptoms and/or signs. The cardiovascular stability and the rapid recovery with intravenous dextrose essentially exclude severe acute illness. Non-islet cell tumour-induced hypoglycaemia usually occurs in the context of large retroperitoneal sarcomas, which may already have been diagnosed and are often palpable on abdominal examination. Further narrowing down of the differential diagnosis requires additional analysis of the blood samples.

Further investigations

Routine biochemistry and liver function tests are normal and salicylate concentrations are not elevated. Serum insulin and C-peptide concentrations are elevated at 70 pmol/L (9.76 mU/mL) and 4 µg/L (4 pg/mL), respectively.

Has the diagnosis been clinched?

Measurements of serum insulin and C-peptide concentrations during the episode of hypoglycaemia are essential in establishing the cause of hypoglycaemia when there is no obvious precipitant. If further information comes to light when the patient recovers from the acute episode, then the samples can be discarded before being assayed. However, unnecessary provocation tests (e.g. prolonged fasting) can be avoided if samples are taken during the acute episode.

The finding of elevated insulin and C-peptide concentrations, taken with the chronic history, points very strongly to this patient having an underlying insulinoma. Exogenous insulin would have caused elevation of only the serum insulin, and other causes of acute hypoglycaemia, e.g. sepsis, liver disease and non-islet cell tumour-induced hypoglycaemia, would have been associated with undetectable levels of both. The only other possibility is sulphonylurea poisoning, but this can be detected in the initial blood sample.

Definitive investigations

There is no detectable sulphonylurea activity in the blood sample. A computed tomography scan (CT) of the pancreas shows no abnormality, but an endoscopic ultrasound scan reveals a 10 mm rounded lesion in the tail of the pancreas (Fig. 50.1). Biopsy confirms the presence of neuroendocrine cells, with heavy staining for insulin.

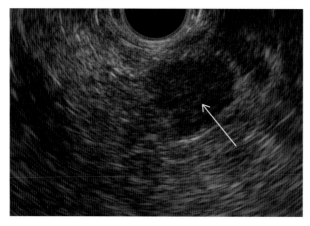

Figure 50.1 Endoscopic ultrasound scan showing 10 mm lesion in the tail of the pancreas (arrow).

How will you treat this patient?

The definitive treatment is surgery. Insulinomas are usually benign and can often be 'shelled out' by an experienced surgeon. While surgery is awaited, or if the patient is not deemed to be fit for an operation, oral diazoxide will suppress insulin secretion and prevent recurrent hypoglycaemia. It is often helpful to teach the patient home blood glucose monitoring and to provide dietary advice on the treatment of hypoglycaemia and the need for regular meals and snacks, particularly prior to exercise.

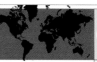

Key points and global issues

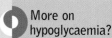

More on hypoglycaemia?

See Chapter 20 of **Davidson's Principles & Practice of Medicine (21st edn)**

- A hypoglycaemic disorder should only ever be diagnosed when all components of Whipple's triad are met.

- Worldwide, insulin and sulphonylurea-treated diabetes are the most common causes of hypoglycaemia.

- In developed countries, alcohol excess is a common cause of hypoglycaemia in non-diabetic individuals.

- Patients with severe *falciparum* malaria should be monitored frequently for the development of hypoglycaemia.

- Toxic hypoglycaemia syndrome can result from the consumption of unripe ackee fruit, which grows in the Caribbean and in West Africa.

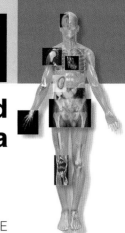

51

Newly discovered hyperglycaemia

SAMAR BANERJEE

Presenting problem

A 26-year-old unmarried school teacher from Kolkata is referred to the diabetes outpatient department with a new diagnosis of diabetes. She has no previous medical history of note, but does describe some mild fatigue, menstrual irregularity and increased frequency of micturition. There is no history of change in her weight, but she has noticed that she has been drinking more fluids each day to quench a thirst. She does not take any medication and she does not smoke or use any recreational drugs. She is from a lower middle-class income group and her father takes tablets to treat type 2 diabetes mellitus.

Prior to referral her GP had performed some investigations. Routine urine examination showed the presence of glucose without pus cells, albumin or ketones. Her fasting plasma glucose was 9 mmol/L (162 mg/dL); 2 h after a 75 g glucose drink, her plasma glucose was 15.5 mmol/L (279 mg/dL).

What would your differential diagnosis include before examining the patient?

A random glucose concentration of ≥11.1 mmol/L (200 mg/dL) and/or a fasting glucose of ≥7.0 mmol/L (126 mg/dL) are diagnostic of diabetes. This young woman also has symptoms that are suggestive of diabetes, notably thirst, polydipsia and polyuria, and so no additional blood tests are required to establish the diagnosis of diabetes, beyond those already performed by her GP. If she had been asymptomatic, then a second 'diagnostic' plasma glucose would be required to confirm the presence of diabetes.

The key question now is 'what type of diabetes does she have?'. Given her age, type 1 diabetes would be most likely, but there were no signs of insulin deficiency, i.e. there was no loss in weight and no ketones were detected in her urine. Type 2 diabetes is being seen more frequently in younger adults (and even in some children) because of increasing obesity in many populations. Type 2 diabetes is more common in certain racial groups, most notably people of South Asian origin. There are rare genetic subtypes of diabetes (maturity onset diabetes of the young, MODY), which are inherited in an autosomal dominant manner and usually present in young adults. Diabetes may also occur secondary to other conditions, especially disorders that effect the pancreas, such as chronic pancreatitis, post-pancreatic surgery, pancreatic tumours, haemochromatosis, cystic fibrosis and fibro-calcific pancreatitis. Endocrine disorders can also cause glucose intolerance, most notably Cushing's syndrome, acromegaly, thyrotoxicosis and phaeochromocytoma. Polycystic ovarian syndrome is associated with central obesity and insulin resistance and so glucose intolerance often coexists. Drugs can also promote the development of diabetes, most notably glucocorticoids, but also agents such as antiretrovirals, thiazide diuretics, antipsychotics and beta adrenoreceptor antagonists.

Examination

On examination, the young woman is 1.63 m tall and her weight is 69 kg, giving a body mass index of 25.6 kg/m². Her waist:hip ratio is 0.94 and she has no signs of dehydration nor a smell of ketones on her breath. She has pigmented velvety skin thickening with rugae and skin tags suggestive of acanthosis nigricans on the back and front of neck and in both axillae. She has no evidence of xanthelasma. She has no facial or other features suggestive of Cushing's syndrome or acromegaly. She has a little facial acne.

Her pulse rate is 80/min and peripheral pulses are present in all four limbs. Her blood pressure is 134/84 mmHg. Neurological examination, including ankle jerks, vibration sense and a monofilament sensation test, is normal. She has no abnormalities in the nails or skin of her feet including the inter-digital spaces. Abdominal and retinal examination reveal no abnormality.

Has examination narrowed down your differential diagnosis?

The history and examination findings rule out the possibility of secondary causes. The presence of acanthosis nigricans and central obesity (increased waist:hip ratio) suggests insulin resistance, which strongly points towards the diagnosis of type 2 diabetes. The presence of acne and menstrual irregularity point towards polycystic ovary syndrome (PCOS), which would also increase the likelihood of her having type 2 diabetes. The family history does not really help. A strong family history is usually seen in patients with MODY (though may not be), but it is often seen too in people with type 2 diabetes.

Initial investigations

A complete blood count is within the normal range. Other investigation results are shown in Box 51.1.

BOX 51.1	
Routine investigations	
Urea	3.9 mmol/L (23.5 mg/dL)
Creatinine	108 µmol/L (1.22 mg/dL)
HbA$_{1C}$	9.9%
Total cholesterol	5.5 mmol/L (213 mg/dL)
LDL cholesterol	3.3 mmol/L (128 mg/dL)
HDL cholesterol	0.85 mmol/L (33 mg/dL)
Triglyceride	2.6 mmol/L (228 mg/dL)
Bilirubin	11 µmol/L (0.65 mg/dL)
ALT	38 U/L
GGT	26 U/L
Alkaline phosphatase	95 U/L
Urine albumin:creatinine ratio	3.9 mg/mmol (normal range 0–3.5)

BOX 51.2	
Therapeutic targets in type 2 diabetes mellitus	
Fasting blood glucose	4–7 mmol/L (72–126 mg/dL)
2-h post-prandial glucose	4–10 mmol/L (72–180 mg/dL)
HbA$_{1C}$	<7%
BP	<130/80 mmHg
LDL	<2.6 mmol/L (100 mg/dL)
HDL	>1.1 mmol/L (40 mg/dL)
Triglyceride	<1.7 mmol/L (150 mg/dL)
Ideal body mass index (BMI)	20–25

Does this narrow down your differential diagnosis?

Type 2 diabetes is associated with central obesity and resistance to the action of insulin at a tissue level. It is usually associated with other factors associated with the 'metabolic syndrome', namely hypertension and dyslipidaemia. This woman has high total and LDL cholesterol levels, high triglycerides and low HDL concentrations; this is the classic pattern seen in the 'Metabolic Syndrome'. Her blood pressure is also higher than might be expected in someone of her age. These findings are all in support of a diagnosis of type 2 diabetes. The raised urine albumin : creatinine ratio suggests the presence of microalbuminuria.

Definitive investigations

Anti-glutamic acid decarboxylase (GAD)-65 antibodies were negative, as were genetic tests for MODY.

How will you treat this patient?

This woman has type 2 diabetes. The antibody and genetic testing were carried out given her young age, but really were 'gilding the lily'. Type 2 diabetes at diagnosis can be associated with neurological, retinal, renal and cardiovascular complications. The presence of dyslipidaemia in type 2 diabetes is a risk factor for macrovascular morbidity and mortality in terms of coronary artery disease and stroke. The woman should be seen by a dietician for a diet plan designed to help her achieve an ideal body weight and to help her to avoid consumption of large amounts of fat and refined carbohydrate. She should also be advised to take regular, moderate exercise. She is a non-smoker.

The patient should be advised to start metformin. This will improve her insulin resistance and optimise her blood glucose. It may also help regularise her menstrual cycle and may improve her fertility. Women with type 2 diabetes are often subfertile, because of the associated PCOS, and it is not uncommon for such women to have had unprotected intercourse with their partners for many years, only to fall pregnant within a few months after starting metformin. Pregnancy in women with poorly-controlled diabetes is associated with an increased risk of miscarriage and fetal anomaly. All women of reproductive age must be counselled about this and be advised to use contraception, until glycaemic control is optimised and any teratogenic drugs are stopped.

If microalbuminuria is confirmed in two further urine samples, then therapy with an angiotensin-converting enzyme inhibitor is usually recommended. However, these drugs are teratogenic and should only be given to women of reproductive age after counselling. If pregnancy is planned in the near future then a non-teratogenic agent, such as nifedipine or methyldopa should be initiated. Statin therapy is usually only advocated in those over the age of 40 years, unless there is evidence of vascular disease.

As diabetes is life-long, she should be reviewed regularly by a multidiscipli-nary diabetes team to assess her therapeutic response and for early detection and treatment of complications in the target organs such as the eyes, kidneys, nerves and heart. As time progresses, she might need other anti-diabetic drugs, including insulin (if beta-cell function worsens further), to maintain good diabetic control. Measurement of HbA$_{1c}$ every 3–6 months will be useful to monitor her diabetes control. The therapeutic targets for type 2 diabetes mellitus are listed in Box 51.2.

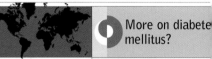

Key points and global issues

<table>
<tr><td>

- Diabetes mellitus is one of the leading causes of death worldwide.

- A considerable geographic variation is observed in the incidences of both type 1 and type 2 diabetes mellitus.

</td><td>

More on diabetes mellitus?

See Chapter 21 of
Davidson's Principles
& **Practice** of
Medicine (21st edn)

</td></tr>
</table>

- The incidence of diabetes mellitus, particularly type 2 diabetes, is increasing globally at a very high rate and more so in Asian countries.

- Type 2 diabetes mellitus typically develops with advancing age but is now being diagnosed frequently in children and young adults.

- Measurement of HbA$_{1c}$ is a useful indicator of the risk of diabetic complications and the quality of diabetes care. At present, its measurement is not recommended for the diagnosis of diabetes mellitus, but that may change in the near future.

- HbA$_{1c}$ is affected by ethnicity and race, independent of glycaemia; higher levels are observed in Afro-Americans compared with whites. Several conditions such as anaemia, recovery from acute blood loss, pregnancy and splenectomy affect its levels.

52

Diabetic ketoacidosis

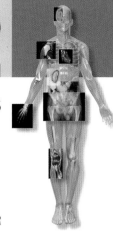

B. M. FRIER

Presenting problem

A 33-year-old Caucasian woman with type 1 diabetes is admitted to hospital with a 2-week history of increasing shortness of breath and a cough, productive of green sputum. She has stopped taking her insulin for 2 days preceding admission because she has lost her appetite, has been feeling nauseated and has not been eating. She has had previous admissions to hospital with diabetes-related problems and seldom attends the diabetes outpatient clinic. In the Emergency Department, a capillary blood sample registers high on the glucose meter, and venous blood samples are sent for urgent laboratory estimations. Urinalysis is also performed. The results are shown in Box 52.1.

What would your differential diagnosis include before examining the patient?

The elevated white cell count and C-reactive protein (CRP), in association with the history of increasing shortness of breath, cough and purulent sputum, suggest that she has a lower respiratory tract infection. The presence of a metabolic acidosis (HCO_3 6.1 mmol/L (mEq/L)) and of ketonuria indicates severe metabolic decompensation.

The Joint British Diabetes Societies Inpatient Care Group has specified criteria for significant diabetic ketoacidosis (DKA):

1. Hyperglycaemia (blood glucose >11 mmol/L (198 mg/dL))
2. Metabolic acidosis with an arterial bicarbonate (HCO_3) concentration of <15 mmol/L (mEq/L) or arterial H^+ of >49 nmol/L (pH <7.31) associated with ketonaemia of 3 mmol/L and over, or significant ketonuria (>2+ on standard urine sticks).

In addition to DKA, the differential diagnosis includes starvation and alcohol-induced ketoacidosis. However, in those circumstances it is rare for the blood glucose to exceed 14 mmol/L (252 mg/dL) and for the plasma

BOX 52.1	
Initial investigations	
Sodium	132 mmol/L (mEq/L)
Potassium	5.5 mmol/L (mEq/L)
Chloride	96 mmol/L (mEq/L)
Bicarbonate	6.1 mmol/L (mEq/L)
Urea	12.2 mmol/L (34.14 mg/dL)
Creatinine	150 μmol/L (1.69 mg/dL)
Glucose	39.2 mmol/L (706 mg/dL)
CRP	248 mg/L
Urinalysis	
Blood	+
Protein	+
Glucose	+++
Ketones	++++
WCC	25.1×10^9/L (10^3/mm^3)
Haemoglobin	149 g/L (14.9 g/dL)
Platelets	322×10^9/L (10^3/mm^3)
MCV	90.3 fL

HCO_3 to fall below 18 mmol/L (mEq/L). If a meter to measure a capillary blood ketone level at the bedside is available, this would confirm the severity of the ketosis.

Examination

On examination, the patient is pyrexial (temperature 38.3°C), tachycardic (120 beats/min), and hypotensive (98/54 mmHg) with an oxygen saturation (SpO_2) of 94% on air. She appears dehydrated with a dry tongue, and her breath has a 'fruity' odour. Heart auscultation and abdominal palpation are unremarkable. Her breathing is noted to be rapid (respiratory rate 30 breaths/min) and deep. Auscultation of her chest reveals upper right-sided coarse crepitations and bronchial breathing.

Has examination narrowed down your differential diagnosis?

In addition to the signs of a right upper lobe infection, some characteristic signs of DKA are present. The relative insulin deficiency and excessive secretion of counter-regulatory hormones that occur in DKA allow uncontrolled lipolysis and result in high circulating levels of free fatty acids, which are metabolised in the liver where they are oxidised to ketone bodies. This produces the classical 'fruity' smell (said to resemble pear drops) on the patient's breath. In an attempt to compensate for the metabolic acidosis of DKA, a respiratory alkalosis is induced via rapid deep breathing (called Kussmaul respirations). A CURB score, commonly used in assessing patients with pneumonia, may be difficult to interpret in this patient because of the presence of dual pathologies.

Further investigations

Arterial blood gases (on air) reveal H^+ 96.9 nmol/L (pH = 7.01), PO_2 9.89 kPa (74.2 mmHg), PCO_2 1.84 kPa (13.8 mmHg), HCO_3 5.9 mmol/L (mEq/L) and base excess −23.0 mmol/L (mEq/L), confirming that she has a severe metabolic acidosis with respiratory compensation. A chest X-ray shows right upper zone opacification (Fig. 52.1).

Has the diagnosis been clinched?

The clinical examination and investigations demonstrate the presence of a lobar pneumonia, and the severe bacterial infection has precipitated DKA in this patient. By stopping her insulin inappropriately, the patient has aggravated the

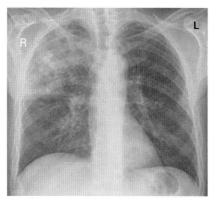

Figure 52.1 Chest X-ray showing right upper lobe pneumonia.

metabolic decompensation. Common precipitating factors of DKA include new untreated type 1 diabetes, intercurrent infection, non-adherence to insulin therapy, psychological factors adversely affecting self-management (especially in adolescents and young adults), myocardial infarction and drugs such as steroids.

How will you treat this patient?

Several different issues need to be considered to treat this patient.

1. *Fluid replacement.* In adults, the water deficit in DKA is usually around 100 mL/kg body weight and the total deficit is often between 5 and 7 L. Between 1 and 2 L of isotonic saline should be administered intravenously in the first hour. Thereafter, 250–500 mL/h of 0.9% saline should be given and continued until the patient is volume-replete. When the blood glucose declines to ~15 mmol/L (270 mg/dL), intravenous 10% dextrose (125 mL/h) should be added to allow intravenous insulin to be continued in sufficiently high concentrations to switch off ketogenesis.

2. *Insulin therapy.* Add 50 U of soluble (short-acting) insulin to 50 mL 0.9% saline and administer intravenously by infusion pump, initially at 6 U/h (approximately 0.1 U/kg per hour). Thereafter, give a continuous intravenous infusion of 1–3 U/h, depending on hourly blood glucose measurements. Aim for a fall in blood glucose of 3–6 mmol/L (54–108 mg/dL) per hour; then maintain blood glucose between 10 and 12 mmol/L (180–216 mg/dL). Continue intravenous infusion for 12–24 h after the ketosis has resolved and the patient is eating and drinking.

3. *Electrolyte replacement.* The initial serum potassium is elevated because of the insulin deficiency and acute renal failure, but patients with DKA usually have profound total body potassium deficits. This patient will need lots of potassium. Give potassium replacement by intravenous infusion, but not in the first litre of fluid, and monitor plasma potassium 2–4-hourly.

4. *Other measures.* The community acquired pneumonia should be treated with a broad-spectrum antibiotic depending on the most likely local organisms and their common sensitivities. In the UK, amoxicillin is often used as the first-line drug, plus or minus a macrolide. In view of the severity of the illness, the antibiotic should be administered intravenously and probably a combination will be required to treat an atypical infection. The patient should be admitted to a high-dependency unit for close observation. Urine output, heart rate and blood pressure should be monitored carefully, and if the patient remains anuric despite volume replacement, a urethral catheter should be inserted. A nasogastric tube is required when the patient is semiconscious to reduce the risk of aspiration. Sodium bicarbonate should not be administered, as it may worsen intracellular acidosis. The use of low molecular weight heparin should be considered and is recommended. Lack of improvement should prompt early involvement of the specialist diabetes team. Intravenous fluid and insulin treatment should not be discontinued until the patient is eating and drinking normally.

Most patients make a complete recovery from DKA and spend only a few days in hospital. Cerebral oedema is a rare but devastating complication that can occur in children and young adults.

Before discharge, she should be reviewed by the diabetes team and reminded about 'sick-day rules', namely the need to monitor blood glucose frequently during intercurrent illness, to increase (rather than decrease) insulin doses and to maintain a high intake of clear fluids. She should be encouraged to re-attend the diabetes clinic.

Key points and global issues

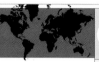

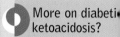
More on diabetic ketoacidosis?

See Chapter 21 of
Davidson's Principles
& **Practice** of
Medicine (21st edn)

- The mortality rate associated with DKA is around 5–10% in Western countries, and is reported to be up to 25% in developing countries where access to intensive clinical and laboratory facilities may not be available.

- While DKA is relatively rare in type 2 diabetes, an increase in incidence has been reported in African-Americans and other ethnic groups with type 2 diabetes.

53

Diabetic foot ulcer

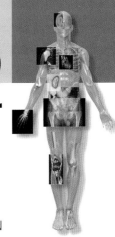

AMBADY RAMACHANDRAN

Presenting problem

A 55-year-old man with type 2 diabetes mellitus of 15 years' duration is hospitalised for control of his diabetes and management of a non-healing ulcer on the left heel, which developed following a thorn prick 2 months earlier. The patient also complains of numbness in his feet. His left first and second toes were amputated 2 years ago and he had laser therapy for diabetic retinopathy last year. He takes several medications, including metformin and glibenclamide for his diabetes, as well as aspirin and enalapril. Prior to referral, his GP had performed some investigations and the results are provided in Box 53.1.

What would your differential diagnosis include before examining the patient?

The foot is a frequent site for complications in patients with diabetes mellitus, and for this reason, footcare is extremely important. Ulcerations in the foot is a common reason for hospital admission in diabetic patients. These admissions tend to be prolonged and may end with amputation. A non-healing foot ulcer in

BOX 53.1	
Initial investigations	
Haemoglobin	72 g/L (7.2 g/dL)
WCC	15.8×10^9/L (10^3/mm^3)
Fasting blood glucose	14.3 mmol/L (258 mg/dL)
Post-prandial blood glucose	25.4 mmol/L (458 mg/dL)
HbA$_{1c}$	13.5%
Urea	12 mmol/L (78 mg/dL)
Creatinine	168 μmol/L (1.9 mg/dL)
Urine examination	
Albumin	++
ECG	T wave inversions in V$_1$–V$_4$ suggestive of anteroseptal ischaemia; normal R–R interval

a patient with diabetes mellitus requires differentiation from other types of neuropathic, ischaemic and neuro-ischaemic ulcers. Since this patient has diabetes and has symptoms suggestive of peripheral neuropathy, the diagnosis favours a neuropathic ulcer.

Examination

The patient is conscious, oriented, febrile and pale. The respiratory rate is 18/min. He is mildly dehydrated and has xanthelasma palpebrarum on the right side. Bilateral pitting oedema is present. His pulse rate is 100/min and regular. Blood pressure readings supine and standing are 160/90 mmHg and 150/80 mmHg, respectively. The pulsations of both carotid and subclavian arteries are equal on both sides. The pulsations of the popliteal, posterior tibial and dorsalis pedis arteries are present in both lower limbs. The first and second toes on the left side are amputated with well-healed scars. The nervous system examination reveals absent ankle jerks and decreased vibration sense and proprioception on both sides. The left foot is swollen and its skin is dry. There is a non-healing ulcer 3×3 cm on the left heel (Fig. 53.1), with foul-smelling pus discharge and erythema and swelling of the surrounding skin. There is flattening of the arch of the left foot with features of Charcot deformity. Non-proliferative diabetic retinopathy, with laser photocoagulation scars, is present in both eyes on fundus examination.

Have examination and initial investigations narrowed down your differential diagnosis?

This man has a royal flush of diabetes complications. He has known retinopathy, while blood and urine tests strongly suggest the presence of diabetic nephropathy. He has electrocardiogram (ECG) evidence of coronary artery disease and clinical evidence of peripheral neuropathy.

Various mechanisms could have produced the initial foot ulceration, including somatic neuropathy (diminished proprioception) and autonomic neuropathy (dry skin, fissures, Charcot neuropathy) Secondary infection of the ulcer has caused surrounding cellulitis.

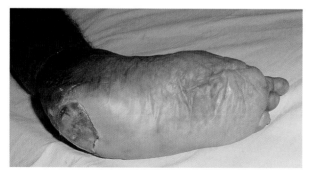

Figure 53.1 Large ulcer on the heel following debridement. Note the Charcot deformity of the foot and the previous toe amputations.

BOX 53.2	
Further investigations	
X-ray left foot	Charcot arthropathy
Doppler test of lower limb	
Right ankle brachial index	1.3
Left ankle brachial index	1.5
Biothesiometry	Severe neuropathy (sensation felt at >40 V of current by vibrating method)
Monofilament test	Protective sensation absent with 10 g monofilament in all areas of foot
Nerve conduction study	Severe sensory motor neuropathy in both lower limbs

In addition to diabetes mellitus, other conditions can also produce persistent foot ulcers and these include Hansen's disease, thromboangiitis obliterans (Buerger's disease) and vasculitis; however, given the overwhelming evidence, diabetes has to be the likely culprit here.

 Further investigations

Box 53.2 provides the results of further investigation of the left foot.

Does this narrow down your differential diagnosis?

The results confirm the clinical impression that this man has severe sensory motor neuropathy. These abnormalities, as well as uncontrolled hyperglycaemia and anaemia, have produced a non-healing ulcer in the left foot. There is secondary infection of the ulcer, surrounding cellulitis and Charcot deformity of the foot.

How will you treat this patient?

Strict glycaemic control should be ensured with conversion of this man's treatment to insulin therapy. Broad-spectrum antibiotics should be administered according to the culture and sensitivity of the organisms grown from a swab taken from the ulcer. Necrotic tissue should be debrided aggressively. Regular dressings and follow-up will be essential; pressure relief is essential – appropriate footwear should be provided, with insoles that redistribute pressure around the foot and away from the ulcerated area. Total contact casting and intravenous bisphosphonate therapy have been advocated for patients with an acute Charcot arthropathy, but the former would be ill advised here, given the presence of active ulceration. The patient should be initiated into a rehabilitation programme comprising education regarding footwear and footcare (e.g. avoiding barefoot walking, regular inspection of the feet for new abnormalities).

The man should be given strong advice and help to stop smoking. He is already taking aspirin and angiotensin-converting enzyme (ACE) inhibitors, but his blood pressure is poorly controlled. This needs to be aggressively targeted (to below 120/70 mmHg), with additional antihypertensive therapy, given his retinopathy and nephropathy. He would also derive prognostic benefit from being commenced on a statin, irrespective of his total cholesterol concentration.

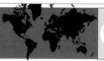
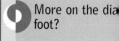
- Diabetic foot disease is one of the most frequent causes of hospitalisation and is one of the most expensive complications of diabetes.

See Chapter 21 of
Davidson's Principles
& **Practice** of
Medicine (21st edn)

- Diabetic foot ulceration is common among people who walk bare foot.

- Diabetic foot disease places a heavy burden on socioeconomic resources of families and countries, particularly developing countries.

- The magnitude of the problem in developing countries calls for epidemiological research to enable and encourage policymakers and health administrators to address the problems caused by this dreaded complication of diabetes mellitus.

54

Dysphagia

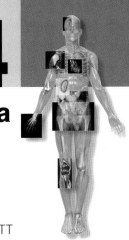

I. D. R. ARNOTT

Presenting problem

A 55-year-old man presents to his GP with a 4-week history of progressive dysphagia. He is able to swallow all liquids, but the ingestion of solid food leads to regurgitation and vomiting. He also complains of some non-specific but occasionally severe retrosternal discomfort that is relieved by regurgitation or vomiting. There is no odynophagia or early satiety. Over the duration of his history, he has lost 3 kg weight and has also noticed a decreased appetite. He has suffered from gastro-oesophageal reflux for many years, being awoken approximately three times a week with symptoms of nocturnal reflux.

His past medical history is notable for a non-ST elevation myocardial infarction 4 years ago. A coronary artery stent was inserted and he has been asymptomatic since then. He is also known to have hypertension. His current medication includes aspirin, atenolol, simvastatin and lisinopril. He lives with his wife and is able to complete all activities of daily living. He gave up smoking following his heart attack, having smoked 15 cigarettes per day since the age of 27. He consumes approximately 32 units of alcohol per week.

What would your differential diagnosis include before examining the patient?

The most important diagnosis to confirm or exclude is oesophageal cancer. The progressive nature of his symptoms makes this most likely. It is of note that he is able to tolerate liquids but not solids. The differential diagnosis includes a benign oesophageal stricture. The history for benign disease is often longer but the same pattern for solids and liquids exists. The other main differential diagnosis is achalasia or other dysmotility syndromes. Again, a longer history would be expected and individuals often experience symptoms with liquids as well as solids. It is common to have some evidence of weight loss with all of the above, but this is much greater with malignant causes. General wellbeing and weight are often maintained in the early stages of oesophageal cancer and so the absence of these does not exclude the diagnosis. Odynophagia is more commonly caused by reflux oesophagitis and infections such as candidiasis, but can also occur in oesophageal cancer.

Examination and initial investigations

There is no evidence of lymphadenopathy or pallor. The patient's body mass index is 30. Pulse is 68/min and venous pressure is not raised. Heart sounds are normal and there is no peripheral oedema. The chest is clear. The abdomen is soft and non-tender, with no masses or organomegaly.

Initial investigations, comprising full blood count, serum biochemistry and liver function tests, are normal and a chest X-ray is also normal.

Have examination and initial investigations narrowed down your differential diagnosis?

No. The differential diagnosis remains the same. Although there are physical findings that do point to a particular diagnosis, it is more common for examination not to influence your decision-making at this stage. An upper gastrointestinal endoscopy is urgently required.

Further investigations

Anatomically, the cricopharyngeus is normally 20 cm from the incisors, and at endoscopy, this marks the proximal extent of the evaluable oesophagus. The gastro-oesophageal junction lies 40 cm from the incisors.

The patient undergoes an upper gastrointestinal endoscopy 4 days following clinic review. There is evidence of columnar lined oesophagus from 32 cm, extending to the gastro-oesophageal junction. At 38 cm, there is an exophytic, macroscopically malignant tumour arising from the oesophageal wall, which causes narrowing of the lumen; the endoscope will not pass through this (Fig. 54.1). Multiple biopsies are taken from the mass and from the columnar lined oesophagus above. Biopsies of the tumour mass reveal adenocarcinoma and those from above reveal specialised intestinal metaplasia, i.e. Barrett's oesophagus.

To stage the patient's oesophageal tumour, a computed tomography (CT) scan of the chest and abdomen is performed. This confirms concentric thickening of the distal oesophagus and some peri-tumour lymph nodes. On the scan, these do not reach size criteria for tumour spread, but they do raise suspicion of lymph node involvement. The scan does not show any solid organ metastatic disease.

CT cannot adequately stage the tumour within the oesophagus and further imaging is therefore required: namely, endoscopic ultrasound (EUS). This confirms the presence of tumour at 38 cm within the oesophagus; although it involves the mucosa and submucosa, it has not breached the muscularis mucosae and is therefore staged as T_2. The lymph nodes noted on CT are enlarged up to 1 cm but there are no enlarged coeliac axis nodes. In view of the relatively early tumour stage, these enlarged nodes have more significance. To classify them further, EUS-guided fine-needle aspiration is undertaken. This reveals malignant cells in two out of three nodes sampled.

Has the diagnosis been clinched?

These investigations have confirmed a distal oesophageal adenocarcinoma arising in an area of Barrett's oesophagus. Investigations have staged this tumour as T2N1M0. The Barrett's oesophagus has occurred as a consequence of long-term acid reflux. Risk factors for oesophageal cancer are shown in Box 54.1 and can be remembered using the mnemonic 'BELCH-SPAT'.

How will you treat this patient?

The priority is to relieve the dysphagia and this is usually achieved by endoscopic balloon dilatation. At endoscopy, a controlled radial expansion balloon may be placed through the stricture under direct vision and then inflated to approximately three atmospheres of pressure. This corresponds to a balloon diameter of 15 mm.

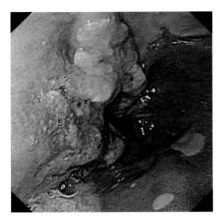

Figure 54.1 An exophytic cancer seen in the distal oesophagus at upper gastrointestinal endoscopy.

Tumours of this stage, specifically because of the lymph node spread, are not generally considered curable by surgery alone. This man should, therefore, undergo two cycles of neoadjuvant chemotherapy with cisplatin and 5-fluorouracil. Current protocols suggest that further staging following this is needed before decisions about surgery can be made. If the restaging CT shows evidence of tumour shrinkage, then the patient should be a good candidate for cardio-oesophagectomy with curative intent. Recovery from such surgery is typically prolonged, and on discharge this man will need strict dietary and nutritional instructions to help him maintain his weight.

Survival rates, despite best treatment, remain low. For oesophageal carcinoma overall, the 1-year survival is 27% and the 5-year survival is approximately 9%. For this man, given best treatment, 2-year survival is in the region of only 45%. A guarded prognosis, therefore, must be conveyed to the patient.

BOX 54.1

Risk factors for oesophageal cancer

- Barrett's oesophagus
- Ethanol abuse
- Lye stricture
- Coeliac disease
- Head and neck tumours
- Smoking
- Plummer–Vinson syndrome
- Achalasia
- Tylosis

Key points and global issues

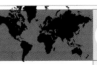 More on dysphagia?

See Chapter 22 of
Davidson's Principles
& **Practice** of
Medicine (21st edn)

- The incidence of oesophageal carcinoma varies worldwide. Squamous cell cancer occurs commonly in parts of China, Iran, Central Asia, Siberia, Mongolia, Afghanistan, parts of Africa, Iceland and Finland, whereas adenocarcinoma occurs in Western populations.

- Invasive oesophageal candidiasis can present with odynophagia, particularly in areas with a high prevalence of human immunodeficiency virus (HIV).

- In developing nations, tuberculosis should be included in the differential diagnosis of odynophagia. Tuberculosis can rarely involve the oesophagus; however, mediastinal lymphadenopathy and a cold abscess can produce similar symptoms.

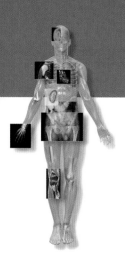

55

Haematemesis

S. M. W. JAFRI

Presenting problem

A 42-year-old man presents to the Accident and Emergency Department with a 1-day history of vomiting fresh blood. He also reports the passing of black-coloured stools for the last 3 days and feeling generally unwell for almost 6 weeks. His main complaint is of easy fatigue and he is unable to carry on his work beyond 3 p.m. He is privately employed as a driver and does not drink alcohol. His past medical history is uneventful, with the exception that he has had three episodes of jaundice: the first when he was 20 years old, then 4–5 years after that and a further episode about 3 years ago. Each time, he was seen by a herbal practitioner, who prescribed some herbs, and after a few days, the patient felt better. He did not have any blood tests. His main reason for not seeking medical attention, other than the herbal practitioner, was financial constraints, as he thought that a doctor would order lots of tests that he could not afford.

What would your differential diagnosis include before examining the patient?

The key facts are that this 42-year-old male patient is presenting with haematemesis and melaena, with at least three previous episodes of jaundice. It is possible that he is suffering from chronic viral hepatitis B or C and has now developed cirrhosis, portal hypertension and bleeding from oesophageal varices, or else he may be suffering from a peptic ulcer, which is bleeding. Other possibilities include oesophageal ulcers from chronic reflux oesophagitis, Mallory–Weiss tears and gastric carcinoma, but with his history, these seem very unlikely.

Examination

Physical examination reveals an icteric and pale patient. His blood pressure is 110/70 mmHg and heart rate 90/min. Although oriented in place and person, he is somewhat confused and, at times, inattentive during examination. The liver is palpable about 2 cm below the costal margin and the spleen is palpable 4 cm below the costal margin. There is no shifting dullness or fluid thrill. On the chest and back, there are a few spider angiomas.

Has examination narrowed down your differential diagnosis?

The mild confusion, hepatosplenomegaly, jaundice and spider angiomas suggest that this patient has portal hypertension secondary to cirrhosis. The haematemesis is most likely due to variceal haemorrhage. However, patients with cirrhosis do have a higher incidence of peptic ulceration, which at this stage cannot be ruled out.

Investigations

Blood test results are shown in Box 55.1. The patient has an emergency ultrasound carried out and this shows mild ascites, splenomegaly, altered echotexture of the liver, a dilated portal vein and varices around the splenic hilum. There is suspicion of a mass in the right lobe of the liver measuring 3.3 cm. As the α-fetoprotein is high in a patient who has a mass in a cirrhotic liver, further investigation with dynamic computed tomography (CT) is performed; this confirms the mass to be a hepatoma.

From the Accident and Emergency Department, and following aggressive resuscitation with intravenous fluids, the patient is transferred to the endoscopy suite, where he has an upper gastrointestinal endoscopy. This reveals bleeding oesophageal varices (Fig. 55.1); the stomach contains about 200 mL of altered blood. There is no ulcer or erosions, but there is significant portal hypertensive gastropathy involving most of the stomach; there are no fundal varices.

Does this narrow down your differential diagnosis?

Yes. This patient has chronic hepatitis C with cirrhosis. He has two further complications: hepatic decompensation (ascites and mild hepatic encephalopathy) and a hepatoma. Hepatitis C is a chronic disease and, if not treated early, can result in cirrhosis in about 30% of patients after a delay of 25–30 years. After a further few years, hepatic decompensation and the development of hepatocellular cancer may occur. There are over 200 million patients with hepatitis C throughout the world and it has evolved as one of the major causes of chronic liver disease and also the major reason for liver transplantation.

How will you treat this patient?

Resuscitation with intravenous crystalloids and, if necessary, blood is essential prior to endoscopy. At endoscopy, the patient should be treated with band ligation

BOX 55.1	
Initial investigations	
Haemoglobin	100 g/L (10 g/dL)
Platelets	54×10^9/L (10^3/mm^3)
WCC	2.3×10^9/L (10^3/mm^3)
Prothrombin time	18 s
Urea	14.3 mmol/L (40.5 mg/dL)
Creatinine	65 μmol/L (0.73 mg/dL)
Bilirubin	74 μmol/L (4.33 mg/dL)
ALT	54 U/L
AST	46 U/L
Alkaline phosphatase	112 U/L
Albumin	28 g/L (2.8 g/dL)
α-Fetoprotein	8 U/L (upper limit of normal 5.5 U/L)
Hepatitis B surface antigen and core antibody	Negative
Hepatitis C virus antibody	Positive

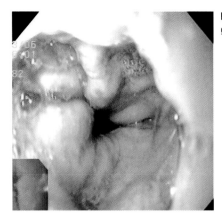
Figure 55.1 Oesophageal varices at upper gastrointestinal endoscopy.

of the oesophageal varices. This would require at least 2–3 endoscopic sessions to achieve complete eradication.

Once his condition has stabilised and the bleeding has been stopped, the patient should be commenced on propranolol at a dose that will lower his heart rate to around ≤60/min. This would reduce portal hypertension, which, in turn, should help his portal hypertensive gastropathy and further bleeding from varices. For mild ascites, he should be treated with a low-salt diet; if that is not enough, he should receive spironolactone at a small dose of 50 mg daily. Resection of the hepatoma is not feasible, as he already has hepatic decompensation. He should therefore receive either percutaneous ethanol injections (PEI), transcutaneous arterial chemo-embolisation (TACE) or radiofrequency ablation, depending on local expertise and facilities. All three modalities have shown comparative results. If he is being treated in a centre where transplant facilities are available, he should be evaluated for a liver transplant, as this would be his best chance for survival.

Key points and global issues

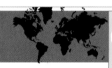

More on chronic liver disease, portal hypertension and variceal bleeding?

See Chapter 23 of **Davidson's Principles & Practice** of **Medicine (21st edn)**

- Chronic liver disease is extremely prevalent throughout the world but has different causes. Viral hepatitis B and C are behind most cases; the other important cause is alcohol.

- Patients with a history of jaundice should be properly evaluated with liver function tests and hepatitis B and C serology. They should be treated without delay if serology is positive.

- Effective treatment is available to control hepatitis B and to cure hepatitis C.

- Patients who have cirrhosis should be treated conservatively. If cirrhosis is complicated by ascites, encephalopathy, bleeding varices or a hepatoma, they should be treated in a specialised centre.

56

Chronic diarrhoea

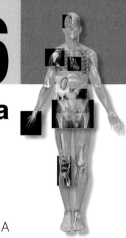

G. K. MAKHARIA

Presenting problem

A 16-year-old boy presents to the outpatient department complaining of diarrhoea, which he has had for 6 years. He passes 4–5 large-volume stools daily, which are frothy, greasy and foul-smelling, and contain undigested food material. The stools do not contain visible blood, mucus or pus. He has post-prandial bloating of the abdomen, generalised weakness and easy fatiguability. He has no abdominal pain, fever or joint pains. His parents mention that he is not growing well.

What would your differential diagnosis include before examining the patient?

The list of causes of chronic diarrhoea (diarrhoea lasting >4 weeks) is extensive. It may be caused not only by diseases of the small and large intestine, but also by systemic diseases such as hyperthyroidism, diabetes mellitus, autonomic neuropathy and drugs (Box 56.1). We need to ask the following questions when approaching this patient:

- Is the diarrhoea due to a functional disease (long-standing symptoms, no nocturnal diarrhoea) or an organic disease (weight loss, fever, short duration)?
- Is the diarrhoea of small-bowel type (large volume, frothy, greasy, foul-smelling stool that contains undigested food material) or large-bowel type (more than six stools per day containing blood, mucus and/or pus, associated with tenesmus)?
- Is the diarrhoea associated with features of malabsorption (bulky, frothy, greasy stool containing undigested food)?
- Is there a systemic inflammatory response (such as fever, sweating or joint pains)?

From the history alone, it seems that the diarrhoea in this boy is chronic and of small-bowel type, and has features suggestive of malabsorption.

> **BOX 56.1**
>
> **Causes of chronic diarrhoea and malabsorption**
>
> **Small-bowel type**
> - Coeliac disease
> - Tropical sprue
> - Parasitic infections
> - Immunodeficiency syndromes
> - Crohn's disease
> - Whipple's disease
> - Abetalipoproteinaemia
>
> **Large-bowel type**
> - Irritable bowel syndrome
> - Inflammatory bowel disease
> - Microscopic colitis

Examination

The height, weight and body mass index of the patient are 150 cm, 32 kg and 14.2 kg/m^2, respectively. He is pale and lacks secondary sexual characteristics. He has angular cheilitis and stomatitis.

Has examination narrowed down your clinical diagnosis?

The physical examination indicates that this patient has short stature (amounting to growth retardation), probable anaemia and nutritional deficiencies. These features support a diagnosis of malabsorption. Malabsorption in turn localises the site of disease to the small intestine. The causes of such chronic diarrhoea include coeliac disease, tropical sprue, parasitic infections *(Giardia lamblia, Cryptosporidium, Strongyloides, Microspora, Isospora)* and Crohn's disease (Box 56.1).

Investigations

The investigations in a patient with chronic diarrhoea with malabsorption include the following:
- Haematological and biochemical tests to determine the type of anaemia and other effects of malabsorption (hypoproteinaemia, hypocalcaemia)
- Tests to confirm the presence of malabsorption: D-xylose test, stool examination for fat globules, measurement of 72-h stool fat excretion
- Endoscopic examination of the upper part of the intestine
- Intestinal mucosal biopsies. In the mucosal biopsies, a note is made on the crypt and villous architecture; these are most often graded using the Modified Marsh classification (grade 0 = normal crypt villous (CV) ratio = 1:3–4; grade 1 = mild increase in intraepithelial lymphocytes (IEL), CV ratio 1:1; grade 2 = moderate villous atrophy, CV ratio <1; grade 3 = flat mucosa with no recognisable villi)
- Tests to determine the precise cause of the chronic diarrhoea and malabsorption, such as stool examination for ova and cysts of parasites, serological tests for coeliac disease (IgA-anti-endomysial antibody, IgA-anti-human tissue transglutaminase antibody, IgA or IgG antigliadin antibody), serum immunoglobulin profile (Iga, IgG and IgM levels), lipid profile and apolipoprotein levels, lactose hydrogen breath test (for lactose intolerance) and glucose hydrogen breath test (for bacterial overgrowth).

This patient's haemoglobin is 70 g/L (7.0 g/dL) and serum protein is 64 g/L (6.4 g/dL) (albumin 31 g/L (3.1 g/dL), globulin 33 g/L (3.3 g/dL)). After 5 g D-xylose ingestion, his 5-h urinary D-xylose excretion is 0.5 g (normal >1 g); his daily stool fat excretion is 8.0 g/day. Upper gastrointestinal endoscopy reveals attenuated and scalloped duodenal mucosal folds. The mucosal biopsy reveals a flat mucosa, an increase in intraepithelial lymphocytes, and infiltration of the lamina propria with chronic inflammatory cells (Fig. 56.1); there are no parasites or abnormal macrophages. Serum IgA anti-human tissue transglutaminase antibody and IgA anti-endomysial antibody are positive. Serum levels of IgG, IgA and IgM are within normal limits. A glucose hydrogen breath test and a lactose hydrogen breath test are normal. Stool examination reveals cysts of *Giardia lamblia*. The serological tests for human immunodeficiency virus (HIV) 1 and 2 are negative.

Does this narrow down your differential diagnosis?

Laboratory investigations show severe villous abnormality and a positive coeliac serological test. The diagnosis of coeliac disease is based on the Modified European Society of Paediatric Gastroenterology Hepatology and Nutrition

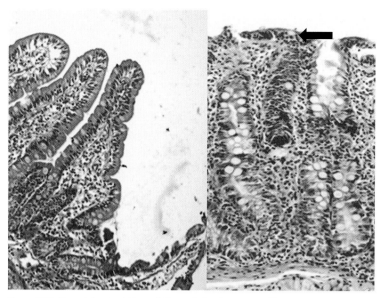

Figure 56.1 Normal duodenal biopsy (left panel) showing a crypt:villus ratio of 1:4. The intraepithelial lymphocyte (IEL) count is <1 in 5 tall columnar mucosal epithelial cells. There are at least 3–4 parallel crypts seen perpendicularly arranged over the muscularis mucosae, signifying that the biopsy is well-orientated. The duodenal biopsy in the right panel is of coeliac disease, with an altered crypt:villus ratio of 4:1, along with crypt hyperplasia and increased IELs (arrow) (H&E ×40).

(ESPGHAN) criteria, which include typical clinical manifestations, and suggestive histology (villous atrophy) and response to gluten-free diet. Therefore, based on clinical, histological and serological features, our patient has coeliac disease. In addition, he has *Giardia lamblia* infection, which might have contributed to his diarrhoea and malabsorption.

How will you treat this patient?

Coeliac disease is a common autoimmune disorder, which occurs in genetically predisposed individuals and is induced by ingestion of a protein called gluten. Gluten is present in cereals such as wheat, barley and rye. The hypersensitivity to gluten in patients with coeliac disease is permanent: 'Once a coeliac, always a coeliac'. Therefore, the treatment of coeliac disease is withdrawal of gluten from the diet, which should continue on a life-long basis. These patients usually have deficiency of several nutrients and therefore a complete nutritional assessment is essential. This man should also be treated with a nitroimidazole for *Giardia lamblia* infection.

Although patients start feeling well 2–4 weeks after the institution of a gluten-free diet, normalisation of the histological picture may take a few months. During the initial days of treatment, vitamins and haematinics should be supplemented. The most important cause of failure to respond to treatment is poor or incomplete dietary compliance. The treatment should be continued under the supervision of a dietitian.

Key points and global issues

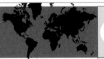

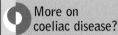

More on
coeliac disease?

See Chapter 22 of
Davidson's Principles
& **Practice** of
Medicine (21st edn)

- Worldwide, coeliac disease affects about 1% of the general population.

- The wide belief that coeliac disease is a disease of childhood is not true. Adult patients with coeliac disease may present with either typical (chronic diarrhoea) or atypical (short stature, refractory anaemia, metabolic bone disease and infertility) manifestations.

- Coeliac disease shows an iceberg phenomenon; for every symptomatic patient, 3–10 patients remain undetected, i.e. are minimally symptomatic or asymptomatic. Such people may be picked up in screening programmes of 'at-risk individuals', such as those with chronic anaemia, short stature, metabolic bone diseases, type 1 diabetes and other autoimmune disorders.

57

Constipation

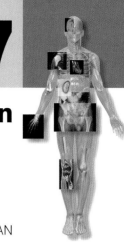

I. D. PENMAN

Presenting problem

A 28-year-old woman is referred with a 2-year history of constipation, passing hard stools with difficulty only once per week. She has to strain, complains of a sensation of incomplete emptying, discomfort around her perianal area on defaecation, and also diffuse lower abdominal discomfort and bloating. In the last few months, she has noticed mucus per rectum and small amounts of bright red blood, mainly on the toilet paper when she wipes herself. On systematic enquiry she reports a lack of energy and fatigue but no fever, sweats, diarrhoea or upper abdominal symptoms. She denies any urinary or gynaecological symptoms.

Past history includes investigations for headaches, but no serious cause was found. She takes codeine intermittently for these headaches and has had a brief period of time off work for anxiety and stress. The patient says her diet is reasonable, but does not contain much fruit. She works in a large office building as an operator in a call centre.

Prior to referral, her GP checked some routine blood tests including urea, electrolytes, glucose, full blood count and erythrocyte sedimentation rate; these were all normal.

What would your differential diagnosis include before examining the patient?

In the majority of young adults with constipation, the problem is one of 'simple' constipation without any underlying structural, inflammatory or other colonic disorder. In the developed world, diet and lifestyle factors are common causes of constipation and many young adults have a diet lacking in sufficient fibre, fruit, vegetable and fluid intake. Medications are a common cause of constipation (Box 57.1); the patient is taking codeine and this could well be contributing. Systemic disease (e.g. endocrine or neurological) can sometimes be associated with constipation and this should be sought. In this woman's case, there may be many explanations for small amounts of blood and mucus per rectum, but it does raise the possibility of colorectal disease such as proctitis

---

BOX 57.1

Drugs commonly associated with constipation

- Opioid analgesics, e.g. codeine, dihydrocodeine, morphine
- 5-HT_3 receptor antagonists, e.g. ondansetron
- Calcium antagonists, e.g. verapamil
- Anticholinergic agents, e.g. amitriptyline
- Diuretics
- Aluminium-containing antacids
- Iron supplements

(which can sometimes be associated with proximal constipation) or with neoplasia. All of these must be considered, but the diagnosis can usually be reached by a careful history, abdominal and rectal examination, and a few relatively simple investigations.

Examination

The patient looks generally well with no signs to suggest a systemic disorder, but is a little overweight. Abdominal examination is normal, rectal examination is tender but otherwise normal, and the rectum is empty. There is no obvious evidence of neurological abnormality.

Has examination narrowed down your differential diagnosis?

As is often the case, clinical examination has ruled out some obvious and serious conditions, but has not significantly narrowed down the differential diagnosis. Colorectal polyps and cancer are rare in people of this age and the patient appears well with no history or examination findings to suggest intestinal obstruction. Proctitis, rectal cancer and other rectal disorders, however, have not been completely excluded. Had proctoscopy or rigid sigmoidoscopy been performed in the clinic, this might have helped. Positive findings are useful (e.g. proctitis, ulcerative colitis, rectal cancer), but in practice the views are often limited and a negative rigid sigmoidoscopy does not adequately exclude problems more proximally in the rectosigmoid or left colon. The bleeding and mucus cannot be ignored and some further investigations are necessary.

Further investigations

A repeat full blood count, along with C-reactive protein (CRP), thyroid function tests and serum calcium, is normal, excluding hypercalcaemia and hypothyroidism; these are unusual but well-known causes of constipation. The patient undergoes a flexible sigmoidoscopy with examination of the colon up to the splenic flexure. Total colonoscopy is not performed, as bright red blood per rectum almost always originates in the distal colon or rectum and colon cancer is very rare at this age and with this presentation. There is considerable stool present despite bowel preparation, something that is often found in patients with chronic constipation. On the anterior wall of the distal rectum is an area of oedematous, friable, inflamed mucosa with ulceration, and this is biopsied. Histology shows non-specific inflammation, excess collagen and muscle thickening, features consistent with solitary rectal ulcer syndrome (SRUS).

Subsequently, an intestinal transit marker study is performed. The patient swallows capsules containing different-shaped pellets on each of three consecutive days and an abdominal X-ray is taken on day 5. While most or all of the pellets should be excreted by day 5, in this patient a large number of pellets are still retained in a uniform distribution throughout the colon (Fig. 57.1). These features are typical of 'slow-transit' constipation and the solitary rectal ulcer has probably resulted from repeated trauma of the rectal mucosa, a consequence of prolapse and ischaemia during straining at defaecation.

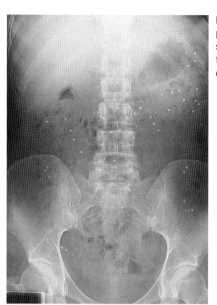

Figure 57.1 Abdominal X-ray (day 5) after the patient ingests capsules containing different-shaped pellets on days 1, 2 and 3. Over 40 of the 60 pellets are still present, diffusely distributed throughout the colon.

Does this narrow down your differential diagnosis?

The clinical picture, normal blood tests and findings from the flexible sigmoidoscopy and intestinal marker study confirm the diagnosis and further investigation is unnecessary.

How will you treat this patient?

By the time patients are referred to specialist clinics with constipation, most of the simple measures have already been tried: stopping any constipating medications, increasing fluid intake to at least 2 L daily, increasing dietary fibre, fruit and vegetable intake and regular exercise. Setting aside a regular, unhurried time for defaecation and availability of adequate toilet facilities and privacy are also important. None of these measures has proved effective in this patient; nor has therapy with a bulking agent (ispaghula), which worsened the bloating. Laxatives, including senna, lactulose and bisacodyl, are also of limited benefit.

In very difficult cases of chronic constipation, several newer methods are sometimes effective. A combination approach may be necessary using agents such as a solution of inert polyethylene glycol salts (e.g. Movicol), which acts as an osmotic agent, glycerol suppositories (which can improve rectal emptying), and prokinetics such as metoclopramide or 5-HT$_4$ agonists such as prucalopride. Other approaches that may be successful include biofeedback, in which a trainer helps the patient to retrain the coordination of rectal sensation and muscular control of defaecation over a number of sessions. It is labour-intensive and not widely available, but good results have been reported. Teaching patients to self-administer a commercially available and irrigation system can also be beneficial. In a minority of severely affected individuals, colectomy with ileorectal anastomosis is necessary, but this is a last resort and requires further careful evaluation and discussion.

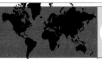
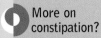

More on constipation?

See Chapter 22 of
**Davidson's Principles
& Practice** of
Medicine (21st edn)

- While more common in the developed world, chronic constipation is a worldwide problem, especially in hot climates.

- In the developing world, tuberculosis and chronic amoebiasis can present with constipation alternating with diarrhoea.

- Complex investigations are rarely necessary and most patients can be managed without resort to expensive medications.

58

Chronic abdominal pain

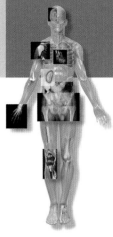

S. M. W. JAFRI

Presenting problem

A 35-year-old woman from Karachi in Pakistan presents to an outpatient clinic with a history of abdominal pain for the last 5 years. The pain generally starts around the umbilicus and radiates to almost the whole of the abdomen. It is colicky in nature and lasts from a few minutes to an hour on most of the occasions it occurs. She has had three or four attacks per year, but in the last 6 months she has had several episodes and now seeks medical advice. On previous occasions, she just attended the Accident and Emergency Department of her local hospital; an injection to lessen the pain was given but few investigations were performed. She belongs to a low socioeconomic class and is the mother of five children; her husband earns a modest salary as a domestic servant. At the age of 14, she was ill for almost 6 months and remembers that she lost a lot of weight and at that time also had a persistent cough with haemoptysis. She was treated by a GP for 18 months and was told that she possibly had tuberculosis. She is mostly constipated and moves her bowels two or three times a week. Her stools are otherwise normal with no mucus or blood. Recently, she has also noticed that she has lost some weight. On further questioning, she admits to having a mild fever but this has not been recorded.

What would your differential diagnosis include before examining the patient?

This woman belongs to a low socioeconomic class and, almost certainly, had tuberculosis at the age of 14, which was treated by her GP. Putting this important historical fact into perspective, her current abdominal pain could be due to abdominal tuberculosis. Mild fever and weight loss, although not documented, would also favour tuberculosis. Other than this diagnosis, she could be suffering from a peptic ulcer, renal or biliary colic, pancreatitis or an intra-abdominal lymphoma. Multiple worm infestation is also a possibility. Crohn's disease is a possibility but the history strongly favours TB.

Examination

On examination, it is apparent that the patient has lost some weight. She is pale. There is no icterus and a few insignificant small lymph nodes are palpable in the cervical region. Chest examination is normal but on abdominal examination there is a palpable mass in the right iliac fossa. The rest of the examination is normal, as is digital examination of the rectum.

Has examination narrowed down your differential diagnosis?

The mass in her right iliac fossa would fit well with the initial probable diagnosis of tuberculosis; however, this needs further evaluation before it is confirmed. There is nothing on examination that points to renal or gallbladder pathology. Crohn's, lymphoma and chronic pancreatitis have still to be excluded.

Further investigations

The patient's haemoglobin is 100 g/L (10 g/dL). White blood cell and platelet counts are normal. The erythrocyte sedimentation rate (ESR) is 66 mm/h. A Mantoux test is positive using 5 tuberculin units. Enzyme-linked immunosorbent assay (ELISA) for *Entamoeba histolytica* is negative. Chest X-ray and stool examinations are normal, ultrasound of the abdomen revealed omental thickening, para-aortic and mesenteric lymphadenopathy. CT scan of the abdomen confirmed the ultrasound findings and also showed stricturing of the terminal ileum (Fig. 58.1). A barium follow-through examination shows evidence of narrowing in the terminal ileum and caecum. Upper gastrointestinal endoscopy is also normal and duodenal biopsies do not show any villous atrophy. Colonoscopy reveals several ulcers in the ascending colon (Fig. 58.2),

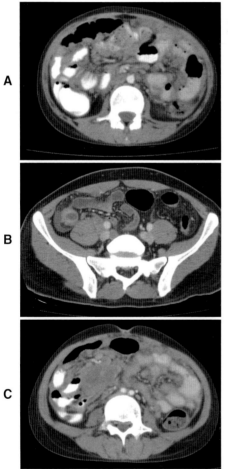

Figure 58.1 Findings at CT. The abdomen shows enlarged lymph nodes, omental thickening and stricturing of the terminal ileum.

A

B

C

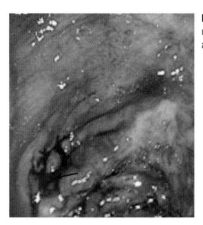

Figure 58.2 Findings at colonoscopy. There is ulceration (arrow) with a surrounding cobblestone appearance.

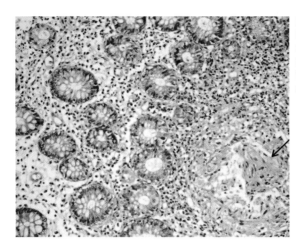

Figure 58.3 Colonic mucosal biopsy. There is a non-caseating granuloma (arrow), suggesting tuberculosis or Crohn's disease.

as well as in the terminal ileum, and biopsies reveal granulomatous inflammation (Fig. 58.3). Stains for acid-fast bacilli and fungi are negative and *Entamoeba histolytica* is not seen. Cultures of the biopsies are negative for acid-fast bacilli.

Does this narrow down your differential diagnosis?

A normal stool examination and the negative ELISA for *E. histolytica* rule out parasitic infestation. The colonic examination and the biopsy reports confirm granulomatous colitis and ileitis; hence the differential diagnosis narrows down to intestinal tuberculosis and Crohn's disease. In South-east Asia, tuberculosis is far more common than Crohn's disease; however, Crohn's disease does exist and should be considered. Unfortunately, it is very difficult to obtain positive cultures for acid-fast bacilli from intestinal biopsies, as abdominal tuberculosis is a paucibacillary disease. If available, polymerase chain reaction (PCR) for myco-bacterial DNA can be performed on tissue biopsies, and this has a higher sensitivity than culture. If in doubt regarding the final diagnosis between tuberculosis and Crohn's disease, then antituberculous treatment should be given before starting steroids for Crohn's disease.

How will you treat this patient?

Given her past history, this patient should be treated with isoniazid, rifampicin, pyrazinamide, ethambutol and streptomycin for a period of 2 months followed by the first four drugs for another month and, thereafter, rifampicin, isoniazid and ethambutol should be continued for a further 5 months (category 11 WHO regimen). The duration of treatment for extrapulmonary tuberculosis is the same as for pulmonary tuberculosis; however, the duration may be extended in individual cases on the basis of clinical evaluation and the results of repeat imaging tests at the end of 8 months. Before starting antituberculosis treatment, liver function tests should be checked and thereafter monitored periodically. Eye examination should be carried out at the start and during treatment with ethambutol. Possible adverse effects of antituberculosis treatment should be thoroughly discussed with the patient before starting treatment. Crohn's disease should be actively considered if her symptoms do not respond to antituberculosis therapy, but even in this situation, the final diagnosis may still be tuberculosis.

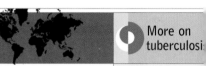

Key points and global issues

More on tuberculosi:

See Chapters 19 and 22 of
Davidson's Principl & **Practice** of
Medicine (21st edr

- Both pulmonary and extrapulmonary tuberculosis are found worldwide.

- With the emergence of human immunodeficiency virus (HIV) infection, tuberculosis has again become one of the world's major health problems.

- In the developing world, tuberculosis still causes major morbidity and significant mortality. The emergence of multidrug resistance makes it important for patients to be investigated properly, not only to confirm the diagnosis but also to assess drug sensitivities.

- In the developing world, amoebomas (localised inflammatory masses due to *E. histolytica*) can be confused with caecal or colonic masses due to tuberculosis. The disease should be treated with anti-amoebic drugs after appropriate investigations.

59

Jaundice during pregnancy

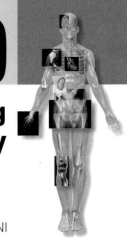

A. L. KAKRANI

Presenting problem

A 20-year-old female working as a farm labourer is admitted to a teaching hospital in India, with a low-grade, intermittent fever, which she has had for 3 days. The onset of fever was followed by yellowish discoloration of her eyes with nausea, vomiting and a decrease in appetite. She is 32 weeks pregnant. This is her second pregnancy; her first was uneventful.

What would your differential diagnosis include before examining the patient?

Several diseases can produce these symptoms during pregnancy. In tropical countries, an acute febrile illness with jaundice should raise the suspicion of acute viral hepatitis (e.g. due to hepatitis viruses A, B, C and E), *falciparum* malaria and leptospirosis. The clinical presentation of hepatitis E is similar to hepatitis A. Both viruses are spread via the faecal–oral route, whereas B and C are transmitted percutaneously. Acute symptoms in hepatitis C virus infection are usually trivial and there is no clue to suggest acute hepatitis B virus infection in this patient. The prodromal symptoms of acute viral hepatitis are systemic and variable. Constitutional symptoms include anorexia, nausea, vomiting, fatigue, malaise, myalgia, headache, photophobia, cough and coryza-like symptoms. These usually precede the onset of jaundice by 1–2 weeks. Fever is usually low-grade. The gastrointestinal symptoms are frequently associated with changes in taste and olfaction. Dark-coloured urine and clay-coloured stools may occur about 1–5 days prior to the onset of clinical jaundice. In *falciparum* malaria, jaundice is common due to haemolysis and hepatic dysfunction, and anaemia develops rapidly. Hypoglycaemia can occur in malaria. Leptospirosis presents with fever, haemorrhages, jaundice and hepatic and renal dysfunction; conjunctival hyperaemia frequently occurs.

Pregnancy-associated liver diseases should also be considered. Intrahepatic cholestasis of pregnancy usually occurs in the 3rd trimester of pregnancy. The condition is characterised by itching and liver function tests (LFTs) suggesting cholestasis; however, the bilirubin may be normal and the liver biochemistry may be hepatic. Acute fatty liver of pregnancy is more common in twin and first pregnancies. Clinical manifestations occur between 31 and 38 weeks of pregnancy, with vomiting and abdominal pain followed by jaundice. Lactic acidosis, coagulopathy, encephalopathy and renal failure may occur in severe cases. These patients have a high serum uric acid and no haemolysis. The HELP (*H*aemolysis, *E*levated *L*iver enzymes and low *P*latelets) syndrome is a variant of pre-eclampsia. The liver disease is associated with hypertension, proteinuria and fluid retention; hepatic infarction and rupture can occur. Gallstone disease with common bile duct (CBD) obstruction also requires consideration, as gallstones are more common during pregnancy and a stone might move into the common bile duct causing biliary colic and cholestatic jaundice.

 ## Examination

On examination, the patient is conscious and alert. She is febrile and has moderate icterus and mild pallor. Her blood pressure is 120/84 mmHg. The uterus is palpable and fetal movements are normal. The liver and spleen are not palpable. No scratch marks are seen on the skin. The patient does not have conjunctival hyperaemia or haemorrhages.

Has examination narrowed down your differential diagnosis?

Acute viral hepatitis and pregnancy-associated liver disease still remain in the differential diagnosis. Infectious causes such as *falciparum* malaria and leptospirosis seem less likely.

Investigations

The results of initial investigations are provided in Box 59.1.

Has the diagnosis been clinched?

A hepatic pattern of LFTs suggests acute viral hepatitis. It is now certain that the hepatitis is due to hepatitis E virus (HEV).

About 24 h after admission, the patient becomes irritable and drowsy. The jaundice deepens and the area of hepatic dullness becomes grossly reduced (less than two percussion spaces). She develops a flapping tremor. Abdominal ultrasound examination performed at this time shows a reduction in hepatic size and increased echogenicity. A computed tomogram (CT) of the brain suggests the presence of cerebral oedema.

HEV normally causes a self-limiting acute hepatitis like hepatitis A and does not lead to chronic disease. However, it differs from hepatitis A because infection during

---

BOX 59.1

Initial investigations

Haemoglobin	90 g/L (9 g/dL)
WCC	10.5×10^9/L (10^3/mm^3)
Differential count	
Neutrophils	70%
Lymphocytes	28%
Eosinophils	2%
Bilirubin	
Total	136 µmol/L (8 mg/dL)
Direct	88.4 µmol/L (5.2 mg/dL)
ALT	2400 U/L
AST	2000 U/L
Alkaline phosphatase	200 U/L
Uric acid	256 mmol/L (4.3 mg/dL)
HbsAg	Negative
Anti-HBc	Negative
IgM-HAV	Negative
IgM-HEV	Positive
Anti-HCV	Negative
Serum HEV RNA	Positive

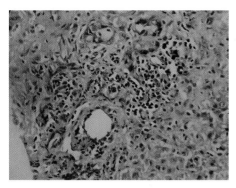

Figure 59.1 Liver necropsy in acute viral hepatitis due to HEV, showing the portal triad with heavy neutrophilic infiltrate and ballooning of hepatocytes in places.

pregnancy can lead to acute liver failure; a mortality of up to 20% is recorded in various studies. In view of the rapid deterioration in the patient's condition, with diminishing consciousness and reduction in liver size, it is clear that she has developed fulminant hepatic failure.

How will you treat this patient?

She is given a bowel washout. A nasogastric tube is inserted and she is given lactulose, 60 mL as a starting dose and later 30 mL 6-hourly, along with vancomycin 250 mL 6-hourly (preferred to neomycin and metronidazole) due to her pregnancy. She is transferred to the intensive care unit and requires intubation, ventilation and inotropic support. Nutrition is provided by a low-protein formulation via the nasogastric tube. Liver transplantation, although ideal in this setting, is not possible in the treating hospital. She continues to pursue a downhill course and dies on the 6th day of hospitalisation. Liver necropsy is performed and the histopathology can be seen in Figure 59.1.

Key points and global issues

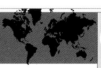

More on viral hepatitis and pregnancy-associated liver disease?

See Chapter 23 of **Davidson's Principles & Practice** of **Medicine (21st edn)**

- HEV infection spreads by the faecal–oral route and is commonly seen in regions with over-crowding and poor sanitation.
- The disease occurs primarily in India, Asia, Africa and Central America. In Europe and USA, infection is usually seen in travellers to an endemic area.
- In developing countries a febrile illness with jaundice should raise the suspicion of acute viral hepatitis due to A and E viruses, *falciparum* malaria and leptospirosis.
- Yellow fever should also be considered in the differential diagnosis in sub-Saharan Africa.
- Large epidemics of hepatitis E can occur after contamination of water supplies from monsoon flooding or contamination of drinking water supply lines with sewage. The disease usually occurs in young adults who are immune to hepatitis A virus (HAV).
- For reasons largely unknown, HEV infection in pregnant females is associated with a poorer outcome, and the risk of developing fulminant hepatic failure is high.
- Presently, there is no commercially available vaccine for the disease.

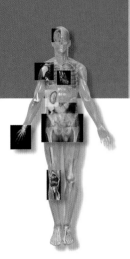

60

Acute hepatitis

C. L. LAI

Presenting problem

A 55-year-old Caucasian businessman is admitted with increasing mental dullness over the preceding 2 days. He has had severe anorexia and nausea, mild diarrhoea and a low-grade fever associated with right upper abdominal discomfort for 2 weeks. For the last 10 days, he has been aware of a gradual darkening of his urine. His wife has noticed progressive yellow discoloration of his skin and sclera. He is a social drinker. He went to Shanghai for a trade conference 6 weeks ago. There is no history of drug-taking.

What would your differential diagnosis include before examining the patient?

The severe prodromal symptoms, followed by jaundice, are typical of acute hepatitis, irrespective of aetiology. The development of mental dullness 2 weeks after the onset of the symptoms of acute hepatitis should alert the physician to the possible complication of acute hepatic failure. The classification of acute liver failure is based on the interval between the development of jaundice and hepatic encephalopathy; <7 days is defined as 'hyper-acute', between 8 and 28 days as 'acute', and between 29 days and 12 weeks as 'subacute'. Our patient falls into the 'acute' category.

The causes of acute hepatitis associated with acute hepatic failure are listed in Box 60.1.

The travel history to Shanghai would indicate a definite risk for acute hepatitis A, Asian countries being endemic for this virus. The other diagnoses are easily excluded. Sexual exposure to hepatitis B is possible, but the short incubation period of 4 weeks makes it highly unlikely. A negative drug history rules out drug-induced hepatitis. Wilson's disease presenting with fulminant hepatitis usually occurs in childhood or adolescence. Autoimmune hepatitis is much more common in women. The patient is not immunocompromised.

BOX 60.1

Common causes of acute hepatitis associated with acute hepatic failure

- Viral hepatitis A–E* (the most common cause globally)
- Drugs (paracetamol overdose being the most common cause in Western countries)
- Fulminant Wilson's disease
- Autoimmune hepatitis
- Pregnancy (including hepatitis E infection)
- Other viruses (mostly in immunocompromised patients): cytomegalovirus, herpes simplex, Epstein–Barr virus
- Other rare causes: extensive malignancy of the liver

*Acute hepatitis C is the least likely to give rise to acute hepatic failure.

Examination

The patient is deeply jaundiced, drowsy and apathetic, though arousable. He has fetor hepaticus and a flapping tremor. His liver is normal in size. A spleen tip is palpable.

Has examination narrowed down your differential diagnosis?

Fetor hepaticus and a flapping tremor are indicative of hepatic encephalopathy, confirming the development of acute hepatic failure as a complication of acute hepatitis. The clinical grading for his encephalopathy is grade 2 out of 4. However, as expected, physical examination does not help in identifying the cause of the acute hepatitis. Analysis of blood samples is required for this. The mild splenomegaly is a common finding in acute hepatitis.

Investigations

The patient's liver function tests are as follows: bilirubin 330 μmol/L (19 mg/dL); alanine aminotransferase (ALT) 5500 U/L; aspartate aminotransferase (AST) 4700 U/L; albumin 37 g/L (3.7 g/dL). Alkaline phosphatase and γ-glutamyl transferase (GGT) are normal. Prothrombin time is prolonged to 70 s. Arterial ammonia is raised to five times above the normal range. His renal function tests and blood glucose level are normal.

IgM anti-hepatitis A virus (anti-HAV) is positive. He is negative for other viral hepatitis markers and antinuclear antibody. He has a normal serum copper and caeruloplasmin.

Has the diagnosis been clinched?

The patient is suffering from acute fulminant viral hepatitis A, complicated by acute hepatic failure. This complication is uncommon, occurring in 0.1% of patients, but the incidence becomes higher with increasing age of infection. ALT and AST levels are of little prognostic value for acute hepatitis, whereas the plasma bilirubin and the prothrombin time reflect the severity of the liver damage. The prothrombin time is dependent on factors V and VII, both of which have short half-lives of <24 h. The prothrombin time is therefore a very reliable prognostic index of the course of the acute hepatic failure, and should be monitored on a daily or twice-daily basis. Arterial ammonia is less sensitive than the prothrombin time as an index of liver failure, but can also be used to monitor the course of the disease.

How will you treat this patient?

The patient should be monitored in the intensive care unit for the development of further complications. If there is any evidence of progressive mental deterioration, intracranial pressure monitoring should be instituted, since cerebral oedema is a known and dreaded complication of acute hepatic failure. Hypoglycaemia is also a common complication. The blood glucose level should be monitored at 2-hourly intervals. Interestingly, cerebral oedema and hypoglycaemia, though common in acute liver failure, are much less likely to develop with liver failure in chronic liver disease such as cirrhosis of the liver.

Renal function and urine output should also be closely monitored for the development of the hepatorenal syndrome. If facilities are available, the surgeons should be alerted early for the consideration of liver transplantation. Patients with poor prognostic criteria (Box 60.2) have ≥90% mortality and should receive liver transplantation at the earliest opportunity, since further clinical deterioration may cause irreversible cerebral oedema as well as increasing the risk of transplantation. This patient has four of the five poor prognostic criteria listed in Box 60.2. Liver transplantation is definitely indicated. The histology of the explanted liver is shown in Figure 60.1.

BOX 60.2

Poor prognostic criteria in acute hepatic failure

Non-paracetamol causes

- Prothrombin time >100 s

  or

- Three of the following five criteria:

  Age <10 or >40 years.

  Time from jaundice to encephalopathy >7 days

  Bilirubin >300 μmol/L (17.6 mg/dL)

  Prothrombin time >50 s.

  Non-viral hepatitis causes

  or

- Factor V level <15% *and* grade 3 or 4 encephalopathy: less commonly used criteria

Paracetamol overdose

- pH <7.3 24 h after the ingestion of paracetamol

  or

- Serum creatinine

  >300 μmol/L (3.38 mg/dL) *and* prothrombin time >100 s *and* grade 3 or 4 encephalopathy

---

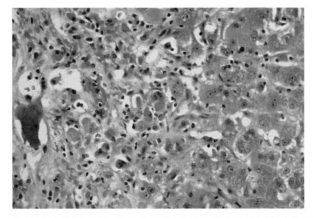

Figure 60.1 The hepatitic changes are predominantly periportal, with inflammatory infiltrate consisting of plasma cells and lymphocytes. Periportal parenchymal necrosis is striking (H&E ×40).

Key points and global issues

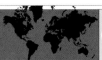

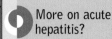
More on acute hepatitis?

See Chapter 23 of
Davidson's Principles
& **Practice** of
Medicine (21st edn)

- In considering the aetiology of acute hepatitis, both the travel history and the drug history are important with the increasing ease of travelling to 'exotic' places and buying of proprietary medicine.

- For all patients admitted with acute hepatitis (or acute exacerbation of chronic hepatitis) of whatever aetiology, it is essential to monitor the disease progression with frequent testing of the prothrombin time to enable timely consideration of liver transplantation.

- The prevalence of hepatitis A is high in Africa, Russia and Central America, intermediate in Asia, and low in North America, Western Europe and Australia.

- Travellers from countries of low endemicity to those of high or intermediate endemicity are at risk of infection and should receive hepatitis A vaccination as prophylaxis.

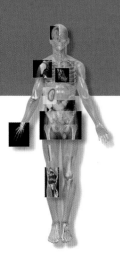

61

Chronic liver disease

J. COLLIER

Presenting problem

A 50-year-old man is referred to the medical admissions unit with a 4-week history of increasing abdominal distension and anorexia, followed by 2 weeks of jaundice. There has been no change in bowel habit or vomiting and he denies any weight loss. His wife has noticed him to be confused over the last 24 h. He takes no regular medication. He has drunk 8 pints of beer a day for about 10 years, but stopped 10 days ago when he started to feel unwell. The GP has checked some blood tests, which are shown in Box 61.1.

What would your differential diagnosis include before examining the patient?

Abdominal distension in the absence of symptoms of bowel obstruction suggests either an abdominal mass or ascites, of which the most common causes in a previously fit man are cirrhosis and malignancy. Cirrhosis is usually asymptomatic until portal hypertension develops and synthetic liver function worsens; then symptoms of chronic liver failure, such as ascites, appear quite quickly.

BOX 61.1

Initial investigations

Sodium	130 mmol/L (mEq/L)
Potassium	3.8 mmol/L (mEq/L)
Urea	0.9 mmol/L (2.56 mg/dL)
Creatinine	89 μmol/L (1.39 mg/dL)
Albumin	25 g/L (2.5 g/dL)
Bilirubin	90 μmol/L (5.29 mg/dL)
Alkaline phosphatase	400 U/L
ALT	150 U/L
AST	180 U/L
Haemoglobin	110 g/d (11 g/dL)
WCC	8×10^9/L (10^3/mm^3)
Platelets	70×10^9/L (10^3/mm^3)
Prothrombin time	20 s

The presence of jaundice indicates either liver disease, which may be acute or chronic, or obstruction to the biliary tree, which is usually due to malignancy.

Acute liver disease can be excluded, as this is not associated with ascites. However, the presence of jaundice with ascites does not differentiate carcinoma of the head of the pancreas with peritoneal metastases from chronic liver failure.

Investigations in this case do narrow down the differential diagnosis, as the presence of pancytopenia suggests chronic liver disease. Platelets are often disproportionately lower than the rest of the blood count in cirrhosis due to a combination of splenomegaly and reduced hepatic thrombopoietic production. The prolonged prothrombin time and low albumin can be seen in both chronic liver failure and biliary obstruction, but in the latter the prolonged clotting is reversible with vitamin K.

It is common for individuals to stop drinking about 2 weeks before jaundice develops in alcoholic liver disease because they feel so unwell; alcohol detoxification will not, therefore, be needed in this man.

Examination

The patient has 5–6 spider naevi on his upper chest wall. He has a 6 cm firm, non-tender palpable liver. Ascites is confirmed on abdominal examination. Asterixis (flapping tremor) is demonstrated.

Does this narrow down your differential diagnosis?

The finding of stigmata of chronic liver disease makes the diagnosis of cirrhosis most likely. However, it is important to remember that not everyone with decompensated chronic liver disease will have these cutaneous stigmata. A large liver is also frequently seen in individuals with cirrhosis due to alcohol.

Alcohol excess increases the risk of progression to cirrhosis in chronic liver disease due to other causes such as chronic viral infection, hepatitis B and C and haemochromatosis. These conditions must also be excluded before concluding that the liver disease is due to alcohol alone.

Jaundice in an alcoholic with cirrhosis may either reflect end-stage liver disease or be due to a superimposed alcoholic hepatitis. The latter can only be confirmed histologically, but in practice, it is usually assumed that alcoholic hepatitis is present if there is jaundice.

The patient's confusion in the presence of a hepatic flap is likely to be due to hepatic encephalopathy. Other causes of confusion in an alcoholic that need to be excluded are subdural haematomas, occurring after a head injury, when there may be focal neurological signs present. Wernicke's encephalopathy can be difficult to exclude, but frequently coexists with nystagmus and is often treated empirically.

Further investigations

Ultrasound shows that the liver is enlarged and has a coarse texture; the spleen is also enlarged but there is no bile duct dilatation. No focal lesions are seen within the liver and the main portal vein is patent. The results of the ascitic tap are shown in Box 61.2 and in Figure 61.1.

BOX 61.2

Ascitic tap

Albumin	4 g/L (0.4 g/dL)
WCC	600×10^9/L (10^3/mm^3)
Neutrophils	90%

The chronic liver disease screen tests indicate that the patient is hepatitis C antibody-positive. It is only on more detailed questioning that he is found to have used intravenous drugs once when he was aged 20.

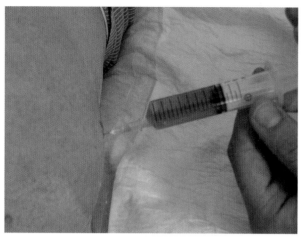

Figure 61.1 Clear ascitic fluid being aspirated at the time of an ascitic tap with a 10 mL syringe.

Does this narrow down your differential diagnosis?

Ultrasound is very good at excluding an obstructive cause for jaundice. A classically irregular cirrhotic liver is not always seen on ultrasound but the liver texture is usually abnormal, as in this case. Splenomegaly suggests portal hypertension and would not be expected with the other causes of ascites. A transudative ascites is also consistent with cirrhosis. This has been complicated by spontaneous bacterial peritonitis, as shown by the elevated ascitic white cell count.

How will you treat this patient?

Spontaneous bacterial peritonitis carries a high mortality. Either intravenous cephalosporins or oral quinolones are effective and should be given while awaiting bacterial culture results. Secondary prophylaxis is then needed to reduce the risk of further infections. Spironolactone, which blocks an activated renin–angiotensin system, should also be started. However, this should be stopped if any evidence of intravascular dehydration occurs, indicated by a rising urea or creatinine or by the serum sodium falling to <125 mmol/L, as this can exacerbate encephalopathy.

The mild hepatic encephalopathy will probably improve with treatment of the infection, but lactulose should also be given orally. Constipation is a common precipitant of hepatic encephalopathy, and if lactulose cannot be given orally because of reduced conscious level, then phosphate enemas are an alternative.

An upper gastrointestinal endoscopy will be needed to look for varices, even though there is no history of bleeding, as β-blocker prophylaxis will reduce the risk of bleeding from asymptomatic large varices.

Long-term abstinence from alcohol is crucial; it will prevent progression of liver disease in most cases and may lead to improvement in liver function over the next 6 months. Treatment of the patient's hepatitis C will need to be considered when his liver function has improved.

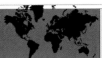

Key points and global issues

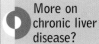

More on chronic liver disease?

See Chapter 23 of **Davidson's Principles & Practice** of **Medicine (21st edn)**

- Chronic hepatitis B and hepatitis C infection remains the most common cause of chronic liver failure worldwide.

- Non-cirrhotic portal hypertension is common in Africa and in other areas where schistosomiasis is prevalent. It usually presents with variceal bleeding. Liver function is preserved and ascites does not occur.

- Tuberculosis is a common cause of ascites in endemic areas.

- Patients with chronic Budd–Chiari syndrome (thrombosis of the large hepatic veins and sometimes the inferior vena cava) may present with features of chronic liver disease and portal hypertension.

- Veno-occlusive disease (occlusion of central hepatic veins) has similar clinical features to Budd–Chiari syndrome. It may result from exposure to pyrrolizidine alkaloids in *Senecio* and *Heliotropium* plants, which are used to make teas, and following administration of cytotoxic drugs and hepatic irradiation.

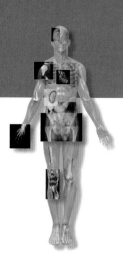

62

Liver abscess

J. A. KER

Presenting problem

A 45-year-old man, married with two children, complains of loss of appetite with subsequent weight loss, nausea and vomiting for 3 weeks. A few days after the nausea and vomiting started, he developed a constant abdominal pain, localised to the right hypochondrium. He is currently unemployed and has not travelled outside his home city of Pretoria, South Africa.

He has never been ill before and does not suffer from any chronic medical problems. He takes alcohol sparingly and only on special occasions. He is a non-smoker. On specific enquiry, he has no other symptoms. A family history is negative for any major illnesses.

What would your differential diagnosis include before examining the patient?

The interpretation of nausea, vomiting and abdominal pain remains a challenging exercise. Great judgement is required, but a meticulously executed history and physical examination will go a long way in assisting the correct approach to such a complaint. An acute surgical abdomen must be excluded. The constant right hypochondrial pain must put pathology of the liver or gallbladder high on the list of causes of this man's symptoms.

Examination

The patient is fully alert, but generally looks ill with signs of weight loss. Oral temperature is 37.5°C. No jaundice, cyanosis or significant pallor is noted and he has no lymphadenopathy. His pulse is 80/min and blood pressure is 160/90 mmHg.

His abdomen is generally tender but there is no obvious rebound tenderness. The liver is tender on palpation and the left lobe is palpable 2 cm below the xiphisternum. The liver span is 15 cm. There is no splenomegaly and no fluid thrill. Bowel sounds and digital rectal examination are normal. No abnormalities are noted in the remainder of the physical examination. Routine urine dipstick testing is normal, with no bilirubin detected.

Has examination narrowed down your differential diagnosis?

The patient does not have an acute surgical abdomen. The examination points to liver pathology and further investigations should focus on this organ. The tender rather than painful abdomen and the absence of fever make cholecystitis unlikely.

BOX 62.1

Initial investigations

Haemoglobin	89 g/L (8.9 g/dL)
MCV	88.1 fL
Platelets	553×10⁹/L (10³/mm³)
WCC	11.1×10⁹/L (10³/mm³)
Neutrophils	90%
Blood smear	Anisocytosis, microcytes, ovalocytes, rouleaux formation and autoagglutination of the red cells
U&E	Normal
Bilirubin	14 μmol/L (0.82 mg/dL)
ALT	34 U/L
Alkaline phosphatase	115 U/L
GGT	103 U/L
Albumin	31 g/L (3.1 g/dL)
Total protein	103 g/L (10.3 g/dL)
Protein electrophoresis	Polyclonal elevation of IgG and IgA

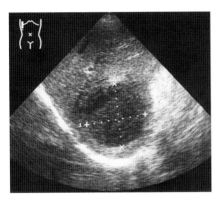

Figure 62.1 Ultrasound of the right lobe of the liver showing an echogenic mass measuring 8×8 cm.

Further basic investigations, particularly liver function tests, are needed. The results are listed in Box 62.1.

Has the diagnosis been clinched?

Not yet. This 45-year-old man has been sick for 3 weeks with nausea, vomiting and abdominal pain, and he has an enlarged tender liver. Blood tests reveal an anaemia of chronic disease and a polyclonal gammopathy. The liver function pattern could fit in with a space-occupying lesion and the most appropriate test at this stage would be an ultrasound scan of the liver. A human immunodeficiency virus (HIV) test should also be carried out to exclude this common cause of polyclonal gammopathy in sub-Saharan Africa.

Further investigations

Liver ultrasonography reveals a large mass (8 cm diameter) in the right lobe of the liver due to either a tumour or an abscess (Fig. 62.1). The HIV test is non-reactive. The most likely diagnosis is a liver abscess (short history, anaemia of chronic disease, elevated white cell count and increased absolute neutrophil count) and in sub-Saharan Africa this is most likely to be due to an amoebic infection.

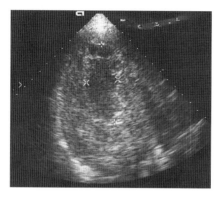

Figure 62.2 Repeat ultrasound examination 16 days later, following therapy with metronidazole. The mass has decreased in size and now measures 3×7 cm.

How will you treat this patient?

Although the diagnosis has not yet been confirmed, time is of the essence and the patient should be started straight away on metronidazole 800 mg per mouth 8-hourly for 10 days. A luminal agent, such as diloxanide furoate 500 mg per mouth 8-hourly for 10 days, should be given to eliminate intestinal colonisation to all patients following completion of metronidazole therapy. Meanwhile, an α-fetoprotein level is checked and found to be in the normal range, making a hepatocellular carcinoma unlikely. Amoebic serology is performed: amoeba haemagglutination test 2.5 ($n<1.0$) with amoeba fluorescent antibody IgG and IgM positive. This confirms recent amoebic infection.

The patient responds to treatment in a dramatic way (he starts eating and his nausea, pain and fever settle), and it is decided that aspiration of the liver abscess is not necessary. The anaemia slowly resolves, as does the polyclonal gammopathy. A repeat ultrasound examination of the mass 16 days later shows significant reduction in the dimensions of the abscess (Fig. 62.2). It is important to note that diarrhoea is often absent in amoebic liver abscess and that the diagnosis can be difficult.

Key points and global issues

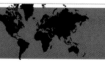

 More on amoebic liv abscess?

See Chapter 13 of
Davidson's Principl
& **Practice** of
Medicine (21st ed▶

- Amoebiasis is an important public health problem and is the second leading cause of death from parasitic diseases worldwide.

- Travellers to endemic areas are at high risk of developing this disease, which can present months to years after travel. Therefore, a careful travel history is essential.

- Amoebic liver abscess is the most common extra-intestinal manifestation of disease. Amoebic liver abscess most commonly affects males between the ages of 18 and 50.

- Amoebic liver abscess usually presents with acute symptoms (<10 days) but a chronic presentation, as with the present case, can occur.

- In some Mexican populations, susceptibility to amoebic liver abscess is associated with HLA-DR3 and complotype SC01.

- At time of writing, no vaccine is available for humans.

63

Malnutrition

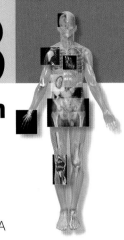

B. S. RAMAKRISHNA

Presenting problem

A 45-year-old man presents to hospital with a history of progressive anorexia, weakness and weight loss for the last 6 months. He complains of difficulty in swallowing solids. He is of extremely poor socioeconomic status and is uneducated, unmarried, unemployed and a chronic alcoholic. When found, the patient was lying curled up and apathetic and had to be lifted and carried as he was unable to stand or walk. He has received no prior therapy.

What would your differential diagnosis include before examining this patient?

Extreme malnutrition in an adult may be secondary to inadequate dietary intake (starvation-related malnutrition) or may be related to disease and inflammation. Starvation-related malnutrition occurs in individuals living in areas of chronic famine, in patients with anorexia nervosa and in individuals who resort to fasting as a means of public protest. It also occurs in alcoholics, who live without families or social support systems, and in those with psychiatric illness. Starvation-related malnutrition results in loss of body fat in the first instance and then loss of lean body mass. Lean body mass may decrease up to 40% over a few months without nutritional intervention. The other major class of malnutrition, disease-related malnutrition (DRM), may occur acutely or chronically (Box 63.1). Acute DRM occurs in relation to conditions such as major infection, burns, trauma and head injury. Chronic DRM occurs in conditions such as internal malignancy (e.g. carcinoma of the pancreas), chronic inflammatory bowel disease, non-gastrointestinal inflammatory conditions such as rheumatoid arthritis, and organ failure. Human immunodeficiency virus (HIV) infection, particularly with super-added opportunistic infection, such as tuberculosis, and those with other chronic gastrointestinal disorders, including idiopathic tropical malabsorption (tropical sprue), are also likely to lead to severe disease-related malnutrition in adults.

Examination and initial investigations

Physical examination reveals generalised cachexia and mild pallor (Fig. 63.1). Pulse rate is 70/min and blood pressure in the supine position is 86/60 mmHg. The patient weighs 30 kg and his height is approximately 165 cm, giving a body mass index of 11.0 kg/m^2. His cheeks and temples are hollow, reflecting loss of fat and muscle, respectively. There is generalised loss of subcutaneous fat and of muscle mass – triceps skinfold thickness is 4 mm and mid-upper arm circumference is 14 cm. His skin is dry and scaly and body hair is sparse. There is mild pitting oedema at the ankles. The abdomen is scaphoid; there are no visible bowel loops or peristalsis, no mass on palpation and bowel

BOX 63.1

Causes of adult malnutrition

Starvation-related malnutrition	Famine and disaster situations
	Hunger strikes
	Anorexia nervosa
	Alcoholism
	Psychosis
	Cerebrovascular disease interfering with deglutition
	Gastrointestinal disorders resulting in poor food intake, e.g. oesophageal stricture, chronic intestinal pseudo-obstruction
Acute disease-related malnutrition	Sepsis
	Surgery
	Burns
	Trauma
	Closed head injury
Chronic disease-related malnutrition	Tuberculosis
	HIV infection
	Internal malignancy
	Malabsorption syndromes
	Inflammatory bowel disease

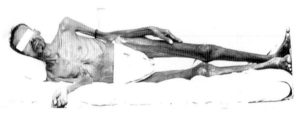

Figure 63.1 The patient was extremely cachectic at presentation.

sounds are normal. Examination of the cardiovascular and respiratory systems is normal. The patient is confused and not oriented in time or place. Examination of the central nervous system reveals normal pupillary reactions to light and accommodation; there is a generalised decrease in muscle tone; deep tendon reflexes are sluggish and plantar reflexes equivocal. Sensation to painful stimuli is preserved. The results of initial investigations are shown in Box 63.2.

Has examination narrowed down your clinical diagnosis?

The circumstances in which this patient was found would suggest a fairly straight-forward diagnosis of starvation-related malnutrition due to alcoholism. Clinical examination and initial investigations did not reveal any pointers to an underlying disease that would give rise to malnutrition. Nevertheless, it is necessary to be alert to predisposing factors, other than alcoholism and social factors that could contribute to poor food intake and malnutrition, even if the circumstantial evidence for the diagnosis in this patient is considerable. Major possibilities among these include concurrent infections, especially tuberculosis and HIV infection.

Further investigations

Further evaluation included investigation of the upper gastrointestinal tract (endoscopy) to exclude oesophageal and gastric malignancy and an abdominal ultrasound to exclude chronic liver disease, both of which were normal. Thyroid function tests and a random serum cortisol (to exclude Addison's disease) were also normal. A brain CT scan was deemed unnecessary.

BOX 63.2

Initial investigations

Haemoglobin	80 g/L (8.5 g/dL)
WCC	15.5×10^9/L (10^3/mm^3)
Platelets	200×10^9/L (10^3/mm^3)
Urea	10.7 mmol/L (30 mg/dL)
Creatinine	80.0 μmol/L (0.9 mg/dL)
Sodium	130 mmol/L (mEq/L)
Potassium	3.4 mmol/L (mEq/L)
Phosphate	0.97 mmol/L (3.0 mg/dL)
Calcium	1.88 mmol/L (7.5 mg/dL)
Magnesium	0.7 mmol/L (1.7 mg/dL)
Glucose	3.7 mmol/L (66.6 mg/dL)
Albumin	30 g/L (3.0 g/dL)
AST	65 IU/L
ALT	60 IU/L
ALP	110 IU/L
Prothrombin time	13 s
Blood culture	No growth
Stool occult blood	Negative
Stool for parasites	Negative examination, including special stains
Chest X-ray	Tubular heart. Lung fields clear

BOX 63.3

Ingredients of the F-75 and F-100 diets prescribed by the WHO for re-feeding severely malnourished individuals

Ingredient	F-75	F-100
Dried skimmed milk	25 g	80 g
Sugar	70 g	50 g
Cereal flour	35 g	–
Vegetable oil	27 g	60 g
Mineral mix	20 mL	20 mL
Vitamin mix	140 mg	140 mg
Water to make	1000 mL	1000 mL

These tests confirmed that the patient had starvation-related malnutrition not complicated by other significant illness.

How will you treat this patient?

Nutritional support for the severely malnourished patient must be provided with appropriate care to correct the critical nutrient deficiencies. Re-feeding should be gradually increased to the necessary level over a period of days in order to minimise metabolic shifts within the body that could have catastrophic consequences. The World Health Organization recommends initial feeding with the F-75 formula diet and continued feeding with the F-100 formula diet shown in Box 63.3. While this is most used in children with malnutrition and in adults in disaster and famine situations, the diet may be adapted for use in most patients with severe malnutrition.

Isotonic versions of F-75, with maltodextrins replacing the cereal flour, are available commercially. The mineral mix supplies potassium, magnesium and other essential minerals. Iron is withheld during the initial re-feeding phase. Hypokalaemia affects cardiac function and gastric emptying and magnesium deficiency potentiates hypokalaemia. Electrolyte and mineral requirements are in the range of 2–4 mmol (mEq)/kg per day for potassium, 0.3–0.6 mmol (mEq)/kg per day for phosphate and 0.4 mmol/kg per day for magnesium. Feeding should be given frequently in small amounts in order to avoid overloading the intestine, liver and kidneys, and may be commenced initially through a nasogastric tube. The requirement is in the range of 40 kcal/kg per day or 2.2 mL/kg per h. However, patients who have starved for considerable periods of time are at risk from the re-feeding syndrome and in such cases it is preferable to start with 10 kcal/g per day and build up to 40 kcal/kg per day over a period of 4–7 days. The re-feeding syndrome consists of cardiac and neurological abnormalities in severely malnourished patients who are fed after long periods of starvation. It is caused by severe electrolyte and fluid shifts associated with metabolic abnormalities. Hypophosphataemia is the key abnormality and may be accompanied by thiamine deficiency, hypokalaemia, hypomagnesaemia and hypoglycaemia. Hypocalcaemia may be corrected if present.

Vitamin A should be given in large doses (200 000 units orally) on the first day, and continued for the next 2 days if the patient has evidence of night blindness, Bitot's spots or corneal xerosis. It may be administered intramuscularly if the patient shows signs of infection. Vitamins of the B group are usually present in the mineral mix. Folic acid and thiamine will need to be supplemented and vitamin B12 deficiency may need to be addressed if present. Thiamine deficiency is a key feature of starvation malnutrition and can lead to neuropsychiatric manifestations including Korsakoff's syndrome (retrograde and anterograde amnesia and confabulation) and Wernicke's encephalopathy (ocular abnormalities, ataxia, confusional state, hypothermia and coma). Thiamine needs to be administered in doses of 200–300 mg/day orally. Electrolyte (potassium, magnesium, calcium and phosphate) levels should be checked daily in the first week and once every 2 or 3 days thereafter. In addition, the patient will need to receive systemic antibiotics in the first week. Hypothermia and hypoglycaemia may occur and need to be managed appropriately. Feeding milk to severely malnourished adults can result in abdominal fullness and diarrhoea as a result of lactose intolerance. In such cases, milk can be partially or completely replaced by yoghurt.

When the patient becomes hungry, it is time to move on to the F-100 formula and then on to a semi-solid and then a solid diet. This usually happens in about a week, when the F-75 diet can be replaced with equal volumes of F-100 diet. The patient may be discharged from hospital when he is feeding well and gaining weight. The social circumstances that precipitated his presentation will clearly need to be addressed.

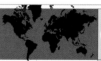

Key points and global issues

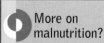

More on malnutrition?

- Severe malnutrition related to starvation occurs on a large scale in settings of famine and disaster.
- Severe malnutrition also occurs sporadically in settings of alcoholism and psychiatric disorders.
- Care must be taken to prevent the re-feeding syndrome during nutritional intervention in these patients.

See Chapter 7 of
**Davidson's Principles
& Practice** of
Medicine (21st edn)

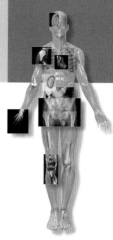

64

Falls in the elderly

M. Y. RAO

Presenting problem

A 75-year-old woman is referred from home complaining of the inability to stand or walk and pain in her left hip, following a fall while getting out of a taxi. On questioning, she says that she has tripped a few times in the recent past without major consequences. She also gives a past history of a stroke at the age of 69, from which she made a complete recovery. There is no history of dizziness or visual disturbance. She is not known to have diabetes, but she has always been frail and was a heavy smoker prior to the stroke. She currently takes aspirin, bendroflumethiazide, ramipril and simvastatin. At 72, she was diagnosed with thyrotoxicosis secondary to a multinodular goitre, following a presentation with atrial fibrillation. This was successfully treated with radio-iodine therapy and she reverted spontaneously to sinus rhythm. The results of laboratory investigations performed by her GP are detailed in Box 64.1.

What would your differential diagnosis include before examining the patient?

Given the predominance of pain, a soft-tissue or bony injury must be excluded – most notably a fractured neck of femur. The key question to be answered is:

BOX 64.1	
Initial investigations	
Haemoglobin	136 g/L (13.6 g/dL)
WCC	14.2×10⁹/L (10³/mm³)
Differential count	
Neutrophils	82%
Lymphocytes	10%
Eosinophils	6%
Monocytes	2%
PCV	0.42
ESR	50 mm/1st hour
Blood glucose (fasting)	4.44 mmol/L (80 mg/dL)
Urea	3.927 mmol/L (11 mg/dL)
Serum creatinine	45.756 μmol/L (0.6 mg/dL)
Sodium	140 mmol/L (140 mEq/L)
Potassium	3.7 mmol/L (3.7 mEq/L)
TSH	0.3 mU/L

'why did this woman fall?'. It might have been a simple trip, but there is a history of this having happened on more than one occasion. Vision is crucial for safe walking gait, especially in the elderly. In this particular case, nothing is known about her vision and this will be an important starting point in our evaluation. With a previous history of stroke, reduced mobility of the affected leg and impaired proprioception would also increase her risk of falling.

In older people who have fallen, another important question to ask is, 'What drugs does this person take?'. The potential for polypharmacy and multiple drug interactions/side-effects to cause falls in this age group, is enormous. This woman is on two antihypertensive agents. Could she have postural hypotension? It is also important to exclude intercurrent illness. Could she have developed a urinary tract infection or a chest infection that has impaired her walking? There is no history of vertigo. The possibilities are almost endless, but careful examination and simple investigations help us get to a possible diagnosis.

Examination

Examination reveals a frail elderly woman, clinically non-icteric and mildly pale. Her left lower limb appears externally rotated and shortened, with tenderness over the greater trochanter. She does not have peripheral oedema or clinically significant lymphadenopathy. Her blood pressure is 130/80 mmHg, with no postural drop, and her pulse is regular at 90 beats/min. She has no murmurs and chest auscultation is clear. Abbreviated mental test score is 10/10. She does not have a visual field defect, but corrected vision is 6/18 in the right eye and 6/24 in the left; fundal examination reveals bilateral cataracts. There is slight reduction in power in the right arm and leg (4+/5), and careful sensory examination reveals impairment of proprioception in the right foot. There are no distal peripheral vascular deficits in either limb, nor any clinical evidence of thyroid overactivity.

Have examination and initial investigations narrowed down your differential diagnosis?

Clinical examination points to a left fractured neck of femur. There is subtle evidence of a residual deficit from the previous cerebrovascular accident, of which the patient was unaware. This might have contributed to the fall, but it seems unlikely that, on its own, this would have been sufficient to cause it. There

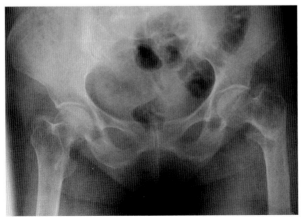

Figure 64.1 X-ray of the hip showing an intertrochanteric fracture of the left femur.

is no postural drop in blood pressure, so on this occasion her medication cannot be blamed. Despite her initial assertion, her vision is not good. She has cataracts and, of course, there may also be an element of age-related macular degeneration. She is clinically and biochemically euthyroid, but her white cell count and erythrocyte sedimentation rate are elevated. Could there be some intercurrent infection?

Further investigations

X-ray of the left hip confirms an intertrochanteric fracture of the left femur (Fig. 64.1). A dual-energy X-ray absorptiometry (DEXA) scan confirms the diagnosis of osteoporosis, with a T-score at the hip of –3.1 and –2.9 in the lumbar vertebrae. A 12-lead electrocardiogram (ECG) and chest X-ray are unremarkable. Urinalysis reveals blood++; protein ++; leucocytes +++ and nitrate +++, and subsequent urine culture grows numerous *Escherichia coli* organisms.

Has the diagnosis been clinched?

Yes. She has a fracture of the left femoral neck. The trauma was relatively trivial and this is in-keeping with it being an insufficiency (osteoporotic) fracture. She has several risk factors for osteoporosis – most notably her postmenopausal status, her previous history of thyrotoxicosis compounded by heavy smoking in the past.

As is often the case in elderly people, the fall was almost certainly multifactorial in nature. The circumstances were crucial; getting out of a car is never easy for older people, who often have back pain or arthritic joints. Add to that, a residual subtle neurological deficit from a previous stroke that will have impaired her joint position sense, poor eyesight and an intercurrent urinary tract infection, we have a veritable *pot pourri* of reasons for her instability and eventual fall. Occam's Razor ('there is usually a unifying diagnosis to explain a person's symptoms') is therefore disproved!

How will you treat this patient?

Diseases with multiple causation need to be tackled with caution with a stress on potentially essential drugs and interventions, starting with the 'life-saving' and then moving on to preventive geriatric strategies. The fractured neck of femur should be treated surgically by closed reduction with internal fixation under spinal block (preferable) or general anaesthesia. If the latter is chosen, the patient will need a good anaesthetist and careful perioperative care. Bisphosphonate therapy and supplemental calcium and vitamin D should be prescribed to reduce the risk of further osteoporotic fractures.

A fractured neck of femur is often a major turning point in an individual's life. It can mark the end of functional independence and may be the start of a general decline in physical (and mental) status. Postoperatively, this woman will need a lot of input from physiotherapists and occupational therapists. A careful assessment of her care needs will be required prior to discharge. Will she be able to return home? If so, will she need aids for bathing and toileting? With regard to her mobility, she will probably need to walk with a stick or walking frame. If her mobility and functional status are poor, she will need support from relatives or 'home helps' as far as shopping and cleaning are concerned; alternatively, she may require placement in sheltered housing or a care home. The implications for this woman are potentially enormous.

With regard to the falls, the urinary tract infection should be treated with appropriate antibiotic therapy. The patient might just need a good pair of glasses to improve her eyesight, but she should be reviewed by an ophthalmologist for consideration of cataract surgery, if her condition following hip replacement makes this appropriate.

Key points and global issues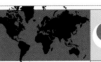

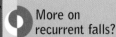 More on recurrent falls?

See Chapter 7 of
Davidson's Principles
& Practice of
Medicine (21st edn)

- Falls are common in the elderly and are usually multifactorial in aetiology, among which limb weakness, dementia and osteoporosis are key factors in determining optimal management.

- One out of three community-dwellers over the age of 65 experience one crippling fall every year.

- Polypharmacy is an increasing problem and is often responsible for falls.

- Osteoporosis prophylaxis should be considered in elderly people, particularly those at high risk, e.g. those with previous insufficiency fractures, premature menopause or a strong family history of osteoporotic fractures.

- Lifestyle modification is an essential component in the management of patients with falls, including patient education and provision of gero-friendly environment.

65

Delirium

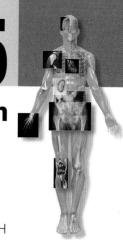

A. M. J. MacLULLICH

Presenting problem

An 86-year-old man is brought to the emergency medical department with a history of acute confusion. He lives with his wife and they have no help from social services. For two nights, the man has been waking up during the night, getting out of bed and wandering in the house, refusing to go back to bed. During the day, he has been intermittently drowsy but at other times he has been restless and agitated. At times, he appears to be seeing people who are not there. His wife states that he has been hot and sweaty over the past day. In the last few months he has been able to go shopping and perform other activities of daily living, but his wife says that he has become more forgetful in the last few months, forgetting what happened earlier in the day, and often repeating himself. He has a past medical history of ischaemic heart disease, hypertension, chronic obstructive pulmonary disease and osteoarthritis. His regular medication is aspirin, enalapril and paracetamol, codeine 30 mg as required and a salbutamol metered dose inhaler to be taken as required. He gave up smoking 10 years ago having smoked 20 cigarettes/day for 60 years, previously. He drinks 20–25 units of alcohol per week.

What would your differential diagnosis include before examining the patient?

The first issue is to determine the diagnosis which best describes the mental status changes. Delirium is characterised by acute onset (hours, days) of deterioration and fluctuation of mental status. The main cognitive change is inattention, where the patient has difficulty in sustaining or focusing attention (Box 65.1). Other acute changes in mental status (such as hallucinations) and also altered arousal (drowsiness, hyperactivity) can occur. Under the broad heading of the term delirium, there are

BOX 65.1

Delirium

- Disturbance of consciousness (i.e. reduced clarity of awareness of the environment) with reduced ability to focus, sustain or shift attention.

- A change in cognition or the development of a perceptual disturbance that is not better accounted for by a pre-existing, established or evolving dementia.

- The disturbance develops over a short period of time (usually hours to days) and tends to fluctuate during the course of the day.

- There is evidence from the history, physical examination or laboratory findings that the disturbance is caused by the direct physiological consequences of a general medical condition.*

Note: studies have shown that in up to 25% of cases of delirium, a clear precipitating cause cannot be determined.

multiple possibilities, as discussed below. Specific aetiologies of delirium are often referred to by specific terms, such as acute hepatic encephalopathy, alcohol withdrawal syndrome, or encephalitis. Dementia is chronic (by definition, the duration should be >6 months), and of insidious onset. The patterns of cognitive deficit seen in dementia are variable, though marked inattention of acute onset is very uncommon as a presenting feature. Depressive illness with psychomotor retardation and late-onset psychotic disorders are the other main diagnoses to consider; again rapid onset and fluctuations in symptoms suggest delirium.

Once a diagnosis of delirium is made, the second issue is to determine the likely precipitating factor(s) and to assess the potential impact of predisposing factors. The differential diagnosis of potential precipitants of delirium is wide, and often more than one is involved. In this case, the history clearly suggests delirium: there is strong evidence from an informant of acute deterioration in mental status. The history also points to several potential precipitating factors, including infection, opioid toxicity and alcohol withdrawal. In terms of predisposing factors, the patient is old, and has a history suggestive of dementia. The alcohol intake is above recommended limits and suggests the possibility of longer-term central nervous system damage. Also, the history of ischaemic heart disease makes cerebrovascular disease, a known risk factor for delirium, more likely.

Examination and initial investigations

The patient is lying back in bed with his eyes closed. He opens his eyes to speech, but closes them again afterwards, and throughout the examination is notably drowsy, only intermittently obeying commands. His peripheries are cool. Temperature is 37.5°C, oxygen saturation is 92% on room air, respiratory rate 20/min, pulse rate 90/min and regular, blood pressure is 102/58 mmHg. There are no stigmata of chronic liver disease, no fine tremor and no asterixis (flapping tremor). Cardiovascular and respiratory examinations are within normal limits. Abdominal examination reveals mild generalised tenderness, which is worse in the right upper quadrant. Neurological examination shows reduced level of alertness, and small pupils. Within the limits of the examination, there are no focal motor or sensory abnormalities. He is able to say his name and address, but is disorientated in place and time. He is unable to count from 20 down to 1 or to state the months of the year in reverse order. He scores 1/3 on immediate recall of three words, and 0/3 on delayed recall. Results of initial investigations are shown in Box 65.2.

Have examination and initial investigations narrowed down your differential diagnosis?

The purpose of the examination is to supplement the information from the history on the possible diagnosis of delirium, and also to give some information on possible precipitating factors. Examination reveals several features of delirium. These include inattention, evident in both his behaviour and on cognitive testing, other cognitive deficits and reduced level of alertness. In terms of precipitating factors, the elevated temperature suggests infection, possibly in the chest or abdomen. The patient is also hypoxic and has a relatively low blood pressure, suggesting reduced CNS perfusion and reduced oxygen supply to the brain as other contributing factors. Finally, the cool peripheries, low blood pressure and pinpoint pupils suggest the possibility of acute renal failure leading to opioid toxicity.

BOX 65.2
Investigations

Sodium	136 mmol/L (mEq/L)
K	5.1 mmol/L (mEq/L)
Urea	11.0 mmol/L (30.8 mg/dL)
Creatinine	164 μmol/L (1.85 mg/dL)
Bicarbonate	20 mmol/L (mEq/L)
Blood glucose	7.6 mmol/L (137 mg/dL)
Ca	2.21 mmol/L (8.9 mg/dL)
Albumin	38 g/L (3.8 g/dL)
Bilirubin	29 μmol/L (1.7 mg/dL)
ALT	55 IU/L
Alkaline phosphatase	164 IU/L
Amylase	280 IU/L
Hb	129 g/L (12.9 g/dL)
MCV	96 fL
WCC	14.3 10^9/L (10^3/mm^3)
Platelets	479 10^9/L (10^3/mm^3)
Arterial blood gases on room air	
H^+	41 9 (pH 7.36)
PaO_2	8.4 kPa (63 mmHg)
$PaCO_2$	5.0 kPa (30 mmHg)
Base excess	−3.3 mmol/L (mEq/L)

Further investigations

The chest X-ray shows expanded lung fields, but no focal areas of con-solidation. Abdominal ultrasound scan shows a thickened gallbladder wall along with multiple gallstones in the gallbladder. A CT head shows generalised atrophy and some white matter periventricular changes.

Does this narrow down the differential diagnosis?

The investigations suggest that this man has acute cholecystitis. This is a likely precipitant of the delirium. However, the investigations also indicate renal failure (acute or chronic, or acute-on-chronic) and type I respiratory failure (duration unknown), both of which could precipitate delirium. The renal failure, combined with the history of use of codeine, suggests the possibility of opioid accumulation and toxicity as a contributing precipitating factor. The generalised cerebral atrophy (Fig. 65.1), though common in this age group and not always linked with chronic cognitive impairment, is a risk factor for delirium.

How will you treat this patient?

Delirium care involves first screening for and treating acute, life-threatening causes of CNS dysfunction. These include hypoxia, hypercapnia, hypoglycaemia and low blood pressure. Along with this, any potential causes of these immediate threats should be screened for, including pneumonia, etc. Here, there are several acute processes which require treatment, including likely cholecystitis, acute renal failure, type I respiratory failure and low blood pressure. Thus, after blood cultures have been taken, the patient should be treated with antibiotics, controlled oxygen (with the appropriate safeguards) and intravenous fluids. The enalapril should be withheld until the renal function has normalised, and the codeine

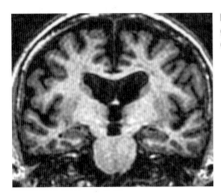
Figure 65.1 Research evidence suggests that generalised cerebral atrophy predisposes to delirium.

should be stopped, and only restarted if necessary. The possibility of alcohol withdrawal should not be overlooked and treatment with parenteral thiamine is required, but at this stage, additional positive evidence (tremor, higher pulse rate) would be required before starting treatment with benzodiazepines.

As well as treating identifiable potential acute precipitants of delirium, it is important to optimise CNS functioning by ensuring good quality oxygenation, hydration and nutrition. Metabolic abnormalities should be treated, constipation treated, and vision and hearing impairments corrected where possible. If appropriate, withdrawing deliriogenic drugs such as amitriptyline would be beneficial, though some drugs require gradual dose reduction rather than sudden withdrawal. Psychological stress should be minimised by providing clear information, repeated frequently. The environment should be kept as stable as possible; involving carers to help with reassurance can be very helpful. Antipsychotic drugs can be used if the patient is extremely agitated and/or distressed and non-pharmacological measures are ineffective. Low dose haloperidol is the first-line drug; low dose lorazepam can be used in patients in whom antipsychotics are contraindicated. Patients with delirium may have undiagnosed dementia and follow-up is essential.

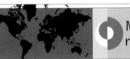
Key points and global issues

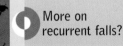
More on recurrent falls?

- Delirium can occur in any age group, although children and older people are more vulnerable.
- Primary CNS causes of delirium, such as TB meningitis, cerebral malaria and encephalitis are common in developing countries.

See Chapters 7 and 26 of **Davidson's Principles & Practice of Medicine (21st edn)**

66

Dizziness

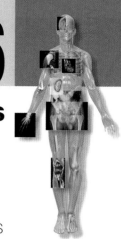

D. DALUS

Presenting problem

A 67-year-old woman is seen in the medical outpatient department, complaining of recurrent dizziness. She has had many episodes in the past, each one lasting for a few hours. When pushed further, the 'dizziness' that she describes has a rotational component consistent with vertigo. For many years she has complained to her family that she has a ringing sensation in her ear and family members have also noticed that she has become increasingly hard of hearing. She is known to have hypertension, but takes her antihypertensive drugs irregularly. Her symptoms are not related to change in posture and she has never blacked out. Her family doctor has checked her blood urea and electrolytes and they are reported as normal.

What would your differential diagnosis include before examining the patient?

Dizziness affects at least 30% of people aged over 65 years. Older people find it difficult to describe the sensation; therefore assessment can be frustrating and time consuming.

The cause of these dizzy spells is frequently multifactorial. An effective way of establishing the cause is to determine which one of the following is the dominant symptom, even if more than one is present. 'Light headedness' suggests presyncope, while the presence of 'vertigo' and 'tinnitus' suggest labyrinthine or brainstem disease; 'unsteadiness' suggests neurological or joint disease.

Labyrinthine disturbances include labyrinthitis, benign paroxysmal positional vertigo (BPPV) and Ménière's disease. Labyrinthitis is the most common cause of vertigo; it usually presents in the third or fourth decade, with vomiting and ataxia, but no tinnitus or deafness; there may be vomiting on walking. It usually has an acute, self-limiting course which clearly is not the case here. BPPV occurs with certain head movements and each attack lasts for seconds; patients often become very distressed and reluctant to move their head, which can in turn produce a tension type of headache. Ménière's disease usually presents first with tinnitus and distorted hearing, and then progresses to paroxysmal attacks of vertigo preceded by a sense of fullness in the ear. Paroxysmal episodes of vertigo and tinnitus with hearing loss in an elderly female suggest Ménière's disease and this must be the presumptive diagnosis in this patient.

There are, however, other possible diagnoses that should be excluded. An acute posterior fossa stroke may also cause vertigo. Brainstem ischaemia can be recognised by the association with other symptoms of brainstem dysfunction such as dysarthria or diplopia. If deafness is present, extra-axial compression of the 8th cranial nerve by an acoustic neuroma should be suspected. Rarely, vertigo originating from the cerebral cortex may be a manifestation of a partial seizure in the temporal lobe. The patient is known to have hypertension, but her compliance in taking anti-hypertensive drugs is poor. Postural hypotension can result from the use of some antihypertensive drugs, notably diuretics and α-blockers. Other drugs producing postural hypotension include antidepressants, phenothiazines, narcotics, barbiturates and calcium channel blockers. Finally, the history here also excludes other underlying causes for the dizziness, such as diabetes mellitus (hypoglycaemia) and Parkinson's disease.

Examination and initial investigations

The patient looks apprehensive. She is obese and has a supine blood pressure of 160/100 mmHg, with no significant postural drop. Neurological examination reveals right sensorineural hearing loss, but there is no nystagmus, nor any other cerebellar or long tract signs. The remainder of the examination is normal.

An ECG is normal and 24-hour ambulatory ECG is deemed unnecessary, in the absence of a history of syncope. A CT scan of the brain is normal. Pure tone audiogram shows low frequency, sensorineural hearing loss (Fig. 66.1).

Have examination and initial investigations narrowed down your differential diagnosis?

Although an MRI scan could be considered to definitively rule out posterior fossa pathology, labyrinthine disturbance seems highly likely and Ménière's disease is top of the list given the triad of vertigo, tinnitus and deafness. In early stages of Ménière's disease, lower hearing frequencies are affected.

Further investigations

Ménière's disease is the result of an abnormality in the endolymph of the inner ear. The membranous labyrinth becomes dilated (hydrops) and this may be because of excess production of endolymph or obstruction of the endolymphatic duct. Most cases are idiopathic. Transtympanic electrocochleography (ECOG) specifically detects distortion of the membranous labyrinth and can be of benefit in

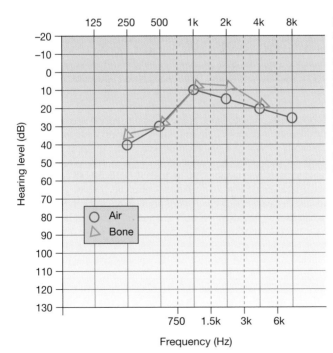

Figure 66.1
Audiogram (right ear only shown) reduced hearing at low frequencies through both air (red circle) and bone (blue triangle), consistent with a sensorineural defect.

making the diagnosis, but in most instances it is a diagnosis of exclusion. It is not performed in this patient. There is an association with thyroid disease, but thyroid function tests are normal.

How will you treat this patient?

Management of Ménière's disease includes medical and surgical options. Medical therapy can be directed towards treating the actual symptoms of the acute attack or directed towards prophylactic prevention of the attacks. If endolymphatic hydrops is attributable to a given disease process (Ménière syndrome), the first-line management is diagnosis and treatment of the primary disease (e.g. thyroid disease).

In an acutely vertiginous patient, vestibular sedatives, such as betahistine, are prescribed. Antiemetics and antihistamines may also be of benefit. In severe episodes, intravenous or intramuscular diazepam provides excellent vestibular suppression and anti-nausea effects. Steroids can be given for their anti-inflammatory effects in the inner ear. Intravenous fluid support helps to prevent dehydration and replaces electrolytes.

Prophylaxis of attacks centres initially around lifestyle measures. Chocolate, caffeine, tobacco and alcohol are triggers for some individuals. A low salt diet may also be of benefit. Reduction in endolymphatic pressure may be achieved by antihistamines, diuretics, anticholinergics and/or steroids. In some centres, early treatment with acyclovir is recommended, as there is a theory that herpes virus infection may trigger the process that leads to Ménière's disease. Many individuals have a poor quality of life and relaxation therapies may be of general benefit.

One innovation in the treatment of Ménière's disease is the 'Meniett' device. It requires the insertion of a tympanostomy tube and alternating pulses of pressure are delivered to the inner ear. Although no-one knows exactly how this works, some patients have symptomatic relief when the device is used on a daily basis. Because it is new, long-term results have not been fully evaluated. Other surgical procedures for Ménière's disease are more destructive and are reserved for medical treatment failures; they are controversial.

The prognosis of Ménière's disease is variable and unpredictable. It is usually unilateral but may progress to bilateral disease. Deafness often worsens but the attacks of vertigo may 'burn-out' with time.

Key points and global issues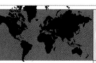

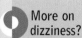 More on dizziness?

- Ménière's disease was first described in 1861 by the French physician Prosper Ménière.

- Although probably underestimated, a prevalence of 1000 cases per 100 000 people is a reasonable approximation.

See Chapters 7 and 26 of **Davidson's Principles & Practice** of **Medicine (21st edn)**

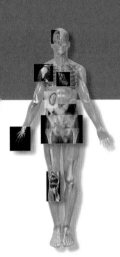

67

Macrocytic anaemia

J. I. O. CRAIG

Presenting problem

A 65-year-old woman is referred to the haematology clinic with a 6-month history of general malaise, tiredness and a 2-month history of shortness of breath on moderate exertion. She has been on thyroxine replacement for 5 years. She has not had any operations. On direct questioning, she admits to a sore tongue and pins and needles in her feet, but has no other complaints. She is on no other medication and has no history of excessive alcohol intake. Her diet is good. She remembers a maternal aunt who required injections for anaemia. The general practitioner has performed a full blood count, which shows a macrocytic anaemia, mild leucopenia and thrombocytopenia (Box 67.1).

What would your differential diagnosis include before examining the patient?

The major cause of a marked macrocytosis with these blood results is megaloblastic anaemia due to vitamin B_{12} or folate deficiency. These occur in quite different clinical circumstances, which can usually be gleaned from the history. The patient's relatively long history of breathlessness on exertion is likely to be due to the slow development of anaemia. Both vitamin B_{12} and folate are required for the synthesis of DNA and will cause systemic symptoms, such as malaise and a sore tongue, in addition to anaemia, leucopenia and thrombocytopenia. Only vitamin B_{12} deficiency, however, is associated with neurological problems. The most common cause of vitamin B_{12} deficiency is pernicious anaemia, an autoimmune disorder causing lack of intrinsic factor and hence vitamin B_{12} malabsorption. It is often associated with other autoimmune disorders in the patient or family. This woman had hypothyroidism and an aunt has probable vitamin B_{12} deficiency ('anaemia requiring injections' – vitamin B_{12} is given by intramuscular injection). Her diet is good: she is not a vegan, eats meat and vegetables and has no symptoms to suggest malabsorption. The stores of folate in the body are short, lasting only a few months, and deficiency is associated with an inadequate diet, in particular, lack of green vegetables. Folate deficiency can be a manifestation of coeliac disease, although she has no overt symptoms of this.

BOX 67.1	
Initial investigations	
Haemoglobin	72 g/L (7.2 g/dL)
MCV	123 fL
WCC	3.5×10^9/L (10^3/mm³)
Platelets	110×10^9/L (10^3/mm³)

Examination

On examination, this woman appears pale, with a hint of jaundice. Her tongue is beefy-red. She is not tachypnoeic, but has an elevated regular pulse of 90/min with a flow murmur on auscultation of her heart. There are no overt signs of cardiac failure. The spleen tip is just palpable on deep inspiration. She has bilateral reduction in pin-prick sensation in her feet to the level of the ankles.

Investigations

The initial full blood count (FBC) results are shown in Box 67.1. Blood film reveals big oval red cells and hypersegmented neutrophils (Fig. 67.1). The bilirubin is elevated at 50 μmol/L (2.93 mg/dL) and is predominantly unconjugated. Other liver function tests and thyroid function tests are normal. Urinalysis shows an increased urobilinogen only. Bone marrow aspirate shows a megaloblastic marrow. Serum B_{12} is low at 50 pg/mL, with normal levels of folate and ferritin.

Have examination and initial investigations narrowed down your differential diagnosis?

The history and the FBC have been the most helpful here in suggesting the diagnosis. Examination confirms a moderate anaemia with pallor, tachycardia and a flow murmur. There are signs of sensory peripheral neuropathy, which would be consistent with vitamin B_{12} deficiency. The mildly enlarged spleen is consistent with haemolysis of the abnormal red cells, confirmed by the findings of increased urinary urobilinogen and unconjugated serum bilirubin.

Further investigations

To determine the cause of B_{12} deficiency, a Schilling test is performed. This test assesses the absorption of radio-labelled vitamin B_{12} (indirectly determined by measuring the amount of radio-labelled vitamin B_{12} in a 24-hour urine collection) before and after administration of intrinsic factor. Normal recovery is 7.5–12%. The following results are obtained: part 1 (without intrinsic factor),

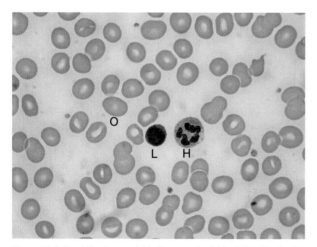

Figure 67.1 Blood film in megaloblastic anaemia. A blood film showing large oval red cells (oval macrocyte, O) and a neutrophil, with many lobes in the nucleus (hypersegmented neutrophil, H). This is typical of megaloblastic anaemia. Usually the red cells are the same size as the nucleus of a lymphocyte (L) and there is a maximum of five lobes in the nucleus of a neutrophil.

<1% recovery of radio-labelled B_{12}; part 2 (with intrinsic factor), 10% recovery of radio-labelled B_{12}. Gastric parietal cell antibodies and intrinsic factor antibodies are positive.

Does this narrow down your differential diagnosis?

The results confirm no absorption of B_{12} until intrinsic factor is given. This confirms that the terminal ileum can absorb B_{12} as long as intrinsic factor is provided. Autoantibodies to gastric parietal cells and to intrinsic factor are positive, confirming the diagnosis of pernicious anaemia.

How will you treat this patient?

She will require life-long supplementation with parenteral vitamin B_{12} (hydroxy-cobalamin). This is given intramuscularly, initially at a dose of 1 mg, 3 times a week for 2 weeks, then life-long every 2–3 months. Response can be confirmed by finding a high reticulocyte count about 1 week after starting treatment.

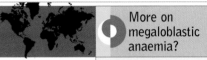

Key points and global issues

More on megaloblastic anaemia?

See Chapter 24 of **Davidson's Principles & Practice** of **Medicine (21st edn)**

- The history is important in determining the cause of a megaloblastic anaemia.
- B_{12} or folate deficiency result in the same blood and marrow findings, but only B_{12} deficiency is associated with neurological abnormalities.
- Nutritional deficiency of vitamin B_{12} is the most common cause of megaloblastic anaemia in Hindu vegetarians and is a significant problem in Mexico, South and Central America and some areas of Africa.
- There is little racial variation in the incidence of pernicious anaemia.

68

Polycythaemia

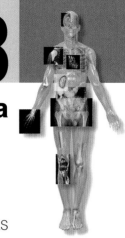

T. DAS

Presenting problem

A 45-year-old man attends the medical outpatient department with a 6-week history of fronto-parietal headache, insomnia, loss of concentration and a generalised itch that is worse after a hot bath. He also complains of a dragging discomfort in the left upper abdomen and early satiety accompanied by weight loss for 1 month. He was treated for pulmonary tuberculosis 4 years ago, but has no other past history of note. He is a fishmonger and does not smoke or drink. Family history is unremarkable.

What would your differential diagnosis include before examining the patient?

Headache, insomnia and loss of concentration are non-specific symptoms. The weight loss and early satiety are of concern and raise the possibility of gastric pathology. Itch after a hot bath is not uncommon, but is a feature of polycythaemia rubra vera (PRV).

Examination

On examination, the patient has stigmata of recent weight loss, but there is no dehydration, cyanosis, jaundice or oedema. His face has a plethoric look and bilateral conjunctival suffusion is present. His pulse is 80/min regular and blood pressure is 130/80 mmHg. Abdominal examination reveals that the spleen is palpable 5 cm below the left costal margin; it is non-tender. The liver is palpable 2 cm below the right costal margin; it is firm and non-tender.

Has examination narrowed down your differential diagnosis?

Examination has been extremely helpful and confirms that this man has a significant systemic disorder. The differential diagnosis at this stage will include causes of hepatosplenomegaly. Chronic liver disease with portal hypertension would be high up the list of potential diagnoses, but there are no peripheral stigmata of liver disease; he is not jaundiced and there are no features of portal hypertension such as ascites and abdominal wall vein distension. Chronic malaria and kala-azar are ruled out because of the absence of fever, and chronic schistosomiasis is excluded because features of portal hypertension are absent.

Haematological causes of hepatosplenomegaly seem more likely. Chronic haemolytic anaemias, such as sickle cell anaemia and the thalassaemia syndromes, are generally associated with jaundice and often, there is a history of repeated blood transfusions in the past; there is frequently a positive family

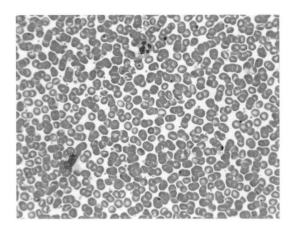

Figure 68.1 Peripheral blood film from a patient with polycythaemia, showing elevated red cell count.

history too. Lymphoma may be characterised by pruritus, but generalised lymphadenopathy is likely to be present. Chronic myeloid leukaemia and myelofibrosis are possibilities, but this man is relatively young and there is no anaemia. Polycythaemia rubra vera is characterised by itch after bathing, plethoric facies and splenomegaly, with or without hepatomegaly, and seems the most likely diagnosis in the present case. Blood tests are clearly required.

Investigations

The blood test results are shown in Box 68.1. The haemoglobin is markedly increased. The red blood cell (RBC) indices are normal. A peripheral blood film (Fig. 68.1) shows numerous RBCs which are normochromic and normocytic. The red cell mass is increased. No abnormal or immature cells of the erythroid series are seen. The urine examination is normal. The chest X-ray and electrocardiogram (ECG) are normal. Biochemical parameters show normal blood glucose, urea, serum creatinine and liver function tests. Serum uric acid is 348 μmol/L (5.8 mg/dL), serum ferritin is 22.9 μg/L (ng/mL). The serum erythropoietin level is at the lower end of the normal range. The oxygen saturation is 95% while breathing ambient air. An ultrasound scan of the abdomen shows mild hepatomegaly and moderate splenomegaly.

Does this narrow down your differential diagnosis?

The striking laboratory finding is the presence of a high haemoglobin, which is defined as haemoglobin values >165 g/L (16.5 g/dL) in females and >180 g/L (18.0 g/dL) in males. The common causes of a high haemoglobin are given in Box 68.2. High haemoglobin may be due to an increase in the number of red blood cells (true polycythaemia) or a reduction in the plasma volume (relative polycythaemia). In this patient, there is no evidence of dehydration, diuretic therapy or alcohol consumption, so haemoconcentration giving rise to relative polycythaemia is ruled out.

True polycythaemia is caused either by increased erythropoiesis in the bone marrow due to increased erythropoietin production (secondary polycythaemia), or

BOX 68.1	
Initial investigations	
Haemoglobin	227 g/L (22.7 g/dL)
Haematocrit	0.69
RBC	7.86×10^{12}/L (10^6/mm³)
WCC	14.3×10^9/L (10^3/mm³)
Differential count	
Neutrophils	87%
Lymphocytes	9%
Monocytes	3%
Eosinophils	1%
Platelets	490×10^9/L (10^3/mm³)
ESR	5 mm/1st hour

by primary increase in marrow activity (primary proliferative polycythaemia). Chronic hypoxaemia can give rise to secondary polycythaemia, but the arterial oxygen saturation is normal in this patient. There is neither a history of living at high altitude nor any evidence of lung or cyanotic heart disease. There are no features of renal disease or other tumours. The serum erythropoietin level is also normal.

The presence of a raised red cell mass and splenomegaly and the absence of any cause of secondary polycythaemia confirms the diagnosis of primary proliferative polycythaemia or PRV. In addition, the raised neutrophil and platelet count are also minor criteria for PRV.

How will you treat this patient?

Periodic phlebotomy (venesection) serves to maintain the red cell mass within normal limits and prevents thrombosis. The target haemoglobin level is ≤140 g/L (14 g/dL) in men and ≤120 g/L (12 g/dL) in women. Between 400 and 500 mL of blood are removed and venesection is initially repeated every 5–7 days until the haematocrit is reduced to below 45%. Thereafter, venesections may be performed at 3-month intervals. Aspirin is indicated to reduce thrombotic risks, unless there is a contraindication to its use. Cytotoxic agents like hydroxyurea or interferon (IFN)-α may be used to treat symptomatic splenomegaly and myeloproliferation, e.g. raised platelets. Intravenous radioactive phosphorus (5 mCi of 32P) may be considered in older patients, but its use is associated with a significant increase in risk of transformation to acute leukaemia. Rarely, massive splenomegaly may require splenectomy. Allogeneic bone marrow transplantation can be curative in the occasional young patient, but there is significant mortality associated with the procedure.

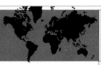 Key points and global issues

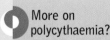
More on polycythaemia?

- PRV, a Philadelphia (Ph)-negative myeloproliferative disorder, is a clonal disorder involving multipotent haematopoietic progenitor cells.

- A single mutation, *V617F* in the *JAK2* gene, has been found in >90% of patients with PRV. Thus, if an individual is positive for this mutation, it obviates the need for red cell mass/bone marrow studies.

- The prevalence is 1–3 cases per 100 000 population.

- There is frequent concomitant iron deficiency. Therefore, these patients may present with a normal haemoglobin, but iron-deficient indices and a raised red cell count.

- PRV appears to be more common in Jews of European origin than in non-Jews. Recently, a higher incidence has been reported from Sweden.

- In many patients with PRV, the leucocyte alkaline phosphatase level is increased and an elevated serum vitamin B_{12} or B_{12}-binding capacity may be present. Bone marrow aspirate and biopsy may reveal an abnormal karyotype and myelofibrosis.

See Chapter 24 of
Davidson's Principles & Practice of
Medicine (21st edn)

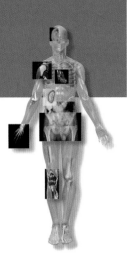

69

Leucopenia

J. I. O. CRAIG

Presenting problem

A 35-year-old woman presents with a 1-week history of a sore throat and a 2-day history of fever. She had coryzal symptoms 2 weeks previously, which settled after 3 days. Her past medical history is unremarkable and there is no family history of note. She had taken paracetamol for the sore throat, but is on no other prescribed medicines; nor has she used any other drugs. A full blood count (FBC) and blood film show a leucopenia with a marked neutropenia and a borderline thrombocytopenia (Box 69.1).

What would your differential diagnosis include before examining the patient?

The main abnormality is a leucopenia, which is as a result of a neutropenia. The patient's sore throat could be either a manifestation of the cause of the neutropenia or a result of neutropenia itself (e.g. a secondary infection with thrush). Isolated neutropenia is commonly associated with viral infections and drugs. During viral infections, it is transient, resolving after a few days. Drugs can cause neutropenia in expected or idiosyncratic ways. Neutropenia is an expected side-effect of chemotherapy and immunosuppressants such as azathioprine. It is known to occur occasionally in patients receiving antithyroid drugs such as carbimazole. Idiosyncratic reactions should be considered with any drug. This woman does not have a significant drug history. Less commonly, neutropenia can be due to lack of production of cells from the bone marrow, which is often associated with abnormalities in the other blood parameters such as haemoglobin and platelets. The patient does have a mildly reduced platelet count in addition to a marked neutropenia; therefore a primary bone marrow cause is a possibility and a bone marrow examination is indicated.

Examination

On examination, this woman appears unwell and has a temperature of 38.5°C. She has white plaques over her soft palate, suggestive of oral candidiasis. There is no cervical lymphadenopathy. She has a tachycardia of 100/min, but her blood pressure is normal. Her

BOX 69.1	
Initial investigations	
Haemoglobin	115 g/L (11.5 g/dL)
WCC	1.6×10^9/L (10^3/mm³)
Neutrophils	0.1×10^9/L (10^3/mm³)
Lymphocytes	1.5×10^9/L (10^3/mm³)
Platelets	140×10^9/L (10^3/mm³)

chest is clear and other examinations normal. There are no signs of skin or mucosal bleeding and funduscopy was normal.

Have examination and initial investigations narrowed down your differential diagnosis?

The examination reveals that this woman is unwell, with fever in the presence of marked neutropenia. She has a normal blood pressure but neutropenic sepsis can be life-threatening. She needs to be admitted to hospital urgently for intravenous broad-spectrum antibiotics and further investigation of the cause of neutropenia, including a bone marrow examination. It seems unlikely in this case that the patient's neutropenia is due to the more common causes such as viral infection or drugs.

Further investigations

A throat swab grows *Candida albicans*. Renal and liver function tests are normal. The bone marrow aspirate shows the marrow to be infiltrated with immature blasts consistent with acute leukaemia. There are many Auer rods in the blasts, which is consistent with acute myeloid leukaemia (AML; Fig. 69.1). The cytogenetics of the leukaemia show a translocation between chromosomes 15 and 17, which is found in acute promyelocytic leukaemia, a subtype of AML with a good prognosis.

Does this narrow down your differential diagnosis?

This establishes the diagnosis of neutropenia as a consequence of acute promyelocytic leukaemia.

How will you treat this patient?

Initially, she requires immediate skilled supportive care, including broad-spectrum antibiotics and oral antifungal treatment, e.g. fluconazole. Neutropenic sepsis is an emergency, and empirical broad-spectrum antibiotics should be started immediately; they can be modified once microbiology results are available.

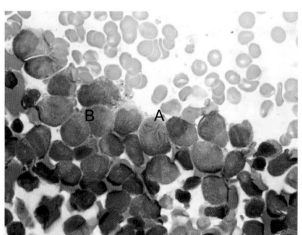

Figure 69.1 Bone marrow aspirate. This bone marrow aspirate shows many granulated blasts (B), some of which contain a number of Auer rods (A). This is typical of acute promyelocytic leukaemia.

To treat the AML specifically, this woman requires chemotherapy and ATRA (all-*trans* retinoic acid) treatment. This differentiating agent has reduced the risks of life-threatening bleeding from the abnormal coagulation associated with this type of leukaemia. The prognosis is good, with an overall survival of around 75% at 5 years.

Key points and global issues

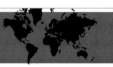

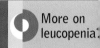

More on leucopenia?

- The normal neutrophil count varies with age and race, and appropriate reference ranges must be used.
- Africans, black Americans and Afro-Caribbeans have a lower neutrophil count than Caucasians.
- A drug history is important when investigating the cause of neutropenia.
- Infection in a neutropenic patient can be life-threatening and should be treated promptly with broad spectrum antibiotics.

See Chapter 24 of **Davidson's Principl** & **Practice** of **Medicine (21st edn**

70

Cervical lymphadenopathy

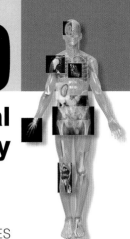

J. M. DAVIES

Presenting problem

A 28-year-old woman is referred urgently by her GP to the Haematology Clinic. She has noticed an enlarging lump on the left hand side of her neck and is extremely anxious about what might be wrong. She describes the lump as being 'in the lower part of my neck above the collar bone'. There is no previous history of note and she takes no regular medication.

She denies any antecedent upper respiratory tract infection and has no oropharyngeal symptoms of note. She does, however, admit to 4 weeks of exertional breathlessness and has noticed unintentional weight loss of approximately 10 kg over the last 6 months. She has not, however, noticed any night sweats and has not, as far as she has been aware, been febrile. There is no family history of note and her parents and brothers and sister have all been well. She is not aware of any contact with any infectious disease and has not travelled outside the UK for 2 years. She has been in a stable relationship for 5 years and has never used drugs recreationally. She is a non-smoker and takes alcohol only very occasionally.

What would your differential diagnosis include before examining the patient?

The differential diagnosis here is wide, but the commonest cause of a persistent neck lump presenting in this context would be cervical lymphadenopathy. Clearly, there are other neck masses which should be considered, including branchial cysts. Of importance here is that the patient is unwell, in that she reports systemic symptoms in association with the neck mass. Both the GP and the patient herself are concerned about haematological malignancy and the referral has been made essentially to confirm or exclude this diagnosis.

Examination and initial investigations

The patient looks pale and there is evidence of recent weight loss. Examination of the scalp, ears and oropharynx is normal. There is a 2.5×3 cm left supraclavicular fossa lymph node mass, which is firm and non-tender. There is no convincing lymphadenopathy in either axilla. Examination of the abdomen reveals no enlargement of the liver or spleen and the inguinal lymph nodes are not palpable. The patient is breathless on minimal exertion and examination of the chest shows signs compatible with a right pleural effusion. There is no evidence of facial or upper limb oedema and the jugular venous pressure is not raised.

The investigations performed by the GP (Box 70.1) confirm the systemic nature of the disorder, with a significant anaemia with normal indices. The white cell count and differential are normal. The erythrocyte sedimentation rate is also elevated, which is a non-specific finding, but does point to the presence of underlying systemic upset. Overall, the blood picture would be compatible with that seen in the anaemia of chronic disease.

Have examination and initial investigations narrowed down your differential diagnosis?

Examining this patient provides two important clues as to what might be going on. First, the left neck mass is an enlarged lymph node. Second, the examination confirms that the patient is unwell and has, in addition to the lymphadenopathy, further pathology involving the chest. Although the differential diagnosis is still wide, the chief possibilities are now lymphoma including both Hodgkin's disease and non-Hodgkin lymphoma or some other disseminated malignancy, e.g. metastatic carcinoma. Not excluded, but less likely would be an infective process, e.g. tuberculosis. What is clear, however, is that urgent further investigation is mandatory.

Further investigations

At the initial clinic visit the anaemia is confirmed. Renal function and liver function are normal. The serum urate is elevated, which may be indicative of increased cell turnover. The lactate dehydrogenase is significantly elevated in-keeping with, but not diagnostic of, a diagnosis of a lymphoproliferative disorder. The serum albumin is low and corrected calcium and phosphate are normal. Tumour markers for germ cell tumours (α-feto-protein and β-HCG) are negative. A chest X-ray shows significant mediastinal widening and a right pleural effusion. A CT scan of chest, abdomen and pelvis reveals massive mediastinal lymphadenopathy, but no abnormality below the diaphragm (Fig. 70.1). Echocardiography shows a pericardial effusion, but with normal left ventricular function.

The pleural fluid is tapped and is an exudate, but contains no demonstrable malignant cells. Culture of the pleural fluid is negative. Fine-needle aspirate of

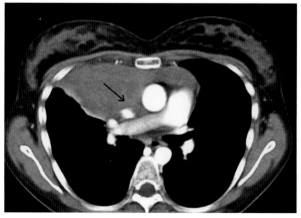

Figure 70.1 CT scan of the chest, showing mediastinal lymphadenopathy (arrow).

the mass shows no evidence of metastatic carcinoma but is highly suggestive of lymphoid malignancy.

The patient is sent for an urgent excision biopsy of the left supraclavicular lymph node. The histology is that of a non-Hodgkin lymphoma of diffuse large B cell (DLBCL) sub-type. Given the clinical presentation, this is considered to represent primary mediastinal (thymic) DLBCL.

Does this narrow down your differential diagnosis?

The diagnosis here was clinched by obtaining tissue for histopathological analysis and this was done by excision biopsy. Where the differential diagnosis is wide or uncertain, then biopsy is essential for a formal diagnosis.

How will you treat this patient?

There are two key components to the management of this woman. First, appropriate psychological support and open and honest communication from the start.

In terms of the lymphoma, the patient is further staged and any appropriate prognostic scoring such as the International Prognostic Index applied.

In patients presenting with DLBCL the current primary treatment is multi-agent chemoimmunotherapy. The incorporation of the monoclonal antibody Rituximab into treatment regimens has been a major advance in this regard. The prognosis in DLBCL depends upon various prognostic factors but the original GELA study demonstrated a 40–60% overall survival in advanced stage older patients at 8 years.

Primary mediastinal DLBCL is an uncommon entity with its own biology. Gene array signatures are different to other DLBCL and are closer to those seen in classical Hodgkin's disease. Dose dense regimens may have a particular role in this entity. Response may be monitored clinically and by cross-sectional imaging. PET scanning may be helpful in evaluation of any residual mediastinal masses and radiotherapy may be used additionally to consolidate chemotherapy responses.

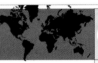

Key points and global issues

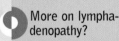

More on lympha-denopathy?

See Chapter 24 of
Davidson's Principles
& **Practice** of
Medicine (21st edn)

- Lymphadenopathy is common. Likely causes may, however, vary by geographical location, with infectious diseases, such as tuberculosis and HIV/AIDS being more common in certain populations than others.

- Where the lymphadenopathy is due to metastatic malignant disease, there again would be variations as to the histopathology within populations, depending on risk exposure.

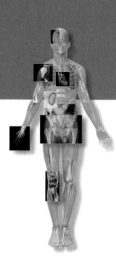

71

Massive splenomegaly

T. AHMED

Presenting problem

A 30-year-old garment worker from Bangladesh is admitted to hospital because of recurrent episodes of fever during the last 18 months and massive splenomegaly. Each episode of fever persists for an average duration of 2–3 weeks and recurs at intervals of about 2–3 weeks. The fever is associated with chills and rigors and usually occurs in the evening, with slight remission in the morning. The patient has taken three courses of chloroquine, without evidence of malarial parasites in the blood film, and several courses of ciprofloxacin on the basis of a positive Widal test. He has anorexia during the febrile episodes, but otherwise has a good appetite and feels well during afebrile periods. He has lost about 9 kg weight during the period of his illness. He has an occasional mild cough. The patient is married and has two healthy children. He has no history of headache, seizures, haematemesis or melaena. The patient has not received any blood transfusions and has no history of extramarital sexual exposure. Recently, he has gone to a traditional healer for the treatment of jaundice. His bowel and bladder habits are normal.

What would your differential diagnosis include before examining the patient?

When a patient from a tropical country presents with recurrent bouts of fever and massive splenomegaly, chronic malaria and visceral leishmaniasis (kala-azar) are at the top of the list in the differential diagnosis. Pancytopenia, with its consequent clinical manifestations, is a common feature in kala-azar. A diagnosis of tropical splenomegaly syndrome might also be entertained, depending on the patient's country of origin. In this syndrome, an exaggerated immune response to malaria, especially in malarious areas, produces splenomegaly. Tuberculosis involvement of liver and spleen should also be considered, as should other chronic infections, such as systemic fungal infections and chronic *brucellosis*.

In untreated patients, the fever of *brucellosis* shows an undulating pattern; the pyrexia persists for weeks before there is a period of apyrexia that may be followed by relapse. This patient is a garment worker and does not give a history of domestic exposure to infected animals or their products. In the absence of an occupational history, therefore, chronic *brucellosis* seems unlikely.

Fungal disease, especially histoplasmosis, can present with fever and hepatosplenomegaly. Fungal infections, although reported in immunocompetent individuals, are much more common in immunocompromised hosts. This patient's history does not provide any clue to immunosuppression. Moreover, chronic fungal infections left untreated for 18 months are often fatal. Therefore, fungal disease is unlikely in this patient.

Cirrhosis with portal hypertension should be considered in a patient with hepatosplenomegaly, but massive splenomegaly occurs rarely, except in extra-hepatic portal hypertension. Hepatosplenomegaly is also a feature of lympho-proliferative or myeloproliferative diseases like lymphoma, chronic myeloid leukemia, chronic lymphatic leukemia, myelofibrosis, polycythaemia rubra vera and, rarely, Waldenström's macroglobulinaemia. Fever is an important symptom in patients with lymphoma; however, in other conditions it is not a

---

BOX 71.1

Initial investigations

Haemoglobin	96 g/L (9.6 g/dL)
WCC	5.5×10^9/L (10^3/mm^3)
Differential count	
Neutrophils	65%
Lymphocytes	28%
Monocytes	05%
Eosinophils	02%
Platelets	250×10^9/L (10^3/mm^3)
ESR	120 mm/1st hour
Peripheral blood smear	Anisochromia, anisocytosis
Thick and thin blood smears	Negative for malarial parasites
Bilirubin (total)	35.7 μmol/L (2.1 mg/dL)
Protein (total)	85 g/L (8.5 g/dL)
Albumin	35 g/L (3.5 g/dL)
ALT	32 U/L

The urine is yellow and on dipstick examination is positive for urobilinogen. Abdominal ultrasonography confirms splenomegaly without evidence of focal abnormalities, but not hepatomegaly. There is no free fluid and no apparent abdominal lymphadenopathy. A formal gel (aldehyde) test shows egg-white opacity within 20 min of adding formalin to the patient's serum (strongly positive). This is a non-specific test which suggests that there are high circulating immunoglobulin levels (Fig. 71.1).

An immunochromatographic test for kala-azar using rK39 antigen is positive. Bone marrow aspiration with examination for amastigotes (Leishman–Donovan (LD) bodies) on Giemsa stain yields a definitive diagnosis in approximately 80% of cases and is carried out here. The sensitivity approaches 100% in splenic aspirates. Despite the safety of splenic aspiration when aspiration is performed very rapidly with a small-bore needle, it is rarely done outside areas where kala-azar is endemic. Alternative but less sensitive diagnostic methods include liver biopsy and lymph node aspiration when lymphadenopathy is present. Culture is a time-consuming and expensive process and is rarely used for clinical purposes.

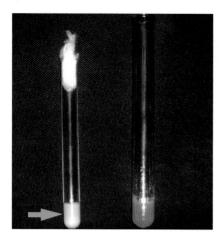

Figure 71.1 Strongly positive formal gel (aldehyde) test (arrow). The tube on the right is a control tube showing no change when aldehyde is added to the patient's serum.

presenting feature but can occur as a result of opportunistic infections. Patients with myelofibrosis and chronic myeloid leukaemia may develop massive splenomegaly.

 Examination

Examination reveals that the patient is mildly anaemic and icteric, but otherwise appears well. His temperature is 40.3°C and pulse rate is 140/mm. Peripheral lymph nodes are not palpable. The spleen is palpable 10 cm from the left anterior axillary line along its long axis. The liver margin is palpable 1.5 cm below the right costal margin. There is no ascites or stigmata of chronic liver disease. Examination of other systems reveals no abnormality.

Has examination narrowed down your differential diagnosis?

The presence of mild jaundice and hepatosplenomegaly favour primary liver disease. However, massive splenomegaly and the absence of other features of chronic hepatic insufficiency and of portal hypertension makes primary liver disease unlikely. Jaundice may also occur in kala-azar (though rarely), chronic lymphocytic leukemia and Hodgkin's disease, but not in chronic myeloid leukemia. The absence of features of hyperviscosity excludes the likelihood of Waldenström's macroglobulinaemia. The absence of peripheral lymphadenopathy makes the diagnosis of chronic lymphocytic leukaemia and lymphoma unlikely but not impossible. Further narrowing down of the differential diagnosis requires a step-wise diagnostic approach starting with simple blood tests.

Initial investigations

Results of peripheral blood investigations are provided in Box 71.1.

Has the diagnosis been clinched?

The presence of LD bodies in bone marrow confirms the diagnosis of kala-azar (Fig. 71.2). However, in a country where malaria, typhoid and tuberculosis are common, the diagnosis of one does not exclude the other.

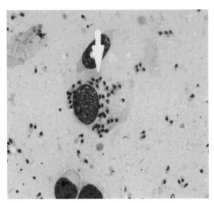

Figure 71.2 Bone marrow aspirate showing intracellular and extracellular Leishman–Donovan (LD) bodies (arrow).

How will you treat this patient?

The standard treatment of kala-azar is with one of the pentavalent antimonial compounds, e.g. sodium stibogluconate (100 mg/mL) or meglumine antimonate (85 mg/mL). The daily dose is 20 mg/kg body weight, given either intravenously or intramuscularly for 28–30 days. The incidence of cardiac toxicity and a haemorrhagic manifestation of unknown mechanism with pentavalent antimonial compounds is significant. Even sudden death during treatment with pentavalent antimonial compounds has been reported. Increasing the duration of stibogluconate therapy, or the use of amphotericin B, pentamidine, paromomycin or oral miltefosine may be required for resistant cases or as the first-line drug, where stibogluconate resistance is high or produces adverse drug reactions.

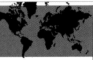

Key points and global issues

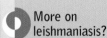

More on leishmaniasis?

See Chapter 13 of
Davidson's Principles
& **Practice** of
Medicine (21st edn)

- Among chronic infectious diseases, chronic kala-azar and malaria are the most common causes of massive splenomegaly in the tropics.

- Travel history and endemicity of the disease are important for the diagnosis of splenomegaly.

- In countries where human immunodeficiency virus (HIV) infection is common, kala-azar is an important opportunistic infection and therefore should be considered in the differential diagnosis of all cases of splenomegaly.

- A few patients develop post-kala-azar dermal leishmaniasis (PKDL), manifest by skin lesions that are most prominent on the face. These lesions develop either during treatment or months to years after treatment. PKDL patients represent a human reservoir of infection and so are epidemiologically important.

- Chronic schistosomiasis due to *Schistosoma mansoni* may produce massive splenomegaly with portal hypertension in the tropics. Endemic areas include Africa, the Middle East, the Caribbean, Brazil and Venezuela.

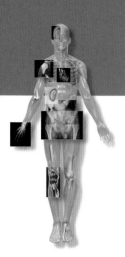

72

Bleeding disorder

C. A. LUDLAM

Presenting problem

A 30-year-old woman with a long history of menorrhagia is being considered for a hysterectomy and is referred for preoperative assessment to establish whether she has a bleeding disorder. She already has a family consisting of two daughters and a son. As a child, she underwent tonsillectomy and required a blood transfusion because of postoperative bleeding. Two wisdom teeth were extracted 7 years previously and bleeding started from one of the sockets 5 h after surgery, and lasted 36 h. A coagulation screen (consisting of an activated partial thromboplastin time (APTT), prothrombin time and fibrinogen) is normal (Box 72.1).

What would your differential diagnosis include before examining the patient?

Judging from the long history of haemorrhagic incidents, a congenital disorder is more likely than an acquired bleeding condition, e.g. secondary to liver or renal failure. This woman probably has a 'mild' bleeding disorder because excess bleeding has only occurred after surgery. A coagulation disorder, due to a reduction in one of the clotting factors, is more likely than a disorder of primary haemostasis (von Willebrand disease or a platelet disorder) because the bleeding started a few hours after, rather than at the time of surgery.

Statistically, von Willebrand disease would be the most likely diagnosis because it is relatively common, although in this condition, bleeding usually starts immediately after trauma. This is because the von Willebrand factor facilitates the arrest of initial haemorrhage by promoting the adhesion of platelets to the damaged vessel wall. In thrombocytopenia or a platelet functional disorder (relatively uncommon) too, bleeding is usually immediate, again because of the poor development of platelet aggregates immediately at the site of trauma. Bleeding which starts a few hours after surgery is more characteristic of a coagulation

BOX 72.1	
Initial investigations	
Platelets	250×10^9/L (10^3/mm³)
Prothrombin time	14 s
APTT	35 s
Fibrinogen	2.1 g/L (0.21 g/dL)
von Willebrand factor (by ristocetin assay)	0.7 U/mL (normal 0.5–1.5)
Factor VIII	0.30 U/mL (normal 0.5–1.5)
Factor IX	0.85 U/mL (normal 0.5–1.5)
Factor XI	0.90 U/mL (normal 0.5–1.5)

factor deficiency, e.g. factor VIII, IX or XI; in this situation, the initial platelet haemostatic plug is poorly reinforced by fibrin strands formed by the coagulation system and it therefore disintegrates a few hours after formation.

Examination

On examination, no bruises or purpura are seen. Joints are normal and there is no evidence of limitation of range of movement or arthritis. No stigmata of chronic liver disease are present and no clinical hepatosplenomegaly is identified.

Has examination narrowed down your differential diagnosis?

Chronic liver disease or thrombocytopenia secondary to hypersplenism is unlikely. Neither is a severe coagulation disorder probable because there is no evidence of joint damage secondary to recurrent haemarthroses.

Further investigations

The platelet count and morphology on a blood film are normal. Heritable platelet functional disorders are uncommon (although that due to aspirin is common). Although the APTT and prothrombin time (PT) are normal, this does not exclude a mild bleeding disorder, as these global coagulation tests are insensitive to mild clotting factor deficiencies and levels have to be below about 25% of normal before the screening tests are prolonged. In this patient, assay of coagulation factors reveals a reduced factor VIII of 0.30 U/mL, but normal factor IX and XI levels.

von Willebrand factor level is normal (Box 72.1), as is the binding of factor VIII to von Willebrand factor. Genetic analysis of the factor VIII gene on the X chromosome reveals that the patient is heterozygous for the intron 22 inversion. This is the most common genetic mutation that causes severe haemophilia A.

Does this narrow down your differential diagnosis?

A low factor VIII level is found in von Willebrand disease, carriers of haemophilia A, acquired haemophilia (unlikely in this case because of the life-long history) and female haemophilia (very rare). Factor IX is measured because it may be reduced in carriers of haemophilia B (factor IX deficiency), which has a prevalence of about one-fifth that of haemophilia A; factor XI deficiency (haemophilia C) is the next most common congenital coagulation factor deficiency. von willebrand factor has the dual function of being both the carrier protein for factor VIII (which it stabilises in the circulation) and the 'adhesive' that sticks platelets to damaged vessel walls. With a deficiency of von Willebrand factor there is a reduction in the factor VIII level (as factor VIII has a shorter half-life in the absence of its carrier protein), and primary platelet plug formation at the site of trauma is defective, resulting in immediate haemorrhage. The von Willebrand factor results exclude von Willebrand disease.

This woman, therefore, is a carrier of severe haemophilia A and has a mild bleeding disorder because of the reduced factor VIII level (secondary to random inactivation of X chromosomes, or lyonisation in early embryogenesis).

How will you treat this patient?

This woman's mild bleeding disorder, due to reduced factor VIII concentrations, may be predisposing her to menorrhagia. Desmopressin (DDAVP) would raise the level to over 0.50 U/mL for up to 12 h. This vasopressin analogue probably releases factor VIII from endothelial cells (along with von Willebrand factor). It can be given either as a nasal spray, or as a subcutaneous or intravenous injection. The nasal spray at the time of menstruation, along with the fibrinolytic inhibitor, tranexamic acid, might lessen the menorrhagia and avoid the need for a hysterectomy.

If this does not reduce the menorrhagia and there is no other correctable gynaecological cause for the excess bleeding, desmopressin could be used preoperatively and the injections continued twice daily to maintain the factor VIII level above 0.50 U/mL after surgery. Tachyphylaxis may develop and it is often not useful to give more than about four injections. As factor VIII is an acute phase reactant, the stress of the surgery will also elevate the factor VIII level and therefore after 1 or 2 days further desmopressin is not likely to be necessary. Desmopressin has potent antidiuretic activity, which lasts about 24 h and may complicate management of fluid balance in the immediate postoperative period. If more than a single injection of desmopressin is given, the plasma sodium and osmolality should be monitored and if significant hyponatraemia develops, fluids should be withheld. Instead of desmopressin, factor VIII concentrate could be used; infusions would need to be given 12-hourly initially, as its half-life is approximately 12 h.

The patient should be informed that she is a carrier of severe haemophilia and counselled about the consequences. As a carrier, each of her daughters will have a one in two chance of being a carrier and a similar chance that each son will have severe haemophilia A.

If she wishes to add to her family, antenatal diagnosis could be offered. Fetal sex could be determined by detecting Y chromosomal DNA in a maternal blood sample after 6 weeks, or by chorion villus biopsy at 11 weeks' gestation. In a male fetus, using the same chorion villus sample, the intron 22 inversion mutation could be sought and, if present, would indicate that the fetus has severe haemophilia.

This woman's existing son should have his factor VIII level measured (even although he has not had any haemorrhagic symptoms), as he has a 50% chance of having severe haemophilia. The daughters should also have their factor VIII measured because each has a 50% chance of being a carrier of severe haemophilia and, like their mother, of having a mild bleeding disorder. A normal factor VIII in a daughter does not exclude carrier status. Genetic testing (to seek the intron 22 inversion and to give a definitive assignment of carrier status) should only be undertaken when the girl is able to understand the implications of the genetic issues and is able to give true informed consent, usually in her early teenage years.

If the woman has sisters and brothers, consideration should be given to offering to measure their factor VIII levels and undertake genetic studies (in the females who might be carriers and in the males if haemophilia is diagnosed).

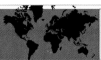

Key points and global issues

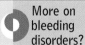

More on
bleeding
disorders?

See Chapter 24 of
Davidson's Principles
& **Practice** of
Medicine (21st edn)

- The incidence of haemophilia is the same throughout the world.

- If desmopressin is contraindicated or it does not raise the factor VIII level sufficiently, factor VIII concentrate could be used. Both recombinant and plasma-derived factor VIII concentrates are available (with the former being preferred). It is usual to offer immunity to hepatitis A and B by vaccination prior to concentrate therapy. If possible, concentrate should be avoided, as there is a small risk of an inhibitory antibody developing to factor VIII, it is more expensive than desmopressin, and a plasma-derived concentrate exposes the recipient to the possibility of transfusion-transmitted infection. Plasma-derived factor VIII concentrates undergo at least one viral inactivation step in manufacture and hence they are exceedingly safe from hepatitis viruses and human immunodeficiency virus (HIV).

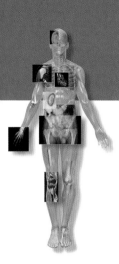

73

Thrombocytopenia

H. A. GOUBRAN

Presenting problem

A 24-year-old woman seeks your advice 2 weeks following the appearance of a rash on her lower limbs. The rash is cherry red in colour, pin-head in size and extensive on her lower extremities and trunk. She has also noted that her gums bleed following brushing of her teeth and, this morning, she observed some reddish spots in her mouth. She denies any unusual bleeding during her last menstrual period 3 weeks ago and does not report any blood in her urine or stools. There is no history of preceding fever or upper respiratory tract infection. She does not take any non-steroidal anti-inflammatory drugs (NSAIDs) or any other medication and has not sought medical care for many years, as she felt she was healthy. She is single, is a cigarette smoker (1 pack/day) and occasionally drinks alcohol.

What would your differential diagnosis include before examining the patient?

When a young patient presents with evidence of cutaneous and mucous membrane bleeds, the diagnostic possibility of a quantitative or a qualitative platelet dysfunction should be raised. Vasculitis should also be considered. A coagulopathy, on the other hand, will result in deep seated haematomata affecting the joints and muscles following surgical interventions and trauma.

Immune thrombocytopenias should come on top of the differential diagnosis list with immune-mediated platelet destruction secondary to a pre-existing autoimmune disease such as systemic lupus erythematosus, or viral infections, e.g. EBV, CMV, hepatitis C or, more frequently, HIV. Dengue and other viral haemorrhagic fevers and malaria can also produce thrombocytopenia and must be ruled out. Our patient does not live in an area where dengue and malaria are common. Infections can have an effect on platelet production and survival. Certain viral infections (infectious mononucleosis and early HIV infection) can affect platelet survival through immune-mediated mechanism. Other mechanisms such as bone marrow suppression due to disease *per se,* opportunistic infections or drugs can all cause thrombocytopenia in the advanced stages of HIV infection. Drug-induced thrombocytopenia should also be considered and for this, the drug treatment history of the patient should be carefully reviewed; in most instances it is reversible after the offending drug is stopped. Primary (idiopathic) immune thrombocytopenic purpura (ITP) is, however, the most common cause of thrombocytopenia in young persons. Increased platelet destruction secondary to splenomegaly and hypersplenism can also result in thrombocytopenia. Consumption of platelets in the context of disseminated intravascular coagulopathy or secondary to a microangiopathic haemolytic process such as the haemolytic uraemic syndrome (HUS) and thrombotic thrombocytopenic purpura (TTP) also results in thrombocytopenia, with renal impairment and neurologic symptoms. Platelet dysfunction could lead to similar symptoms. This may either be congenital such as Glanzmann's thrombasthenia or von Willebrand's disease, or secondary to drugs such as anti-platelet agents or NSAIDs. Thrombocytopenia resulting from reduced production of platelets by the bone marrow due to aplasia, myelodysplasia or replacement by neoplastic cells, should also be contemplated. Acute leukemias result in marrow infiltration with subsequent development of thrombocytopenia, concomitantly seen with anaemia and evidence of neutropenia, with fever and infections.

Vascular defects can also present with purpuric eruptions. Henoch–Schönlein purpura presents with a vasculitic rash mimicking purpura on the buttocks and back, whereas leukocytoclastic vasculitis and cryoglobulinaemic rash is usually seen on the lower extremities. The rash, however, will be palpable. Scurvy can also present with a perifollicular purpuric eruption, mostly on the trunk, whereas amyloidosis may underlie periorbital purpuric lesions.

Examination and initial investigations

On general physical examination, the patient appears healthy, conscious and well-oriented, though anxious.

She is of average body weight and height. Her blood pressure is 110/70 mmHg, her pulse is 84/min, regular and she is afebrile. Her hands, lips and conjunctivae are not pale and she does not have jaundice. There are no palpable lymph nodes in her neck, axillae or groins. Examination of her mouth reveals some evidence of gum bleeds with no hyperplasia, with a red spot on the inner aspect of her left cheek. Examination of her lower limbs and trunk reveals an extensive non-palpable purpuric eruption. Examination of her chest, heart and abdomen reveals no abnormalities and neurological examination is normal.

The results of the initial laboratory work-up are shown in Box 73.1.

Have examination and initial investigations narrowed down your differential diagnosis?

The pattern (non-vasculitic) and distribution of the rash is characteristic of a primary haemostatic defect.

The absence of anaemia or evidence of infection points to a probable isolated thrombocytopenia. The absence of jaundice, anaemia and evident neurological symptoms reduces the diagnostic probability of HUS or TTP, whereas the absence of splenomegaly rules out hypersplenism, narrowing the differential diagnosis to immune thrombocytopenia.

Further investigations

Serology for HIV, EBV, CMV and hepatitis C are negative; an autoimmune screen, including antinuclear antibodies, is negative. Anti-platelet antibodies are positive.

BOX 73.1

Initial investigations

Haemoglobin	135 g/L (13.5 g/dL)
Total leukocyte count	7.2×10^9/L (10^3/mm³)
Differential count	
Neutrophils	85%
Lymphocytes	11%
Eosinophils	2%
Basophils	0%
Monocytes	2%
Blood smear	Severe thrombocytopenia, normal haemoglobin, white cell count and differential count with no abnormal cells
Platelet count	22×10^9/L (10^3/mm³)
INR	1
Activated partial thromboplastin time	30 s

Does this narrow down your differential diagnosis?

The aim of the further investigations is to differentiate primary from secondary disease. The presence of antiplatelet antibodies, in the absence of positive viral and standard autoimmune serology, helps to consolidate the diagnosis of primary (idiopathic) immune thrombocytopenic purpura, although a negative antiplatelet antibody test would not have excluded the diagnosis.

There is no true consensus about the need to examine the bone marrow in the context of ITP in young patients and children. The test is, however, mandatory in patients above the age of 60, to rule out myelodysplasia or leukaemia, and before splenectomy.

How will you treat this patient?

The principal therapeutic options for ITP include glucocorticoids, intravenous immunoglobulins, intravenous anti-Rho (D), splenectomy and, more recently, thrombopoietin analogues. A wide palette of management options is reserved for patients who fail to maintain an acceptable platelet count after splenectomy (refractory); they include immunosuppressive agents, rituximab and plasmapheresis.

In the absence of life-threatening bleeding, a trial of steroids (prednisone) administered orally in a dose of 1 mg/kg for 4 weeks is often offered as the first line of therapy. The dose may be tapered once a response is achieved. Intravenous immunoglobulins are administered in the context of life-threatening bleeding with an expected response in 4–7 days. Platelet transfusion should only be used in severe, life-threatening bleeding, when the platelet count is below 10×10^9/L (10^3/mm³) and are usually given in conjunction with intravenous immunoglobulins. Thrombopoietin analogues (TPO-like agents) have been used recently as second-line drugs or may be given to refractory patients. Splenectomy is reserved for steroid-resistant patients. Immunosuppressive/immune-modulatory agents are used only in refractory patients who fail to maintain an acceptable count

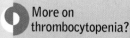

(usually a count of $20 \times 10^9/L$ ($10^3/mm^3$)) following splenectomy. These include azathioprine, cyclophosphamide, vinca alkaloids, ciclosporin and more recently, rituximab (anti-CD20, expressed on B lymphocytes).

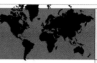

Key points and global issues

More on thrombocytopenia?

See Chapter 24 of
Davidson's Principles & Practice of **Medicine (21st edn)**

- Several viral infections (cytomegalovirus, infectious mononucleosis, mumps and rubella) can produce thrombocytopenia through immune mechanisms and produce a clinical picture identical to acute ITP. In the majority of cases, thrombocytopenia remits spontaneously.

- Viral haemorrhagic fevers, including dengue, should be considered in areas known to have periodic outbreaks of these infections.

- Malaria should always be considered in the differential diagnosis in endemic areas in patients presenting with fever and thrombocytopenia.

- HIV should also be considered in the differential diagnosis.

- Drug history should be thoroughly reviewed in patients presenting with thrombocytopenia.

- Idiopathic immune thrombocytopenic purpura is not uncommon; it has a low mortality rate from bleeding.

- The target platelet count that should be maintained in refractory cases is around $20 \times 10^9/L$ ($10^3/mm^3$).

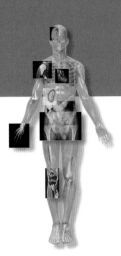

74

Thrombocytosis

P. SHEPHERD

Presenting problem

A 75-year-old woman is admitted for an elective total knee joint replacement. Postoperatively, she requires monitoring for a short period in the high-dependency unit and on discharge is noted to have a haemoglobin of 75 g/L (7.5 g/dL), white cell count of 20.3×10⁹/L (10³/mm³) and platelets of 690×10⁹/L (10³/mm³). Two months later, she is referred to the local haematology clinic. Her blood count now shows: haemoglobin 135 g/L (13.5 g/dL), WCC 11.4×10⁹/L (10³/mm³) and platelets 1346×10⁹/L (10³/mm³). She is well and has had no previous problems with strokes, transient ischaemic attacks (TIAs), or cardiac or peripheral vascular disease.

What would your differential diagnosis include before examining the patient?

Thrombocytosis may be reactive or due to an underlying myeloproliferative disorder. The initial results after her knee joint replacement could well be reactive in nature due to either bleeding or inflammation/infection. Other markers of inflammation may be present, such as an increase in the C-reactive protein (CRP) or the erythrocyte sedimentation rate (ESR). Most cases of thrombocytosis, particularly in the acute setting, are reactive in nature. However, if the thrombocytosis persists for a period of months in the absence of an ongoing inflammatory/infectious or neoplastic cause, then a myeloproliferative disorder should be suspected. There are no specific diagnostic features to separate a reactive thrombocytosis from a myeloproliferative disorder. In fact, the diagnosis of a myeloproliferative disorder is one of exclusion of reactive causes. The major causes of reactive thrombocytosis and of myeloproliferative disorders associated with increased platelets are shown in Box 74.1. The most common myeloproliferative disorder is primary thrombocythaemia, but other disorders should be excluded.

BOX 74.1

Causes of thrombocytosis

Reactive disorders

- Infection, acute or chronic
- Bleeding, acute or chronic
- Neoplasia
- Inflammation, e.g. rheumatoid arthritis, connective tissue disease
- Post-splenectomy

Myeloproliferative disorders

- Primary thrombocythaemia
- Primary polycythaemia
- Chronic myeloid leukaemia
- Myelofibrosis
- Myelodysplasia with raised platelets

Examination and initial investigations

Examination shows a woman who looks well with no obvious problems. Her weight is steady and cardiorespiratory examination is normal. There is no hepatosplenomegaly. There is no obvious problem with her knee replacement and there are no features of inflammatory arthritis. Peripheral pulses are present and there is good capillary circulation in the feet.

The blood count is repeated and is similar to that above. The mean cell volume (MCV) is at the lower end of the normal range (79 fl). The blood film shows a normal white cell differential and no abnormal red or white cells. ESR is 14 mm/h and CRP is 3 mg/L. Urea and electrolytes are normal, apart from a slightly elevated potassium of 5.6 mmol/L. Lactate dehydrogenase (LDH) is high at 840 U/L and urate is normal. The chest X-ray is normal.

Have examination and initial investigations narrowed down your differential diagnosis?

There are no positive findings on examination that support or refute the differential diagnosis. However, the duration of the thrombocytosis and the absence of any systemic symptoms or an underlying obvious inflammatory/infective/neoplastic lesion would support an underlying myeloproliferative disorder. If splenomegaly was present, this would be a strong pointer to a myeloproliferative disorder. However, with the ready availability of blood counts and possibly earlier diagnosis, this is frequently not present in many myeloproliferative disorders. In addition, the normal ESR, normal CRP and elevated LDH and potassium would point towards a myeloproliferative disorder. The particular type of myeloproliferative disorder is probably primary thrombocythaemia. There are no features on the blood film to suggest myelodysplasia or myelofibrosis. The normal haemoglobin generally excludes primary polycythaemia, provided there is no associated iron deficiency.

Further investigations

Bone marrow examination shows a hypercellular marrow with increased megakaryocytes, many of which are large and clustered in the marrow spaces (Fig. 74.1). Erythropoiesis and myelopoiesis appear to be maturing normally.

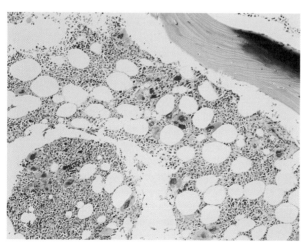

Figure 74.1 Bone marrow biopsy Giemsa stain (×100), showing large clustered megakaryocytes.

Fine reticulin fibres are present throughout (grade 2). Iron stores are absent. Cytogenetic examination shows a normal female karyotype, and molecular studies using probes for *BCR* and *ABL* exclude a *BCR-ABL* fusion gene. *JAK2 V617F* mutation screening is negative.

Does this narrow down your differential diagnosis?

The blood and bone marrow findings exclude chronic myeloid leukaemia, myelofibrosis and myelodysplasia as a cause of the increased platelets. Iron-deficient primary polycythaemia can present with normal or low haemoglobin. In many of these cases, the red cell count will be increased and the cells may be hypochromic and microcytic. If indicated, a short trial of iron therapy may suggest the true diagnosis of primary polycythaemia and the haemoglobin will exceed the normal range. In this case, the likely diagnosis is primary thrombocythaemia. A single mutation in the *JAK2* gene (*V617F*) on chromosome 9 is frequently found in myeloproliferative disorders, being present in over 90% of cases of primary polycythaemia and 50% of cases of primary thrombocythaemia and myelofibrosis. If positive, the test is helpful in diagnosing myeloproliferative disorders; if negative, it does not refute the diagnosis.

How will you treat this patient?

The major risk with primary thrombocythaemia is that of occlusive arterial events such as a stroke, TIAs or digital ischaemia. Venous thrombosis can also occur. The risk of thrombosis does not correlate with the level of the platelet count. Some patients, particularly those with platelet counts over 1500×10^9/L (10^3/mm^3), may have bleeding problems due to abnormal platelet function. Such patients may present with retroperitoneal haemorrhage or excessive tissue bleeding, e.g. after trephine biopsy of the bone marrow. For most patients, aspirin 75 mg daily is indicated to inhibit platelet activation. This often relieves digital pain or erythromelalgia (red, hot and painful extremities on exposure to heat) due to platelet aggregation in the capillary circulation. Aspirin should in general not be used until the platelet count is $<1500 \times 10^9$/L (10^3/mm^3). Other contributing factors to arterial occlusion should be looked for and treated appropriately, e.g. hypertension, hypercholesterolaemia, smoking history, diabetes and so on. The risk of occlusive events is related to age, particularly over the age of 60, and the presence of other contributing factors. If a thrombotic history is present or the patient is over 60 years, cytoreductive therapy should be offered with hydroxycarbamide (hydroxyurea), an RNA inhibitor, which aims to reduce the platelet count to below 400×10^9/L (10^3/mm^3). Monitoring of the blood count at regular intervals is required to determine the optimum dose and efficacy. This agent, given orally, is usually very well tolerated. Since this is a clonal stem cell disorder, there is a low risk ($<5\%$) that further abnormalities in the stem cell compartment can occur and lead to transformation to acute leukaemia over the years. The use of chemotherapy can increase this risk, particularly with alkylating agents such as busulfan, and the use of radioactive phosphorus (32P). The risk of this occurring with hydroxycarbamide alone is significantly lower, but may be slightly above the baseline risk. Reducing the platelet count does, however, reduce the risk of occlusive events significantly and is recommended for this high-risk group. For those under 60 years old, who have had no occlusive events and have a platelet count $<1500 \times 10^9$/L (10^3/mm^3), the use of chemotherapy to reduce the count is unproven, although trials are in progress. For young people under

40 years with no thrombotic history and with platelets $<1500\times10^9$/L (10^3/mm^3), aspirin alone is recommended.

Other agents can be used, particularly if treatment is indicated for younger people or those who are intolerant of hydroxycarbamide. These include anagrelide, a vasodilator that reduces platelet production from megakaryocytes, and interferon-α, neither of which is leukaemogenic. However, a randomised study comparing anagrelide with hydroxycarbamide showed a higher rate of occlusive events and a higher rate of myelofibrotic transformation in those treated with anagrelide. Thus, hydroxycarbamide is currently used as first-line treatment in the UK (and is markedly cheaper than anagrelide or interferon). Interferon-α has to be given by injection and has many side-effects. It is particularly useful when patients need treatment when other drugs are contraindicated, e.g. in pregnancy.

Key points and global issues

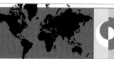

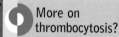

More on thrombocytosis?

See Chapter 24 of
Davidson's Principles
& Practice of
Medicine (21st edn)

- Reactive causes of thrombocytosis are more common than myeloproliferative disorders, particularly where chronic infections such as tuberculosis are present.

- *JAK2* mutation screening is not necessary for diagnosis of myeloproliferative disorders, but if positive, strongly indicates a myeloproliferative disorder.

- In future, selective JAK2 inhibitors may be a clinical option for therapy.

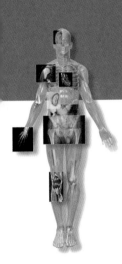

75

Blood transfusion reaction

M. L. TURNER

Presenting problem

A 69-year-old woman with myelodysplastic syndrome receives a transfusion of 2–3 units of red cell concentrate every 4 weeks to maintain her haemoglobin. During the current admission, she receives her first unit of red cell concentrate (Fig. 75.1) without incident, but halfway through her second unit she complains of feeling unwell; in particular, she feels cold and slightly sick, and complains of back pain. The nurse temporarily stops the transfusion and asks you to review the patient urgently.

What would your differential diagnosis include before examining the patient?

A wide variety of different reactions can occur during red cell transfusion. A modest rise in temperature (<1.5°C) with no other clinical signs would suggest a febrile non-haemolytic transfusion reaction, while an urticarial rash would suggest a mild allergic reaction. More serious possibilities include ABO incompatibility or a haemolytic reaction to other red cell alloantibodies, a severe allergic reaction, or bacterial contamination of the red cell unit. Finally, there is the possibility of fluid overload or transfusion-related acute lung injury (TRALI).

Examination

The patient has a temperature of 39°C and looks flushed. General examination reveals no evidence of urticaria or other generalised rash. Her cardiovascular examination reveals a modest tachycardia at 100/min and a drop in her blood pressure to 100/60 mmHg, but is otherwise normal. Respiratory examination is normal; in particular, there is no evidence of dyspnoea or wheeze. Her abdomen is soft and non-tender.

Has examination narrowed down your differential diagnosis?

It is clear that this cannot be dismissed as a mild allergic or febrile non-haemolytic transfusion reaction, and there is no evidence of fluid overload. There is no evidence of acute respiratory distress and therefore TRALI can also be dismissed. A severe allergic reaction would be expected to demonstrate relevant signs such as bronchospasm, angioedema or urticaria, along with hypotension. ABO incompatibility, other red cell alloantibody incompatibility and bacterial contamination all remain high on the list of differential diagnoses.

Figure 75.1 A unit of red cell concentrate.

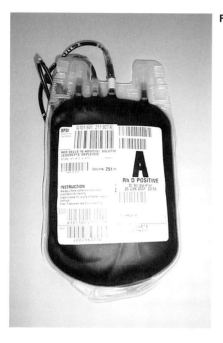

Further investigations

Close inspection of the red cell pack and prescription sheet show a discrepancy in the date of birth and hospital number with the patient's wristband. A patient with a similar name is also regularly transfused within the same ward.

Does this narrow down your differential diagnosis?

It seems most likely that the blood sample from this patient has been inadvertently mixed up with that of another patient with a similar name. Major ABO incompatibility can cause these symptoms and signs as a result of acute haemolysis. A reaction to other red cell alloantibodies and bacterial contamination cannot be formally excluded at present.

How will you treat this patient?

The unit of blood should be taken down and returned intact to the hospital blood bank, along with a fresh blood sample from the patient correctly labelled for repeat ABO grouping, red cell alloantibody screen, direct antiglobulin test and cross-match. Intravenous saline infusion should be commenced and the urine output carefully monitored by catheterisation, if necessary. It is important to maintain urine output at >100 mL/h and diuretics should be used if necessary. The full blood count and coagulation screen should be monitored for evidence of disseminated intravascular coagulation, and the renal function and biochemistry for any evidence of renal failure. Blood cultures should be taken. The hospital blood bank should be alerted immediately. Steps clearly need to be taken to prevent a recurrence of this incident and the precise measures to be implemented would be determined by local policy. In the UK, the transfusion should be reported through the Hospital and Blood Service's incident reporting systems to both the Serious Hazards of Transfusion (SHOT) and the Medicines and Healthcare Products Regulatory Agency (MHRA). Audit of hospital practice and educational intervention/retraining might be necessary.

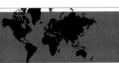

Key points and global issues

More on transfusion reactions?

See Chapter 24 of **Davidson's Principl** & **Practice** of **Medicine (21st ed**

- ABO-incompatible blood transfusion remains the most common serious hazard of transfusion, with an overall incidence of around 1 per 100 000 transfusions.

- Most are due to errors in identification of the patient at the time of labelling the sample tube for pre-transfusion testing and/or in identifying the patient correctly against the blood pack at the time of transfusion.

- If the diagnosis is missed during the early stage of the transfusion and it continues, then the risk of severe morbidity or mortality is high.

76

Unilateral swollen leg

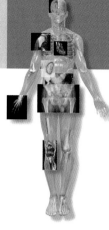

C. F. GORDON

Presenting problem

A 57-year-old woman is sent up to an assessment unit by her GP for evaluation of her painful, swollen right leg. She first noticed the pain on waking up two mornings ago and assumed that she had pulled her calf muscle slightly while out walking. However, she became concerned that the pain had not settled and now thinks that her right leg is more swollen than the left – her trousers are now tight at the ankle on the right. She feels well otherwise and has no significant past medical history. She does not smoke, drinks 16 units of alcohol per week and works part-time as a physiotherapist. She has no recent history of foreign travel. Her son has just been diagnosed with a deep venous thrombosis (DVT) after fracturing his leg while skiing. She is not on any routine medication and has no allergies. She has not applied any topical medications or cosmetic preparations to the leg. Systemic enquiry is unremarkable and she confirms that she is post-menopausal.

What would your differential diagnosis include before examining the patient?

Unilateral leg swelling is a common presenting complaint to acute medical services. The differential diagnosis includes: DVT, cellulitis, ruptured Baker's (or popliteal) cyst, venous obstruction in the pelvis, impairment of lymphatic drainage, venous insufficiency, allergic contact dermatitis to some local application, filariasis, trauma and reflex sympathetic dystrophy. Interestingly, peripheral oedema, due to congestive heart failure for example, can be asymmetric.

Examination

The patient looks fit and well, with no evidence of jaundice, pallor, cyanosis, clubbing or lymphadenopathy. Her temperature is 37.1°C, pulse rate is 60/min and blood pressure is 130/80 mmHg. Heart sounds are normal and respiratory rate is 16/min, with oxygen saturation of 99% breathing room air. No abnormality is detected on examination of the chest or abdomen. The neurological examination is also normal. Her right leg is slightly erythematous and warm to touch (Fig. 76.1). There is pitting oedema confined to the right leg. She is tender over the distribution of the deep venous system to the mid-thigh on the right. The circumference of her right calf, 10 cm below the tibial tuberosity, is 38 cm; the circumference at a similar point on the left calf is 34 cm. There is no evidence of trauma or break to the skin and no suggestion of tinea pedis. Peripheral pulses are intact and hair distribution is normal for the patient (she gets her legs waxed regularly with no recent change to hair growth).

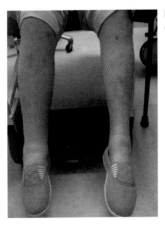

Figure 76.1 The right calf is swollen and slightly erythematous.

BOX 76.1	
Wells' score for DVT	
Active cancer (patient receiving treatment for cancer within the previous 6 months or currently receiving palliative treatment)	1
Paralysis, paresis or recent plaster immobilisation of the lower extremities	1
Recently bedridden for ≥3 days, or major surgery within the previous 4 weeks	1
Localised tenderness along the distribution of the deep venous system	1
Entire leg swollen	1
Calf swelling at least 3 cm larger than that of the asymptomatic side (measure 10 cm below tibial tuberosity)	1
Pitting oedema confined to the symptomatic leg	1
Collateral superficial veins (non-varicose)	1
Previously documented deep vein thrombosis or pulmonary embolus	1
Alternative diagnosis at least as likely as deep vein thrombosis	−2

Has examination narrowed down your differential diagnosis?

Examination has not excluded any of the differential diagnoses so far, although reflex sympathetic dystrophy would appear unlikely.

Initial investigations

Exclusion of DVT should be the first priority. Her Wells' score is 3 (Box 76.1). The clinical probability of DVT is high if the score is 3 or more. Most authorities would recommend Doppler ultrasound of the leg as a first-line investigation in this case. A typical investigation algorithm is provided in the Figure 76.2. Blood tests are not indicated at present in this case. A Doppler ultrasound scan is duly performed and shows venous thrombosis in the posterior tibial vein of the right leg, extending to, but not above, the popliteal vein.

Does this narrow down your differential diagnosis?

A DVT is confirmed. She has no obvious risk factors for DVT (Box 76.2) except the family history and she should be tested for the common familial disorders

---

BOX 76.2

Risk factors for DVT

- Increasing age
- Obesity: BMI >30 kg/m^2 (3× risk)
- Varicose veins (1.5× risk)
- Malignancy (7× risk)
- Previous DVT/PE
- Family history (especially of proven VTE at young age)
- Known hypercoagulable states including polycythaemia rubra vera, essential thrombocythaemia, deficiency of anticoagulants (antithrombin, protein C, protein S), paroxysmal nocturnal haemoglobinuria, gain of function mutations (factor V Leiden, prothrombin gene G20210A), myelofibrosis, anti-phospholipid syndrome (lupus anticoagulant, anticardiolipin antibodies)
- Pregnancy and the puerperium
- Immobility (e.g. long distance travel >4 h duration)
- Hormone therapy (3× risk with combined oral contraceptive (COC), HRT, raloxifene, tamoxifen; 6× risk with high dose progesterone for indications other than contraception)
- Intravenous drug use involving femoral veins
- Major surgery (especially >30 min duration)
- Other medical conditions:
  Recent myocardial infarction (3 months)
  Severe infection
  Inflammatory bowel disease
  Nephrotic syndrome
  Polycythaemia
  Paroxysmal nocturnal haemoglobinaemia
  Behçet's disease
  Neurological conditions associated with immobility
  Paraproteinaemia

---

after she has completed 3 months of anticoagulation and had a further 4 weeks with no anticoagulation. A thrombophilia screen includes: coagulation screen, antithrombin activity, protein C levels, protein S levels (free and total), factor V Leiden mutation, prothrombin 20210 G-A mutation and lupus anticoagulant screening tests (lupus sensitive APTT, lupus anticoagulant screen and an anticardiolipin assay). This may vary locally.

A thorough history and examination to look for occult neoplasm or pelvic vein compression should be performed, but no further investigations are required at present in this regard.

How will you treat this patient?

She should be managed initially with low molecular weight heparin for 5 days and then commenced on warfarin for 3 months with a target INR of 2.5. After 3 months, her warfarin should be stopped and she should be seen by a haematologist 4 weeks later.

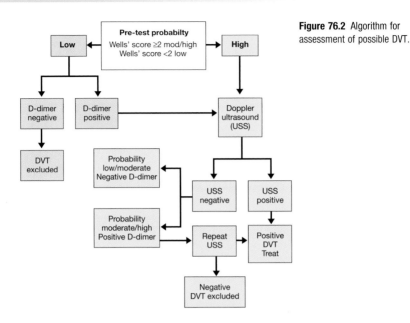

Figure 76.2 Algorithm for assessment of possible DVT.

Following cessation of the warfarin therapy, the patient was found to be heterozygous for the factor V Leiden mutation (her son was also heterozygous for this gene). She was not advised treatment with warfarin on a long-term basis (although if she had a further VTE event, this would be indicated), but she was advised regarding prophylactic measures should she require an operation, have prolonged bed rest or take a long haul flight.

Key points and global issues

More on deep vein thrombosis

See Chapter 24 of **Davidson's Princip** & **Practice** of **Medicine (21st ed»**

- Unilateral limb swelling is a common presentation to acute medical services.

- In areas where filariasis is common, this should be considered in the differential diagnosis and ruled out by appropriate blood tests.

- DVT is best diagnosed by Doppler ultrasound. If the initial Doppler ultrasound is negative, but clinical suspicion remains high, then the Doppler ultrasound should be repeated after an interval of 1 week.

- Screening for thrombophilia should be undertaken where there is no obvious cause for DVT in a patient under the age of 60 years, or if there is a positive family history (one 1st-degree relative or more than two 2nd-degree relatives). This should not be undertaken in the event of acute thrombosis or while on anticoagulation.

77

Acute monoarthritis

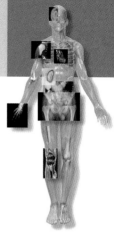

R. GUPTA

Presenting problem

A 70-year-old woman with known diabetes mellitus presents to the Accident and Emergency Department with pain and swelling of the right knee joint for the preceding 24 h. Yesterday morning, she got out of bed without difficulty, but by the afternoon noticed a mild pain and swelling in the right knee joint which rapidly became unbearable and made her virtually immobile. She now feels unwell and has developed a fever. She denies any history of trauma. Five years ago, the woman was diagnosed with osteoarthritis of the knees and was prescribed anti-inflammatory drugs by her GP; she has been taking these from time to time. She has had type 2 diabetes for the last 10 years and takes oral hypoglycaemic drugs on a daily basis. Her recent records show good glycaemic control.

What would your differential diagnosis include before examining the patient?

The two most important causes of monoarthritis in someone of this age are septic arthritis and a crystal-associated arthritis (gout and pseudogout). Other causes of monoarthritis include monoarticular presentation of oligo-articular or polyarticular arthritis (e.g. reactive, psoriatic or other seronegative spondarthritides and rheumatoid arthritis), but these usually present at a younger age. Trauma or haemarthrosis associated with clotting abnormalities will also cause an acute monoarthritis, but there is no history to make either of these likely possibilities.

Examination

The patient looks slightly pale. She is febrile (38.3°C), with a pulse rate of 92/min and blood pressure of 140/80 mmHg. Her right knee joint is warm, swollen and tender with a moderate effusion. She has severe limitation of movements of the right knee joint and is unable to flex the joint because of pain. Other joints are normal, except for the presence of Heberden's nodes in the second, third and fifth fingers of both hands. Systematic examination is otherwise unremarkable.

Has the examination narrowed down your differential diagnosis?

Not really! The prime possibilities of septic arthritis and crystal arthropathy still remain. Fever can occur with either cause and the examination may not be discriminatory. It is crucial that septic arthritis is actively considered, as this condition can be easily treated with antibiotics, but is potentially devastating if untreated. Gout seldom involves the knee joint in a first attack and is unlikely in

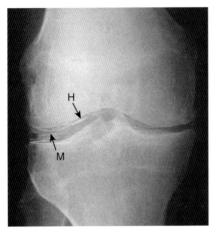

Figure 77.1 X-ray of the right knee showing calcification of the fibrocartilaginous menisci (M) and articular hyaline cartilage (H).

patients over the age of 65, without a prior history of primary gout or chronic diuretic therapy. Pseudogout is the most common cause of acute monoarthritis in the elderly and the knee joint is the most commonly affected site. Synovial fluid analysis is the pivotal investigation in patients suspected of having septic arthritis or crystal-associated arthritis, and should be performed in all patients with acute monoarthritis, especially if there is overlying erythema.

Investigations

An X-ray of the right knee joint shows features of osteoarthritis with calcification of the cartilage (Fig. 77.1). The right knee is aspirated under aseptic conditions. Examination of the synovial fluid, using compensated polarised light microscopy, shows a weakly positive birefringence for calcium pyrophosphate dihydrate (CPPD) crystals (Fig. 77.2). Moreover, an urgent Gram stain of the synovial fluid is negative and culture of the synovial fluid after 48 h is sterile. Results of other less discriminating laboratory tests show: haemoglobin 112 g/L (11.2 g/dL), white cell count 11.6×10^9/L (10^3/mm^3) with 80% polymorphs, and an erythrocyte sedimentation rate (ESR) of 70 mm/h. A blood culture is sterile. Rheumatoid factor and antinuclear antibodies (ANA) are negative.

Has the diagnosis been clinched?

Yes. The presence of characteristic crystals and the absence of organisms in the synovial fluid suggest a diagnosis of pseudogout, which results from the deposition of CPPD crystals. It is important to wait for the synovial fluid culture report, as the presence of PPD crystals and calcification of the cartilage may be coincidental in someone of this age. It is also important to remember that a high neutrophil count in synovial fluid does not necessarily indicate infection.

How will you treat this patient?

The patient should be treated with non-steroidal anti-inflammatory drugs (NSAIDs), such as indometacin or diclofenac. If the symptoms are not controlled with

BOX 77.1

Conditions associated with CPPD crystal arthritis

- Ageing
- Osteoarthritis
- Metabolic disease
  Haemochromatosis
  Hyperparathyroidism
  Hypophosphatasia
  Hypomagnesaemia
  Wilson's disease
- Familial predisposition

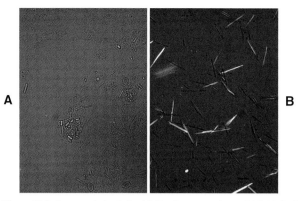

Figure 77.2 Compensated polarised light microscopy of synovial fluid. (A) Calcium pyrophosphate crystals showing weak birefringence. (B) Compare with monosodium urate crystals, which show bright birefringence and needle-shaped morphology.

NSAIDs alone, then the patient may be given an intra-articular injection of corticosteroids, provided infection has been confidently excluded. Pseudogout is associated with a wide array of underlying causes (Box 77.1). It is important that these are considered and investigated; in particular, serum calcium should be measured to exclude primary hyperparathyroidism.

BOX 77.2

Causes of chronic monoarthritis

- Infections (tuberculosis and fungi)
- Chronic sarcoidosis
- Monoarticular presentation of:
  Rheumatoid arthritis
  Seronegative spondarthritis

Enteropathic arthritis (e.g. Crohn's disease)
Juvenile idiopathic arthritis
- Pigmented villonodular synovitis
- Foreign body (e.g. plant thorn)
- Synovial chondromatosis

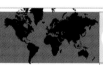

Key points and global issues

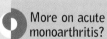

More on acute monoarthritis?

See Chapter 25 of **Davidson's Principles & Practice** of **Medicine (21st edn)**

- Arthritis due to tuberculosis may present as a chronic monoarthritis (Box 77.2) and is not unusual in developing countries where tuberculosis is still a common problem. This may be more important in countries where human immunodeficiency virus (HIV) is a major public health problem. Tuberculosis commonly involves the spine, hip and knee joints.

- The incidence of pseudogout is highest in the elderly (>65 years) and increases with advancing age.

- Osteoarthritis is the most common joint disease worldwide and the knee joint is the most common site of involvement. CPPD crystal deposition is favoured in a joint with osteoarthritis.

- Pseudogout (CPPD deposition disease) is very rare at a young age; if it is diagnosed, the associated conditions mentioned in Box 77.1 should be sought.

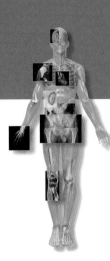

78

Polyarthropathy

E. R. McRORIE

Presenting problem

A 30-year-old woman presents with a 3-month history of joint pain and swelling affecting her hands, feet and right knee. She is stiff in the morning for around 1 h and also tends to stiffen up in the evening. Due to the severity of her symptoms, she has been experiencing increasing difficulty with fine hand function and mobility, and has been off work (she is a primary school teacher) for the past 4 weeks. Medication is ibuprofen 400 mg 12-hourly and occasional paracetamol. Past medical history is unremarkable, save for the diagnosis of a duodenal ulcer at endoscopy 5 years previously. Her mother had an unspecified form of arthritis that resulted in a right hip replacement. There is no family history of psoriasis. On direct questioning, she reports recent grittiness of the eyes and has noticed that her fingers turn pale in cold weather. There is no history of rashes, photosensitivity, orogenital ulceration, alopecia or recurrent miscarriages. She smokes 10 cigarettes per day.

What would your differential diagnosis include before examining the patient?

The character of her symptoms, i.e. joint pain and stiffness, the latter with a diurnal variation, and the reported definite joint swelling, is suggestive of an inflammatory arthropathy. Rheumatoid arthritis (RA) with associated Raynaud's phenomenon and keratoconjunctivitis sicca is the most likely diagnosis, given the distribution and relative symmetry of her symptoms. A connective tissue disease (CTD), such as systemic lupus erythematosus (SLE), is another possibility, as is psoriatic arthritis; although typically asymmetrical, this can occur in a symmetrical form. Parvovirus arthropathy is also part of the differential diagnosis, particularly as this woman's employment puts her at increased risk of parvovirus exposure. The persistence of her symptoms, however, makes this diagnosis less likely. The duration of the symptoms also effectively excludes septic arthritis, which is typically an acute monoarticular illness. The absence of preceding infective symptoms such as diarrhoea or urethritis, as well as the pattern of joint involvement, makes a reactive arthritis unlikely. A crystal arthropathy is very unlikely, given her age and gender.

Examination

On examination, the patient is found to be apyrexial. There is tenderness and slight swelling of the proximal interphalangeal joints and the metacarpophalangeal joints, and a tense effusion in the right knee, where flexion is restricted to 120°. The metatarsal squeeze test is positive. There is no psoriasis, subcutaneous nodules, cutaneous vasculitis, sclerodactyly or nailfold capillary dilatation. Cardiorespiratory and abdominal examination is normal and there are no neurological signs. Urinalysis is clear. Schirmer tear testing reveals 3 mm of moisture after 5 min.

Initial investigations

X-rays of the hands, wrists and feet reveal peri-articular osteoporosis and periarticular erosions (Fig. 78.1). Blood test results are shown in Box 78.1.

Have examination and initial investigations narrowed down your differential diagnosis?

The diagnosis of an inflammatory arthritis that is likely to be persistent has been established by the duration of the patient's symptoms and the presence of erosions. The negative family history and absence of psoriasis on examination exclude psoriatic arthritis. The absence of prominent extra-articular features, along with the raised C-reactive protein and the findings on autoimmune serology and X-rays, makes RA a more likely diagnosis than a CTD such as SLE or systemic sclerosis.

Further investigations

If available, a positive test for anticyclic citrullinated peptide antibodies offers increased specificity, compared with rheumatoid factor (RF) testing in RA. Other autoimmune serology, such as antibodies to double-stranded DNA or extractable nuclear antigens, is likely to be negative, given the clinical picture and the presence of erosions.

BOX 78.1

Initial investigations

Haemoglobin	108 g/L (10.8 g/dL)
MCV	88 fL
WCC	11.1×10⁹/L (10³/mm³)
Neutrophils	90%
Platelets	289×10⁹/L (10³/mm³)
ESR	50 mm/1st hour (Westergren)
CRP	24 mg/L
U&E, serum creatinine and LFTs	Normal
RF	Positive, 110 U/mL (0–20)
ANF	Positive, 1:80

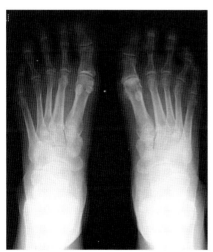

Figure 78.1 X-ray of the feet showing periarticular erosions. No periarticular osteoporosis is evident on these films, but it is often observed in people with rheumatoid arthritis.

How will you treat this patient?

Treatment with second-line (disease-modifying antirheumatic drug, DMARD) therapy should be commenced. This is likely not only to lead to a significant improvement in symptoms, but also to retard radiological progression and thus improve the long-term outcome. Opinion varies as to whether this should be sequential DMARD monotherapy, combination DMARD therapy, or step-up combination DMARD therapy, based on disease activity. Examples of DMARDs include methotrexate, sulfasalazine and leflunomide. Treatment using therapy directed against tumour-necrosis factor-α (TNF-α) is increasingly used in early disease if local resources permit, particularly if initial DMARD treatment is ineffective or not tolerated. The early development of radiological erosions is a poor prognostic sign and emphasises the need for rapid disease control. As a temporising measure, the right knee should be aspirated and injected with a long-acting steroid. Treatment with plain analgesics will afford some additional pain relief but non-steroidal anti-inflammatory drugs (NSAIDs) should be avoided, if at all possible, as the past history of duodenal ulcer increases the risk of NSAID-induced peptic ulcer disease. As Schirmer tear testing has revealed inadequate tear production, treatment with artificial tears is likely to be of benefit. Disease education is also an important part of the management. The patient should be referred to occupational therapy for advice on joint protection and physiotherapy for instruction in quadriceps exercises. Stopping smoking is important not only as a general health measure, but also because it is likely to improve the symptoms of Raynaud's phenomenon. In addition, modification of vascular risk factors is an important part of the long-term management of individuals with RA.

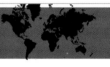

Key points and global issues

More on polyarthriti

See Chapter 25 of **Davidson's Princip** & **Practice** of **Medicine (21st ed**

- Many of the DMARDs used to treat inflammatory arthritis carry a risk of acquiring opportunistic infection, or reactivating previous latent infection.

- Autoimmune serology could be considered a luxury! Remember that the diagnosis of a CTD is primarily clinical and supported by the results of autoimmune serology, not the other way round. If in doubt, treat with a DMARD but keep your diagnostic eyes open. Most of the extra-articular manifestations of inflammatory arthritis, other than renal involvement, cause symptoms, so continue to monitor urinalysis and blood pressure if the possibility of a CTD remains.

- Treatment with anti-TNF-α biological agents is highly effective; however, access to these agents in resource-poor nations may be limited due to their high cost.

- Patients being considered for anti-TNF-α therapy should be carefully selected and should not have active tuberculosis. Patients with latent tuberculosis infection (LTBI) should ideally be screened with interferon-γ release assays (IGRAs), but in developing nations, the tuberculin skin test (TST) may be more cost-effective.

79

Osteoporosis

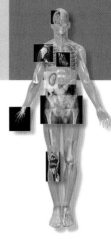

S. H. RALSTON

Presenting problem

A 76-year-old Caucasian woman is referred to the outpatient clinic with gradual onset of back pain of several months' duration. She has angina and hypertension, which are well controlled with atenolol, bendroflumethiazide and simvastatin. She has a past history of breast cancer, which has been in clinical remission for 15 years following surgery, radiotherapy and tamoxifen, which she took for 5 years but which has now been stopped. She suffered a wrist fracture about 10 years previously, which occurred when she tripped and fell while out shopping with her daughter. She does not smoke or drink alcohol, has a normal diet, her menopause occurred at the age of 42 years and there is no family history of note. Prior to referral, her GP checked some routine blood tests (Box 79.1).

BOX 79.1	
Initial investigations	
Haemoglobin	125 g/L (12.5 g/dL)
ESR	15 mm/h
Creatinine	110 μmol/L (1.24 mg/dL)
Sodium	140 mmol/L (mEq/L)
Potassium	3.6 mmol/L (mEq/L)
Calcium	2.45 mmol/L (9.46 mg/dL)
Albumin	45 g/L (4.5 g/dL)

What would your differential diagnosis include before examining the patient?

Back pain is a common complaint and could be due to a variety of conditions, including osteoarthritis of the lumbar spine, soft tissue rheumatism, ankylosing spondylitis and osteoporotic vertebral fracture. Bone metastases from breast cancer would also be possible, although the history of early menopause increases the likelihood of osteoporosis as a cause for the patient's symptoms. Aortic aneurysm would also enter into the differential diagnosis in view of the history of hypertension, but the chronic nature of the pain would make this less likely.

Examination

The patient is apyrexial and looks well. Her height is 1.53 m and weight is 52 kg. When informed of these measurements, the patient reports that her weight is steady but she thinks that her height has fallen by about 6 cm from when she was younger. There is an obvious kyphosis mainly affecting the upper thoracic spine, but physical examination is otherwise unremarkable.

Has the examination narrowed down your differential diagnosis?

The height loss and kyphosis point strongly towards vertebral osteoporosis as the cause of this woman's symptoms. Bone metastases from breast cancer would be possible but are less likely in view of the fact that the patient looks well and has not lost weight. Ankylosing spondylitis can be associated with height loss, due to fixed flexion deformity of the spine, but it would be very unusual for ankylosing spondylitis to present at this age. Soft tissue rheumatism and osteoarthritis remain possible diagnoses and could be contributing to the back pain, but neither condition would explain the height loss and kyphosis.

Further investigations

Dual energy X-ray absorptiometry (DEXA) reveals that bone mineral density (BMD) values are reduced to within the osteoporotic range at the lumbar spine (T-score −3.7), and the femoral neck (T-score −2.6). The lateral imaging DEXA shows evidence of vertebral compression fractures (Fig. 79.1). Entering her data into the FRAX risk assessment tool (www.frax.shef.ac.uk) reveals that she has an estimated 10-year risk of major osteoporotic fracture of 25% and hip fracture of 10%. Radiographs of the thoracic and lumbar spine reveal evidence of osteoporosis with several wedge compression fractures in the thoracic and lumbar spine. Degenerative changes are also noted in the lumbar spine and at the thoracolumbar junction. An isotope bone scan reveals linear areas of increased tracer uptake in the thoracic spine consistent with benign vertebral collapse. Further biochemistry is performed to exclude secondary causes of osteoporosis, including thyroid function tests, calcium, phosphate and immunoglobulins, but these are normal.

Does this narrow down your differential diagnosis?

These investigations would be consistent with a diagnosis of osteoporosis and vertebral fractures as the cause of this patient's back pain and height loss.

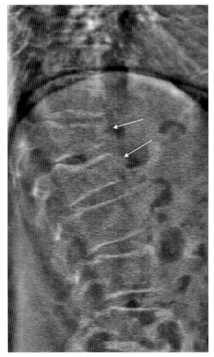

Figure 79.1 Lateral DEXA scan image showing vertebral wedge fractures (arrows).

Osteoarthritis of the spine could be contributing to the back pain but could not explain such dramatic height loss or the kyphosis, and the isotope bone scan appearances make metastatic disease unlikely. The normal biochemistry and haematology are consistent with post-menopausal osteoporosis and are helpful in excluding secondary causes of osteoporosis, such as thyrotoxicosis, myeloma and primary hyperparathyroidism.

How will you treat this patient?

This woman has established osteoporosis of the spine and hip, and fragility fractures affecting the spine and wrist. She is at increased risk of future fractures and the aims of therapy are to reduce this risk. The first choice would be oral alendronate 70 mg once weekly in combination with calcium and vitamin D supplements. Alternative treatments would include risedronate 35 mg once weekly or strontium ranelate (2 g daily). If the patient developed gastrointestinal side-effects with oral treatments, parathyroid hormone (20 μg daily subcutaneously for 24 months), Zoledronic acid 5 mg intravenously on an annual basis or Denosumab 60 mg subcutaneously every 6 months would be suitable alternatives. All of these treatments have been shown to reduce the risk of both vertebral and non-vertebral fractures. Raloxifene, calcitonin or ibandronate would be further alternatives but the evidence that these agents protect against non-vertebral fracture is less robust than that for the treatments mentioned above. Hormone replacement therapy is known to provide protection against osteoporotic fractures but would be contraindicated in view of the history of breast cancer.

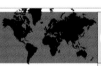

Key points and global issues

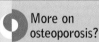

More on osteoporosis?

See Chapter 25 of **Davidson's Principles & Practice** of **Medicine (21st edn)**

- Post-menopausal osteoporosis is a common problem worldwide, although the disease is less common in some ethnic groups such as African-Americans, probably because of genetic factors.

- DEXA may not be available in low-resource settings. Although it has confirmed the diagnosis of osteoporosis in this case, the presence of vertebral fractures and radiological osteopenia in this patient would have been sufficient to clinch the diagnosis, even without a DEXA examination.

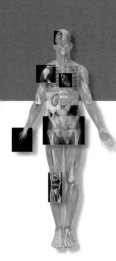

80

Antiphospholipid antibody syndrome

R. GUPTA

Presenting problem

A 32-year-old woman presents to the Emergency Department with a 4-h history of acute onset shortness of breath and left-side chest pain. Her symptoms started while working in the kitchen. She was diagnosed with systemic lupus erythematosus (SLE) 3 years ago when she presented to another hospital with fever, thrombocytopenia with proteinuria. Her ANA and dsDNA were positive and kidney biopsy revealed mesangioproliferative glomerulonephritis (WHO grade II). She was started on prednisolone along with azathioprine. At the time of this presentation, she is taking prednisolone 5 mg/day and azathioprine 100 mg/day. She has been married for 10 years and has one boy aged 9 years; that pregnancy was followed by two spontaneous 1st trimester abortions at the age of 25 and 27 years.

What would your differential diagnosis include before examining the patient?

The differential diagnosis of acute onset dyspnoea in a patient with SLE is extensive (Box 80.1). The most likely cause of breathlessness in this woman is pulmonary thromboembolism (PTE). When embolism is suspected, a source of emboli from a deep venous thrombosis should be sought. The antiphospholipid antibody syndrome should be considered as a possibility in view of her poor obstetric history and SLE with nephritis. Other causes of breathlessness in SLE to be considered are pneumonia, myocardial infarction, serositis, pneumothorax, myositis and diffuse alveolar haemorrhage. The absence of other clinical features makes pneumonia and myositis in this young woman most unlikely. Myocardial infarction, serositis and diffuse alveolar haemorrhage need to be further investigated.

BOX 80.1
Common causes of acute onset dyspnoea in SLE
• Pulmonary thromboembolism
• Pneumonia
• Lupus pneumonia
• Myocardial infarction
• Pleural effusion serositis
• Pneumothorax
• Myositis
• Diffuse alveolar haemorrhage

Examination and initial investigations

The patient is apyrexial and looks dyspnoeic; her pulse is 116/min, blood pressure is 100/76 mmHg and respiratory rate is 28/min. There are no skin lesions, oral ulcers or alopecia. Cardiovascular examination reveals normal peripheral pulses and no obvious abnormality of the heart except tachycardia.

Chest examination is unremarkable; there is no evidence of consolidation or a significant pleural effusion. She does have polyphonic rhonchi.

Some urgent investigations are necessary. Initial blood tests show: haemoglobin 135 g/L (13.5 g/dL); white cell count 7.8×10^9/L (10^3/mm^3); platelet count 98×10^9/L (10^3/mm^3); and erythrocyte sedimentation rate (ESR) 24 mm/h. Renal and liver function tests are normal. Dipstick examination of urine reveals 3+ protein. Arterial blood gas analysis reveals: PaO_2 8.7 kPa (65 mmHg) and $PaCO_2$ 2.4 kPa (18 mmHg) on 40% oxygen. A 12-lead electrocardiogram (ECG) shows sinus tachycardia and a chest X-ray reveals blunting of left costophrenic angle. A D-dimer test is strongly positive and an emergency computed tomography pulmonary angiography scan (CTPA) reveals thrombus in the left main pulmonary artery (Fig. 80.1). A subsequent Doppler ultrasound of the legs is normal.

Have examination and initial investigations narrowed down your differential diagnosis?

PTE has been identified in a young woman with SLE, but the cause of the PTE needs to be investigated further. Since examination did not reveal any heart abnormality or source of embolism, the most likely cause will be a systemic vasculitis or thrombophilia. To narrow the differential diagnosis further investigations are required.

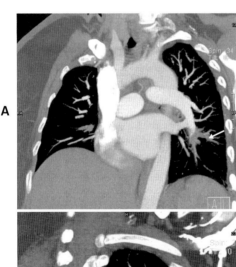

Figure 80.1 CT pulmonary angiogram showing extensive thrombus in the left main pulmonary artery (arrows), in coronal (A) and sagittal (B) views.

Further investigations

A repeat full blood count again shows mild thrombocytopenia. An echocardiogram of the heart and Doppler studies of the carotid arteries are normal. Serological test for autoantibodies show antinuclear antibody (ANA) – positive (1:320 homogenous pattern); antinuclear cytoplasmic antibody (ANCA) – negative; anticardiolipin antibody (aCL) IgG – 52 GPL U/mL (normal <12 GPL U/mL), aCL IgM – 26 MPL U/mL (normal <12 MPL U/mL) and anti-β_2-glycoprotein I antibody (IgG) – 22 U/mL (normal <8 U/mL). Her lupus anticoagulant is positive, but protein C, protein S and antithrombin III concentrations are normal.

Has the diagnosis been clinched?

Yes. The presence of strongly positive antiphospholipid antibodies in this young woman with recurrent abortion and PTE has confirmed the diagnosis of antiphospholipid antibody syndrome. Antiphospholipid antibody syndrome may be primary or secondary. Secondary antiphospholipid syndrome is common in patients with connective tissue disease like SLE. In primary antiphospholipid syndrome, no such cause is usually seen. There are many phospholipid antibodies. Most commonly used in clinical practice are anticardiolipin antibodies (IgG and IgM) and lupus anticoagulant. Recently, antibodies against the cofactor β_2-glycoprotein I have become available to aid diagnosis of antiphospholipid syndrome. It is important to remember that these antibodies may be present transiently in low titre in many other conditions, such as infections, drugs, etc., and so testing should be repeated after 6 weeks to confirm the diagnosis.

How will you treat this patient?

Initially she needs parenteral anticoagulation with unfractionated or low molecular weight heparin and subsequent oral anticoagulation with warfarin. The dose of warfarin should be adjusted to maintain an INR 2–3. The aim of therapy is to prevent further thrombosis. She will need lifelong anticoagulation. At the time of any future pregnancy, warfarin should be replaced with heparin or low molecular weight heparin. She is also at increased risk of arterial thromboembolic disease, and antiphospholipid syndrome should be considered in young patients presenting with acute stroke. Some clinicians would recommend additional antiplatelet therapy, such as aspirin, although the risks of bleeding would be increased.

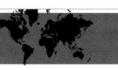

Key points and global issues

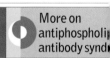

More on antiphospholip antibody synd

- Antiphospholipid syndrome is still under-diagnosed worldwide because of lack of proper investigation facilities, especially in developing countries.

  See Chapter 24 of **Davidson's Principles** & **Practice** of **Medicine (21st edn)**

- Antiphospholipid syndrome should be considered in all patients who present with arterial or venous thrombosis and/or recurrent abortion. The lupus anticoagulant test cannot be done once anticoagulation has been started.

- None of the currently available tests is sensitive enough to diagnose antiphospholipid syndrome in all patients. Increasing availability of more sensitive tests, such as β_2-glycoprotein I, should enable the diagnosis to be made in many more cases.

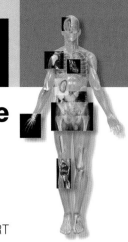

81

Acute headache

R. J. DAVENPORT

Presenting problem

A 65-year-old man develops a sudden-onset headache (i.e. of maximal intensity immediately) while masturbating, at the point of orgasm. There are no other symptoms other than nausea. He is otherwise well, apart from treated hypertension, and his only medication is bendroflumethiazide and aspirin. Embarrassment prevents him from seeking immediate medical attention, but 48 h later he is seen in the Emergency Department, where the examination is normal; he is discharged with simple analgesia. Ten days later the headache and nausea persist, and he re-attends.

What would your differential diagnosis include before examining the patient?

The concern here is that this is a secondary rather than primary headache syndrome, and the most obvious worry is subarachnoid haemorrhage (SAH). SAH is no more likely to occur during physical activity (including sex) than other benign primary headache syndromes, and this may turn out to be either thunderclap headache or headache associated with sexual activity (previously called benign sex headache or coital cephalalgia). The problem is that the history is insufficient to distinguish benign from potentially sinister headaches and thus, all sudden-onset headaches (maximal immediately or within minutes) must be assumed to be sinister until proved otherwise and require investigation. SAH may present with headache alone in between 10% and 20% of cases. Cigarette smoking, hypertension, a family history (1st-degree) and alcohol intake of more than 2 units/day are all independent risk factors for SAH. SAH is not the only potential serious cause, however, and other diagnoses, including: cerebral venous thrombosis; arterial dissection; infectious meningoencephalitis; subdural haematoma and pituitary apoplexy, should all be included in the differential diagnosis. Temporal arteritis is a potentially treatable cause of headache in older patients (usually over 60 years), but an abrupt onset such as this would be very unusual.

Examination

The patient is orientated and his Glasgow Coma Score is 15. He looks tired and fed up but not unwell. His blood pressure is 190/100 mmHg, pulse 85/min and there are no physical signs of illness. His neurological examination

BOX 81.1

Initial investigations

Full blood count	Normal
ESR	30 mm/1st hour
U&E, glucose	Normal
12-lead ECG	Voltage criteria for left ventricular hypertrophy; otherwise normal
CT brain scan (unenhanced)	Normal

BOX 81.2

Further investigations

Opening pressure	28 cm CSF
Cell count	312 red blood cells, 1 white cell/mm^3
Protein	700 mg/L (0.07 g/dL)
CSF appearance	Yellow compared against white background to naked eye
Spectrophotometric analysis	Positive for oxyhaemoglobin and bilirubin

is normal and there is no neck stiffness. The results of the initial investigations are shown in Box 81.1.

Have examination and initial investigations narrowed down your differential diagnosis?

No. Blood tests are rarely helpful in identifying serious intracranial disease in this scenario, although hyponatraemia (due to cerebral salt wasting rather than inappropriate antidiuretic hormone secretion) is common in SAH. The electrocardiogram (ECG) is consistent with the history of hypertension, although it is not an accurate guide to left ventricular hypertrophy; never assume that headache is due to hypertension outside of hypertensive encephalopathy (which is clearly not the case here, as the patient is not encephalopathic). ECG changes of ischaemia may be seen in SAH, but this is very non-specific. The normal computed tomography (CT) brain scan would have been much more reassuring if it had been performed within 48 h of the initial onset, but after that, the sensitivity of CT for subarachnoid blood falls rapidly and a normal scan never excludes SAH. Given the delayed presentation and the suspicion of SAH from the history, this man requires a lumbar puncture to exclude SAH.

Further investigations

A lumbar puncture is performed by an experienced operator and is successful at first pass. The sample is hand-delivered to the laboratory without delay. The results are shown in Box 81.2.

Does this narrow down your differential diagnosis?

The lumbar puncture has confirmed a diagnosis of SAH. At this late stage of presentation (10 days after the initial onset) and with a normal brain CT, the cell count is unlikely to be relevant and we are more concerned with the pigment analysis. As the red blood cells lyse, they lend a yellowish tinge to the cerebrospinal fluid (CSF; xanthochromia); this can be seen with the naked eye, although samples should also be sent to the laboratory (by hand, as soon as possible, and protected from light if there is any delay). Oxyhaemoglobin alone can be seen after traumatic taps, as it may form *in vitro*, but the presence of bilirubin is much more persuasive because this only occurs *in vivo* (provided the sample has not been left to degrade in light, when deoxyhaemoglobin can be broken down into bilirubin).

The next step is to identify the underlying cause, with intracranial aneurysms found in at least 85% of SAH; the remainder are due to perimesencephalic bleeds (good prognosis), and rarer vascular malformations such as arteriovenous malformations. Although conventional catheter angiography has been the preferred test in the past, many centres now undertake CT angiography as the initial test. In this case, it confirms an anterior communicating artery aneurysm (Fig. 81.1).

How will you treat this patient?

He should be transferred immediately to a neuroscience centre, if not already there. Analgesia and stool softeners should be prescribed, along with antiemetics if required. He should rest in bed and a careful fluid balance chart should be recorded, with regular monitoring of his electrolytes. He should receive 3 L of normal saline/24 h and be prescribed nimodipine 60 mg 4-hourly. His aneurysm should be secured as soon as practicable, either by endovascular coiling or surgical clipping (Figs 81.2, 81.3).

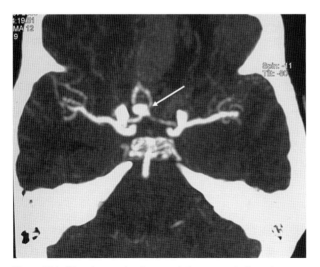

Figure 81.1 CT angiogram showing an anterior communicating artery aneurysm (arrow).

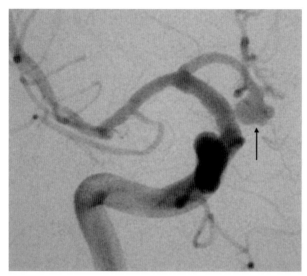

Figure 81.2
Conventional catheter angiogram of the aneurysm before treatment (arrow).

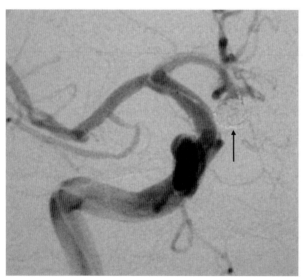

Figure 81.3 Catheter angiogram after endovascular coiling is completed, showing total occlusion of the aneurysm (arrow).

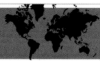

Key points and global issues

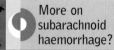

More on
subarachnoid
haemorrhage?

See Chapter 26 of
Davidson's Principles
& **Practice** of
Medicine (21st edn)

- The overall incidence of SAH is 6–8 per 100 000 people per annum.

- The risk of SAH is about twice as high for black people compared with white.

- Studies from Finland and Japan have produced much higher incidences of SAH: over 20/100 000 per annum.

82
Chronic headache

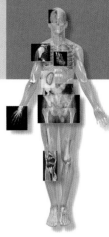

R. AL-SHAHI SALMAN

Presenting problem

You are asked to see a 47-year-old counsellor who has been referred by her GP because she has had headaches on most days of the month for the last 6 months. When you assess her, the headaches are occurring on alternate days; she finds them worst early in the morning when they wake her from sleep. She is feeling depressed.

Since her 30s she has tended to have a day-long headache around the time of every wedding anniversary; these headaches are severe and unilateral, are preceded by visual fortification spectra lasting for an hour, and are accompanied by photophobia and vomiting, all of which compel her to lie down in a darkened room. Over the year prior to your assessment, she has suffered hot flushes and her periods have become infrequent. Her annual headaches have now become much more frequent, but oral sumatriptan has not been particularly effective in relieving them. She has resorted to over-the-counter (OTC) combination analgesics, obtained from her daughter who suffers from frequent migraine.

What would your differential diagnosis include before examining the patient?

This woman has chronic daily headache, which is either 'secondary' to an underlying neurological or systemic disorder, or due to a 'primary' headache syndrome (in other words, a recognisable pattern of headache and accompanying symptoms, without underlying structural pathology). Your patient is naturally worried that she has a brain tumour. Although you must always eliminate secondary headaches from the differential diagnosis first, a brain tumour is an unlikely explanation in her case because she has no suggestive symptoms: e.g. cognitive dysfunction or focal neurological symptoms. She has early morning headaches but these are not a reliable indicator of raised intracranial pressure. In the absence of symptoms indicating other causes of secondary headache (e.g. head injury or fever), this woman is most likely to have a primary headache disorder.

Primary headaches can be subdivided according to their associated symptoms, as well as the duration of pain. Cluster headaches and other rare 'trigeminal autonomic cephalgias' tend to last 90 min at most, whereas migraine headaches tend to last for at least 4 h. Because of the difference in treatment, it is important to distinguish between tension-type headaches, which account for almost three-quarters of chronic primary headache disorders in the population, and chronic

BOX 82.1

The International Headache Society's diagnostic criteria for migraine without aura from the International Classification of Headache Disorders II

A At least 5 attacks fulfilling criteria B–D

B Headache attacks lasting 4–72 h (untreated or unsuccessfully treated)

C Headache has at least two of the following characteristics:

- Unilateral location
- Pulsating quality
- Moderate or severe pain intensity
- Aggravation by or causing avoidance of routine physical activity (e.g. walking or climbing stairs)

D During headache at least one of the following:

- Nausea and/or vomiting
- Photophobia and phonophobia

E Not attributed to another disorder

---

migraine, which is the more prevalent diagnosis in hospital outpatient clinics. Nausea, photophobia, phonophobia, aggravation of pain by movement, throbbing headache and a need to lie down in a darkened room are key pointers to migraine (Box 82.1). This woman's headaches fulfil these criteria for migraine, and their occurrence on ≥15 days/month for >3 months make chronic migraine the most likely diagnosis in this case.

BOX 82.2

Initial investigations

ESR	17 mm/1st hour
TFTs	Normal
U&E, calcium	Normal

Examination

Neurological examination, including funduscopy, is normal, but the patient looks tired and depressed. Blood pressure is 132/64 mmHg. When you palpate her cervical paraspinal muscles, they are tender. Her GP performed some simple blood tests and these are shown in Box 82.2.

Have examination and initial investigations narrowed down your differential diagnosis?

Examination has provided further reassurance that there are no signs to indicate structural pathology within the central nervous system. Furthermore, neck examination has revealed another potential factor that might be contributing to this woman's chronic migraine. It was important to check her thyroid function and calcium level, given her low mood and chronic headache, but measuring the erythrocyte sedimentation rate (ESR) was unnecessary. The ESR certainly needs to be checked in anyone *over the age of 50 years* with a new daily persistent headache, to look for giant cell arteritis (which very rarely occurs under the age of 50 years).

Further investigations

Although you might be tempted to organise a brain scan to 'rule out' a secondary cause of the headache, especially if the patient requests it, the yield of anything but incidental abnormalities on a brain scan is negligible in patients with chronic headache and a normal neurological examination. A careful drug history, including an enquiry about OTC medicines, is the crucial next step here.

Does this narrow down your differential diagnosis?

Further questioning and examination of the pill packets in the woman's handbag reveal that she has been taking at least two tablets of an OTC preparation of paracetamol and codeine on a daily basis for most of the last 6 months. On a background of infrequent migraine with visual aura, she has developed chronic migraine, compounded by analgesic overuse and cervical muscle tension. If her headaches resolve or revert to their previous pattern within 2 months of discontinuing analgesics, they would then fulfil the diagnostic criteria for 'medication-overuse headache'.

How will you treat this patient?

Gradual or sudden withdrawal of analgesics will eventually lead to a resolution of the headaches related to medication misuse. During drug withdrawal, a non-steroidal anti-inflammatory drug (NSAID) can safely provide some relief. Following analgesic withdrawal, the underlying headache disorder usually persists, and it is possible that this woman is suffering a perimenopausal exacerbation of migraine. Lifestyle measures can ameliorate migraine, and you should encourage a regular sleep pattern, regular meals, avoidance of over-exertion and minimal stress; some people find that dietary exclusion of certain foodstuffs prevents some migraines. Chronic migraine can respond to amitriptyline (10–75 mg), sodium valproate (up to 1500 mg daily) or topiramate (up to 50 mg 12-hourly), the doses of which should be titrated according to their beneficial effects and/or side-effects.

Key points and global issues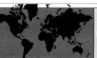

 More on migraine?

- The most prevalent neurological disorders worldwide are migraine (10% prevalence) and CDH (5% prevalence).
- Patterns of analgesic overuse depend on the regional availability of OTC analgesia.
- There are numerous potential causes of headache in patients with human immunodeficiency virus/acquired immunodeficiency syndrome (HIV/AIDS), and such individuals should be investigated thoroughly.

See Chapter 26 of
Davidson's Principles
& **Practice** of
Medicine (21st edn)

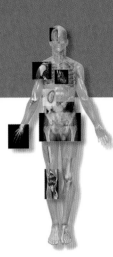

83

Peripheral neuropathy

S. B. GUNATILAKE

Presenting problem

A 25-year-old woman is seen in a neurology clinic in Colombo, Sri Lanka, with a history of numbness and loss of sensation over the left small and ring fingers. She first developed numbness about 6 months ago, and a few days prior to the clinic visit, she burnt her small finger while cooking but felt no pain. The numbness has gradually worsened and now affects the whole of the two fingers, as well as part of the palm. She has also noticed that the two affected fingers tend to bend without her being aware and that it is difficult to keep them straight with the other fingers.

What would your differential diagnosis include before examining the patient?

Numbness and loss of sensation affecting the ulnar border of the hand can be due to an ulnar nerve lesion, a C8/T1 root lesion, or even a lesion within the lower cervical cord such as syringomyelia. Ulnar neuropathies at the elbow typically present with complaints of numbness and tingling of the fourth and fifth fingers. In severe cases, there is weakness and wasting of the ulnar innervated small muscles of the hand: namely, the abductor digiti minimi and the first dorsal interosseous muscle. Ulnar neuropathy can occur from excessive and repeated leaning on the elbow, entrapment of the nerve just below the elbow by the aponeurosis joining the two heads of the flexor carpi ulnaris muscle, and following fractures and dislocation of the elbow. Ulnar neuropathy can also be a presentation of a mononeuritis multiplex such as seen in vasculitides, systemic lupus erythematosus and leprosy (Box 83.1).

> **BOX 83.1**
>
> **Vasculitides affecting peripheral nerves**
>
> - Polyarteritis nodosa
> - Churg–Strauss syndrome
> - Wegener's granulomatosis
> - Rheumatoid arthritis
> - Systemic lupus erythematosus

Examination

The patient's higher functions, speech and cranial nerves are normal. She has an ulnar claw hand on the left side and a large hypopigmented patch over the skin of the left ulnar border of the forearm (Fig. 83.1). There are burn scars on the small finger. Wasting of the first dorsal interosseous and abductor digiti minimi is present, and abduction of the second finger and flexion of the fourth and fifth fingers are weak. There is sensory loss to touch, pain and temperature over the ulnar nerve territory and over the hypopigmented patch.

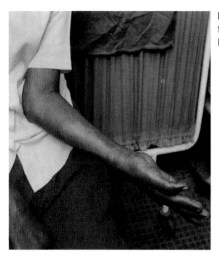

Figure 83.1 The patient's left forearm showing the ulnar claw and the hypopigmented skin lesion.

The left ulnar nerve is grossly thickened at the elbow groove. The right ulnar nerve is not thickened, but on general examination, the patient has a prominent greater auricular nerve on the left side. Lower limb examination is normal, with normal tendon reflexes and plantar responses.

Has examination narrowed your differential diagnosis?

Thickened, hypertrophic nerves are seen in hereditary motor sensory demyelinating neuropathy type 1 (Charcot–Marie–Tooth type 1). However, the absence of family history and normal findings in the lower limbs make this diagnosis very unlikely. Leprosy can be diagnosed with confidence in a patient with hypopigmented anaesthetic skin lesions and thickened ulnar and greater auricular nerves from a region where leprosy is still seen or endemic (Box 83.2). Histological examination with skin biopsy or nerve biopsy is not required when all these features are present. Leprosy is a chronic granulomatous infection of the skin and peripheral nerves with the intracellular bacterium *Mycobacterium leprae*.

BOX 83.2
Diagnostic signs of leprosy
• Hypopigmented or reddish patches with definite loss of sensation
• Thickened peripheral nerves
• Acid-fast bacilli on slit skin smears or biopsy material

Investigations

Routine blood tests are normal. The erythrocyte sedimentation rate (ESR) is 10 mm in the 1st hour. A vasculitis screen is negative and antinuclear antibody (ANA) is absent. Nerve conduction studies show absent sensory action potentials in the fourth and fifth digits and evidence of axonal damage in the ulnar nerve.

How will you treat this patient?

The diagnosis needs to be carefully explained to the patient and, as social stigma is still attached to the disease, counselling and reassurance are necessary. Multi-drug therapy is now the standard treatment. As this patient has paucibacillary (1–5 skin lesions) or tuberculoid leprosy, she does not discharge any viable organisms and therefore is not a risk to others. Treatment is with rifampicin 600 mg once a month for 6 months and dapsone 100 mg daily for 6 months. For multibacillary or lepromatous leprosy, treatment consists of rifampicin 600 mg once a month, dapsone 100 mg daily, clofazimine 50 mg daily combined with 300 mg once a month for 1 or 2 years. For the ulnar claw hand, the patient will require a splint to keep the fingers in the neutral position and advice on proper hand care because of the sensory loss.

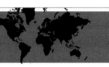

Key points and global issues

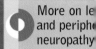

More on le
and periphe
neuropathy

See Chapters 13 and 26 of
Davidson's Principl
& **Practice** of
Medicine (21st ed

- Leprosy is still one of the major health problems of developing countries.

- When the features are typical and the patient is from a country where leprosy is still endemic (India, Brazil, Mozambique, Nepal and Madagascar) or known to occur, skin and nerve biopsies are not required.

- Leprosy should be considered in any unfamiliar skin lesion or a peripheral nerve lesion in a patient from an endemic area.

84

Acute coma

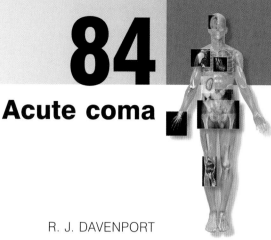

R. J. DAVENPORT

Presenting problem

You are called to the Emergency Department (ED) to see a 49-year-old man who was admitted 2 h previously. He is now unconscious and intubated, and thus unable to provide a history. The (rather vague) history is that he is a businessman who requested a doctor while in his hotel. He told the doctor that he felt unwell and dizzy, and had vomited once with some mild headache. While the doctor was speaking to him, he developed a left-sided weakness and slurred speech, and an ambulance was called. He told the staff at the ED when he arrived that he was usually well, and his only medication was a 'water pill'. He is a heavy smoker, and was able to request a cigarette in the ED. His left-sided weakness improved during his transfer to hospital, but he still complained of headache and felt unwell, and also complained that his vision was not right. He then developed a rapidly evolving right-sided weakness, and while a brain scan was being organised, his left side became weak again. He became increasingly drowsy and proceeded to have a respiratory arrest. He was rapidly resuscitated, with no cardiac arrest, and was given short-acting sedation and paralysing agents prior to endotracheal intubation and ventilation.

What would your differential diagnosis include before examining the patient?

The differential for coma is wide and, as always, the key lies in the history. By definition, this is never directly available from a patient in coma, but you must pursue family, carers, GPs, ambulance crew and anyone who might be able to provide a history. Vital questions to ask are when was the patient last well, what pre-existing comorbidities are known, and what medications are being taken? In this case, you should seek to identify the patient's next of kin as soon as possible to obtain more information, and you should also speak directly to the doctors who attended to him before he lapsed into coma.

Coma is (somewhat arbitrarily) defined as a Glasgow Coma Score (GCS) of ≤8, made up of failure to open the eyes to verbal command (≤E2), abnormal flexion (≤M4) and making unrecognisable sounds in response to pain (≤V2). You should always use the GCS to measure consciousness, and avoid terms like stuporose, obtunded or drowsy, which mean little. Never quote a sum score but describe the three components of the scale; to describe someone as eye opening to speech (E3), localising to pain (M5), with confused speech (V4) paints a much clearer picture than simply GCS = 12.

Coma requires either diffuse bilateral hemispheric damage, or damage to the ascending reticular activating system within the brainstem. Thus, unilateral hemispheric damage does not cause coma, unless there is associated brainstem compression, which is why early (within 24 h of onset of symptoms) coma due to an ischaemic hemispheric stroke is most unlikely.

It is useful to consider three clinical appearances of coma (Box 84.1), which will suggest possible underlying causes. Always consider head injury, which is usually obvious from the history but may not be, particularly in patients found unconscious with no witnesses. Beware of ascribing coma solely to alcohol. When considering 'medical' (i.e. non-traumatic) coma, stroke accounts for about 50% of all cases, with 20% due to anoxic–ischaemic injury, and metabolic and infective encephalopathies accounting for most of the rest.

In this case, the focal symptoms and signs clearly suggest a primary intracranial cause, rather than a global brain problem such as a toxic or metabolic insult. The onset is clearly abrupt, suggesting a stroke, and the alternating hemipareses and early disturbance of consciousness exclude a hemispheric ischaemic or haemorrhagic stroke, and localise the lesion to the brainstem. Thus, an ischaemic brainstem stroke is the most likely diagnosis; haemorrhage is less likely due to the fluctuating nature. The unequivocal focal signs exclude a psychogenic coma. An anoxic–ischaemic complication of this man's brief respiratory arrest is not plausible, as he clearly was developing a neurological syndrome with coma before his arrest. Rather, it was a consequence of his syndrome, not the cause.

Examination and initial investigations

Prior to this man's respiratory arrest, his coma score was recorded as eye opening to pain (E2), not speaking (V1) and extending to pain (M2), a sum score of 5/15. No details relating to other neurological signs were recorded. On examination now, he is intubated with no gag response and has not received any anaesthetic drugs for about 30 min (and the anaesthetist tells you that the drugs she used at the time of his emergency intubation will have worn off by now). There is no rash or other skin signs, and no neck stiffness. His pulse is 90/min regular, blood pressure is 205/115 mmHg, and he is hyperventilating spontaneously. He is obese with heavy nicotine staining of his fingers.

He has no eye opening to pain (E1) and extends to painful stimuli on the left, with abnormal flexion of the right (i.e. his best motor response is M3). His pupils are 3 mm and equal, and reacting sluggishly. His oculocephalic reflexes

BOX 84.2

Initial investigations

FBC, U&E	Normal
Blood glucose	12.1 mmol/L (218 mg/dL)
12-lead ECG	Sinus rhythm, voltage criteria for left ventricular hypertrophy, otherwise normal
Chest X-ray	Normal
CT brain	Reported as normal (Fig. 84.1)

(doll's eye response) are absent. His reflexes are uniformly brisk, and both plantar responses are extensor.

The results of initial investigations are shown in Box 84.2.

Have examination and initial investigations narrowed down your differential diagnosis?

Yes. The 'normal' computed tomography scan (CT) of the brain has excluded a haemorrhagic stroke or subarachnoid haemorrhage (although neither of these was the most likely diagnosis). The most likely diagnosis remains a brainstem ischaemic stroke, and early CT in such cases is often normal. In fact, closer review of the CT reveals that it was not normal. There was a 'hyperdense' basilar artery (suggesting intraluminal thrombosis) and early ischaemic change within the left occipital region; these subtle signs of early ischaemic stroke are often missed. The raised blood glucose indicates either hitherto unknown diabetes or an acute stress response.

Further investigations

The following day, the patient undergoes repeat CT imaging and CT angiography. This confirms widespread infarction of the brainstem and an occluded basilar artery (Figs 84.2, 84.3).

Does this narrow down your differential diagnosis?

This confirms the initial clinical diagnosis of an ischaemic brainstem stroke due to an occluded basilar artery.

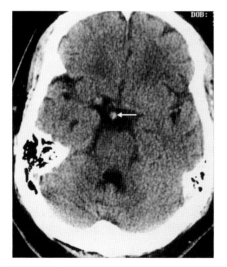

Figure 84.1 Initial CT brain scan interpreted as normal. Closer inspection reveals a hyper-dense basilar artery (arrow), suggestive of thrombosis.

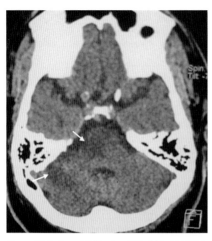

Figure 84.2 Repeat CT brain within 24 h. Established brainstem and right cerebellar hemisphere infarction (arrows).

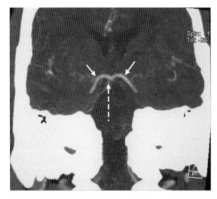

Figure 84.3 CT angiogram revealing no flow within the basilar artery (broken arrow). The posterior cerebral arteries are filling from the anterior circulation via the circle of Willis (solid arrows).

How will you treat this patient?

Where available and licensed, intravenous thrombolysis within 3–4.5 h of presentation, or randomisation into any ongoing trials would be appropriate considerations. Other more experimental techniques, such as intra-arterial thrombolysis with stenting or endovascular clot removal, might also be considered in some centres. Otherwise, standard stroke care, on an organised stroke unit, is the most appropriate management.

Neurologists are sometimes asked to see such patients several days or weeks after their presentation as persisting 'coma', whereas in fact they are 'locked in' (i.e. fully conscious but paralysed, able to communicate only with eye opening and vertical eye movements). The identification of this syndrome and discriminating it from coma is essential, and the patient described above is precisely the sort of case that may recover to such a state.

Key points and global issues

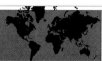

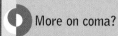
More on coma?

- Infectious diseases account for a higher proportion of coma patients in the developing than the developed world.

- The frequency of traumatic causes of coma (i.e. traumatic brain injury) has been successfully reduced in some developed countries following the introduction of safety measures, but paradoxically is increasing in many developing countries as road traffic intensifies.

See Chapter 26 of
Davidson's Principles
& **Practice** of
Medicine (21st edn)

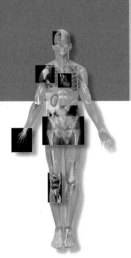

85

First fit

J. STONE

Presenting problem

A 30-year-old woman is admitted to hospital following an episode at home where, according to ambulance staff, she became unresponsive and apparently 'shook all over' for 'quite a long time'. There is a history of a previous episode 4 weeks before. She has a history of depression and is seeing a psychiatrist. She takes fluoxetine 20 mg once daily. By the time you see her, she is feeling physically back to normal, but is upset and wants to go home.

What would your differential diagnosis include before taking a further history from the patient and a witness?

The main causes of loss of consciousness with shaking in adults are epilepsy, syncope and non-epileptic attack disorder (also called psychogenic/dissociative non-epileptic attacks/seizures). Separating these relies mostly on a detailed history of the attack from the patient and a witness (Box 85.1), and much less on examination or investigations.

First, ask the patient about any warning symptoms. In syncope, there may be ringing in the ears or darkening of vision. In epilepsy, there may be no warning or an indescribable 'aura'. How did she feel afterwards? Rapid recovery is more common in syncope. Patients with a long generalised seizure usually want to sleep and may have a headache. Did she bite her tongue (Fig. 85.1)? This is common in epilepsy, can happen in non-epileptic attacks but is rare in syncope. Urinary incontinence on the other hand happens in epilepsy, non-epileptic attacks and syncope.

BOX 85.1

Features in the history that are helpful in distinguishing epilepsy from syncope		
	Epilepsy	**Syncope**
Tongue-biting	Common	Rare
Duration of shaking, if present	60–90 s	5–20 s
Post-ictal confusion	Common	Rare
Post-ictal headache	Common	Rare
Rapid recovery	Occasional	Usual

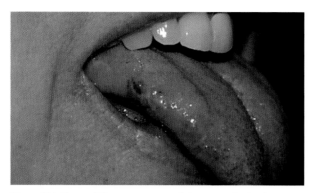

Figure 85.1 Tongue-biting occurs commonly in a generalised seizure, rarely in non-epileptic attacks and hardly ever in syncope. When the lateral tongue is visibly bitten like this, epilepsy is most likely.

Second, spend time trying to speak to a witness. Use the telephone if you have to. Remember that the witness may overestimate the duration of the attack. Could the shaking have lasted <30 s? If it did, then it could easily be the kind of brief twitching that is not infrequently seen after syncope (and which is not epilepsy). In a tonic–clonic seizure there should be a tonic phase (when the patient is rigid) followed by a clonic phase (in which the patient jerks). Typically, generalised tonic–clonic seizures last around 2 min. If the shaking attack lasts longer than 5 min, then this should raise suspicion of a non-epileptic attack, although you may need a specialist to make this diagnosis. Other clues to non-epileptic attacks include closed eyes, resistance to eyelid opening, weeping after the attack and tremor-like movements of limbs (rather than jerking).

In someone with suspected epilepsy, ask about a family history of epilepsy, childhood seizures, head injury or meningitis. Look hard for provoking factors, such as sleep deprivation and alcohol use (which are associated with a lowered seizure threshold the following day), as this may influence treatment. Do not let a psychiatric history put you off a diagnosis of epilepsy. However, the presence of multiple symptoms unexplained by disease would point more towards non-epileptic attack disorder. The presence of focal neurological symptoms or signs indicates the need for urgent investigations.

Further history

The history obtained is that both attacks occurred the day after 'binge' alcohol consumption. There was no warning, tongue-biting or incontinence, and afterwards the patient was drowsy. Although the terrified witness initially reports an attack lasting 10 min, after discussion he says that it was probably more like 2 min, but definitely longer than 30 s. The witness also comments that the woman's body was 'stiff' at the beginning of the attack. The previous attack was similar. Examination is normal.

Has the further history narrowed down your differential diagnosis?

The history is most suggestive of two generalised tonic–clonic seizures provoked by alcohol abuse. Although limbs can sometimes stiffen briefly in syncope, the duration is too long for this. There are no positive features of non-epileptic attack disorder. The use of fluoxetine in standard doses is now not thought to lower seizure threshold further, and antidepressants are not contraindicated in people with epilepsy.

Further investigations

For any adult with suspected epilepsy cerebral imaging with computed tomography (CT), and preferably magnetic resonance imaging (MRI), is usually advisable, whether or not there have been provoking factors. This is especially true for patients with focal (partial) seizures. EEG is sometimes useful in distinguishing the type of epilepsy but is rarely helpful in determining the diagnosis. Around 50% of patients with epilepsy have a normal inter-ictal EEG and there may be non-specific EEG abnormalities in patients without epilepsy. In this case, both MRI of the head and EEG were normal.

Does this narrow down your differential diagnosis?

No. Usually, the diagnosis of attacks like this depends on the history.

How will you treat this patient?

The patient has had two seizures, both apparently provoked by alcohol. First, she needs general advice about driving (depending on local regulations) and avoiding risk in day-to-day activities.

Usually, drug treatment is advised after two unprovoked generalised seizures. The decision to start anticonvulsants is a major one and should be taken collaboratively with the patient. This case is more difficult, as both seizures were provoked. The decision to treat depends on:

1. Whether the patient is likely to continue to have binge drinking sessions
2. Whether she drives or not
3. How 'risk-averse' she is.

The choice of anticonvulsant depends on the type of epilepsy, age, gender and comorbidity. First-line agents include carbamazepine, lamotrigine levetiracetam and sodium valfroate. Sodium valproate should be avoided in women of childbearing age. If this patient is prescribed anticorowcelsants than a drug without hepatic side-effects may be preferable. The patient may also need treatment for alcohol overuse.

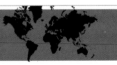

Key points and global issues

More on epilepsy?

See Chapter 26 of **Davidson's Princip** & **Practice** of **Medicine (21st ed»**

- There are many infective causes of epilepsy to consider worldwide, including neurocysticercosis, human immunodeficiency virus (HIV), toxoplasmosis, tuberculoma and encephalitis.

- An accurate diagnosis of epilepsy should be possible in most cases on the basis of a detailed history. Investigations are there to find out the cause of epilepsy, not to decide whether it is epilepsy or not.

- Phenytoin and phenobarbital have inferior pharmacokinetics and side-effects profile to newer drugs, but they are just as effective and may be more readily available in some parts of the world.

86

Progressive uniocular visual loss

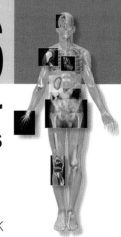

C. J. LUECK

Presenting problem

A 25-year-old woman is referred to an Accident and Emergency Department with a 12-h history of progressive visual loss in her right eye. She has been completely well until 2 days ago, when she developed a mild ache behind her right eye which was worse when she moved her eyes. The evening before presentation, she thought the vision in her right eye was a bit blurred, but it was late and she went to bed hoping that it would clear up. The next morning, the vision was markedly worse and it has continued to deteriorate ever since. She has no significant past medical history. In particular, there is no history of recent infection or of any cardiovascular risk factor. There is no relevant family history and she is not taking any medication. She is still experiencing mild discomfort behind her right eye when she looks around. She can still detect movement and shapes in the periphery of her vision, but she cannot see faces. Vision out of the left eye is normal.

What would your differential diagnosis include before examining the patient?

The fact that only her right eye is involved means that the pathology must lie in the right eye, the right optic nerve or just possibly the optic chiasm. Ocular vascular disorders, such as a central retinal artery occlusion (CRAO) or anterior ischaemic optic neuropathy (AION), would be unlikely, as the evolution has been gradual. A central retinal vein occlusion (CRVO) is a possibility, as are other ocular causes such as infections or central serous retinopathy, but these should all be obvious on ophthalmic examination.

In Europe, North America or Australia, optic neuritis (ON) is the most likely diagnosis in a woman of this age with this history, but it is important to consider other possibilities. For example, nutritional optic neuropathy or optic nerve compression from an intra-orbital mass, infection, inflammation or thyroid eye disease should be considered. The history in this case is very short, making all these possibilities very unlikely.

It is also important to remember that involvement of the optic chiasm can (rarely) cause symptoms referable to only one eye. Compression of the anterior part of the chiasm where the optic nerve joins it can catch crossing fibres from the other eye and result in a small upper temporal visual field loss, of which the patient might not be aware.

Examination

General examination is normal. The patient's visual acuity is 6/60 on the right and 6/4 on the left. On confrontation, the left visual field is normal but there is an obvious right central scotoma, and this is borne out by subsequent visual field testing. Colour vision (assessed using Ishihara charts) is markedly impaired on the right. There is an obvious right relative afferent pupillary defect (Marcus Gunn pupil). Funduscopy is normal.

Has examination narrowed down your differential diagnosis?

The fact that funduscopy is normal means that ocular vascular disorders (CRAO, CRVO, AION) and macular disease are very unlikely. There is no suggestion of involvement of the left eye, making a chiasmal lesion extremely unlikely, and there is no sign of orbital disease, making thyroid disease most unlikely. It is just possible that there may be a small compressive lesion in the orbit (e.g. an optic nerve sheath meningioma), but this would be most unlikely to present so quickly.

The examination findings are those of acute ON. If the optic disc had been swollen, this would have been labelled 'papillitis'. As it is not, this is referred to as 'retrobulbar neuritis'.

Further investigations

Some practitioners would perform a magnetic resonance (MR) scan of the brain and orbits at this point. This is not essential to making the diagnosis. (Many cases of ON show no abnormality on MR imaging.) However, a great concern is whether this episode of ON might represent the first episode of what will become multiple sclerosis (MS). Another less likely possibility is that the ON might be a feature of neuromyelitis optica (NMO).

MS *cannot* be diagnosed on the basis of just one episode. Thus, the MR scan will make no difference to the immediate diagnosis. A diagnosis of MS will only be made if the patient goes on to have a further episode of central nervous system inflammation or if an MR scan performed in at least 3 months' time demonstrates the development of new lesions. The MR scan is, however, useful for prognostication. If it is normal, the chance of the patient developing MS is <20%. If it shows abnormalities typically seen in MS (Fig. 86.1), there is at least a 50% chance that the patient will develop MS within the next 5 years.

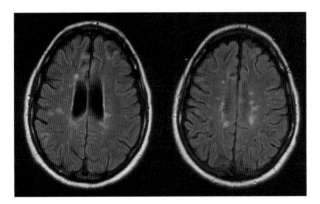

Figure 86.1 Fluid-attenuated inversion-recovery (FLAIR) MR scan showing the typical areas of periventricular high signal seen in MS.

NMO is a condition in which optic neuritis, often bilateral, is associated with transverse myelitis, although these need not occur simultaneously. The optic neuritis is often more severe with less recovery than that seen in MS. The condition has an autoimmune basis and many patients can be shown to have antibodies to a cellular water channel, aquaporin 4.

How will you treat this patient?

Most patients with ON recover vision over a few months, though their recovery may not be completely back to normal. The only available treatment for acute ON is corticosteroids but these make no difference to the long-term outcome and are only indicated if:

1. There is severe pain
2. Vision in the other eye is already impaired, *or*
3. Binocular function is crucial.

Interferon-β (IFN-β) (or glatiramer acetate) should be considered in those patients with abnormal MR scans, as there is evidence that it delays the onset of MS after ON, and it may eventually be shown to reduce disability in MS if it is started early. However, IFN-β is not available for this indication in many countries.

NMO is likely to require more aggressive immunosuppression; however, there are, as yet, no clinical trials to guide optimum therapy. Corticosteroids with steroid-sparing agents such as cyclophosphamide are often used.

Whether an MR scan is performed or not, the patient will need a review in 4–6 weeks to make sure that vision is recovering, at least partially. If there is no recovery at all, the diagnosis of ON may still be correct, but other diagnoses including NMO will need consideration. Hence, a diagnosis of ON should always be seen as 'conditional' until the patient has been reviewed.

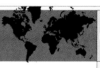

Key points and global issues

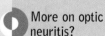

More on optic neuritis?

- ON and MS are uncommon in more equatorial countries.

- Not all countries have licensed IFN-β (or glatiramer acetate) for use after isolated ON.

See Chapter 26 of **Davidson's Principles & Practice** of **Medicine (21st edn)**

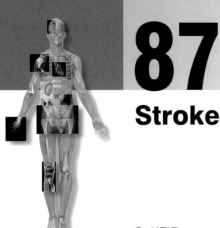

87

Stroke

S. KEIR

Presenting problem

A 72-year-old man presents with sudden left-sided weakness. He was outside walking when his legs suddenly gave way beneath him. A passer-by came to his assistance. They noticed his speech was slurred, his face looked asymmetrical and he was unable to lift his left arm up for very long. An ambulance was called and he was brought to hospital. He is a smoker and has a history of hypertension for which he takes medication, including aspirin.

What would your differential diagnosis include before examining the patient?

The presence of any one of the findings the passer-by noticed with regards to the man's face, arm and speech makes stroke by far the most likely diagnosis. About 90% of strokes are due to acute arterial occlusion (ischaemic infarct) and the remaining 10% to intracerebral haemorrhage. Contrary to popular belief, intracerebral haemorrhages can cause relatively mild symptoms. Hemispheric weakness can occur during a migraine, following a seizure and, in an elderly person, during acute hypoglycaemia. Other important causes to consider would be intracerebral tumour, subdural haemorrhage and intracerebral infection (e.g. abscess).

Examination

The man is examined an hour after the onset of his weakness. He is apyrexial and has a regular pulse rate of 84/min. His blood pressure is high at 174/102 mmHg. He is alert, orientated and able to respond to commands. His visual fields are intact. He has a moderate left-sided facial weakness with sparing of the muscles of the forehead. On being asked to extend his arms out in front of him, his left arm drifts down and his hand grip is noticeably weak. He is unable to lift his left leg off the bed for more than a few seconds. There is sensory inattention on the left side.

Has examination narrowed down your differential diagnosis?

The history is one of the strongest pointers to the precise diagnosis; few conditions can provoke significant neurological findings without warning, in the absence of triggers such as epilepsy or hypoglycaemia. Intracranial tumours usually have a more insidious history of events that individually may seem rather inconsequential – perhaps a slight increase in the frequency of headaches, atypical clumsiness or paraesthesia. Subdural haemorrhage can also present with a prodrome of non-specific signs; families may describe the person as 'just not

BOX 87.1

Initial investigations

Full blood count	Normal
U&E	Normal
Clotting screen	Normal
ESR	18 mm/h
Blood glucose	7.3 mmol/L (132 mg/dL)
Serum total cholesterol	5.8 mmol/L (224 mg/dL)
ECG	Sinus rhythm; no acute changes

being themselves'. There may also be a history of fall some time previously, which may have precipitated the start of the subdural haemorrhage.

There are no signs to suggest the man has had a fit, such as tongue-biting or incontinence. We already know he is not a diabetic and there are no signs to suggest he drinks large amounts of alcohol, which could predispose him to hypoglycaemia. He is known to have hypertension, a risk factor for stroke. Ischaemic stroke remains the most likely diagnosis.

Investigations

The man has presented within the time window for thrombolysis treatment. All investigations must be requested urgently, including CT brain. Initial investigations are shown in Box 87.1. The CT brain excludes haemorrhage and other space-occupying lesions and demonstrates the subtle signs of early ischaemic change (Fig. 87.1A).

Does this narrow down your differential diagnosis?

Hypoglycaemia has been ruled out. There are no signs to suggest infection. The CT has shown evidence of an evolving ischaemic stroke in the area of the brain consistent with the man's symptoms and signs. The pattern of signs demonstrating involvement of the cortex (inattention), along with motor symptoms, makes the aetiology of thromboembolism a strong possibility. A normal erythrocyte sedimentation rate (ESR) makes a vasculitic cause of the stroke highly unlikely.

It is important to note that CT of the brain may be normal in some patients with ischaemic stroke, particularly if performed very early on after the onset of symptoms. Abnormalities may be demonstrable with magnetic resonance imaging (MRI; Fig. 87.1B), but even if this is not available, it is still possible to make a positive diagnosis of ischaemic stroke if the other differential diagnoses have been confidently excluded.

How will you treat this patient?

This man is a candidate for thrombolysis with recombinant tissue plasminogen activator. This is a clot-busting drug that increases the chances of reperfusing the affected area quickly enough to minimise the amount of permanently damaged brain. However, it is also associated with an increased risk of potentially fatal intracerebral haemorrhage. There are firm criteria for its use, with a number of exclusions including excessively high blood pressure (>180/110 mmHg) and age (over 80 years). Maximum benefit is derived with 3 h of onset of symptoms (some benefit is seen in some patients beyond 3 h and studies are ongoing to explore this).

Doppler ultrasound of the internal carotid arteries should be performed, as carotid artery stenosis represents an important source of thromboembolism. If carotid Dopplers demonstrate a stenosis of >70% in the internal carotid on the same side as the hemisphere responsible for the symptoms, and there is excellent recovery, consideration should be given for carotid endarterectomy. This can markedly reduce the risk of further stroke, but does carry with it a chance of

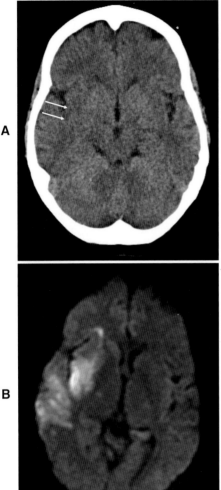

Figure 87.1 (A) CT scan of the brain showing an area of hypodensity in the right hemisphere consistent with an area of subacute infarction (arrows). The right lateral cerebral ventricle is distorted by the mass effect of the infarct and surrounding oedema. (B) Diffusion-weighted MRI. The ischaemic damage is more obvious than on CT as an area of hyperintensity in the right hemisphere.

A

B

provoking a stroke at the time of operation. Whether this is considered should be determined locally and depends on when the operation could be performed. Usually, the sooner it can be done, the most benefit is gained. However, operating on people who have just recovered due to thrombolysis is relatively uncharted territory.

Transthoracic echocardiography should also be considered to investigate cardiac sources of embolism (if carotid Doppler studies do not identify a causative lesion); if normal, however, this does not necessarily exclude a cardiac source. If clinical suspicion remains high, transoesophageal echocardiography should be performed.

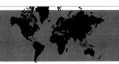

Key points and global issues

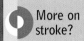

More on stroke?

See Chapter 26 of **Davidson's Principles** & **Practice** of **Medicine (21st edn)**

- Stroke is the third most common cause of death worldwide after heart disease and all cancers combined.

- Stroke is one of the leading causes of adult disability.

- Takayasu's arteritis in young females is an uncommon but important cause of stroke, especially in Asia.

- Vasculitis secondary to tuberculosis meningitis is an important cause of stroke in those countries where tuberculosis and human immunodeficiency virus (HIV) are common.

- Moyamoya syndrome is a rare cause of stroke characterised by occlusion of one or both internal carotid arteries with accompanying new vessel formation. (Moyamoya is Japanese for 'puff of smoke'; the new vessels are said to resemble this on cerebral angiography.) It has a number of causes, including clotting and endothelial abnormalities. It can cause ischaemic and haemorrhagic strokes. It was originally noted in Japan and is more common in the Asian population, but it can be seen in any population group.

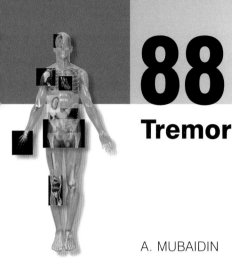

88

Tremor

A. MUBAIDIN

Presenting problem

A 67-year-old Jordanian engineer, who is a non-smoker and a non-drinker, is referred to the neurology clinic with a 3-year history of tremor. The tremor began in both hands almost simultaneously, predominantly at rest. More recently, he has also noticed difficulty in maintaining his posture and in performing some simple actions. In the last several months, he has felt his tremor getting worse and it is now severe enough that he feels embarrassed holding a cup of tea, drinking soup from a spoon and pouring water from a jug. There is no change in his speech or swallowing. He also has recent problems with his bank regarding his small signature. He denies any history of diarrhoea, weight loss, heat intolerance or frequent falls. His wife says that the tremor is now noticeable when he stands up and even when he is walking; she recently noticed some shivering movement of his lower jaw. She does not report any fluctuation in her husband's cognition. His past history is remarkable for hypothyroidism diagnosed 4 years ago; he has also experienced recurrent vertiginous attacks, along with tinnitus affecting both ears, for many years. He has taken levothyroxine 100 μg daily for the last 4 years and cinnarizine 75 mg daily for the last 5 years; he also takes aspirin, 100 mg once daily. There is no family history of a similar condition. He has seen four different doctors for this problem and has received a different diagnosis each time.

What would your differential diagnosis include before examining the patient?

He is describing a mixture of resting and action (kinetic and postural) tremor. Since the tremor occurs predominantly when resting, one should think first of idiopathic Parkinson's disease. Other diseases that can present with tremor at rest include essential tremor, drug-induced Parkinson's disease, Wilson's disease, akinetic rigid syndromes, and certain type of dementia, such as Lewy body dementia. This patient also has an action tremor, which is seen in conditions such as exaggerated physiological tremor, essential tremor, Parkinson's disease and Wilson's disease. The issue of simultaneous onset in both hands is somewhat unusual for idiopathic Parkinson's disease, and this raises the possibility of drug-induced Parkinson's disease, essential tremor, multiple system atrophy (MSA) or Wilson's disease, although the latter is unlikely to present at this age. The 'shivering movement' of his lower jaw is most likely a jaw tremor, which can be seen in a variety of diseases such as essential tremor, Parkinson's disease, dystonia, hereditary geniospasm or Whipple's disease. The absence of dystonic posturing, GI complaints and a negative family history of geniospasm, makes the latter two improbable. Essential tremor is often inherited, but can present without a family history. Review his drug history to exclude medications causing tremor, e.g. cinnarizine can cause extrapyramidal manifestation as one of its side-effects, especially with prolonged use, as in this patient.

The absence of diarrhoea, weight loss or heat intolerance makes hyperthyroidism, related to excess levothyroxine intake, an unlikely cause for his tremor. The absence of memory problems and fluctuation in cognition makes Lewy body dementia unlikely.

Examination and initial investigations

His blood pressure is 130/70 mmHg, with no postural drop. He has intact higher cerebral function including normal memory and speech. Cranial nerve examination is normal. His head posture is slightly flexed and his neck is quite rigid. A resting, postural and kinetic tremor is intermittently present in both hands along with tremor of his jaw. There is no evidence of pyramidal weakness and coordination and sensation are normal. He walks somewhat slowly and has mild postural instability. He has bradykinesia and rigidity in both upper limbs. His arm swing is decreased on both sides, and his pace is short. Thyroid function tests are all within normal range.

Have examination and initial investigations narrowed down your differential diagnosis?

The presence of tremor at rest raises the possibility of idiopathic Parkinson's disease, drug-induced Parkinson's disease, Wilson's disease, essential tremor or one of the akinetic rigid syndromes. Although essential tremor may manifest with tremor at rest in addition to actional (postural, kinetic) components, especially in advanced disease, and may even present with purely isolated rest tremor, the presence of bradykinesia and rigidity exclude it from the diagnosis.

The absence of postural drop in the blood pressure, early instability, rapid progression and bulbar dysfunction makes MSA unlikely. Patients with MSA tend to have an unusual irregular, arrhythmic tremor with myoclonic characteristics, both at rest and with intention.

The presence of bradykinesia, rigidity, postural instability and resting tremor limits our diagnosis to idiopathic Parkinson's disease, drug-induced Parkinson's disease or Wilson's disease. However, the simultaneous onset of tremor in both hands is rather unusual for idiopathic Parkinson's disease.

Further investigations

The 24-h urine copper, serum ceruloplasmin, liver function tests and slit lamp examination of the eyes were all normal. A brain MRI was normal, with no evidence of a basal ganglia or mid-brain lesion.

Does this narrow down your differential diagnosis?

Wilson's disease is now excluded. In view of the simultaneous onset of tremor at rest in both hands, with bradykinesia and rigidity, and in the presence of several years' exposure to cinnarizine, drug-induced Parkinson's disease is the most likely diagnosis.

This condition begins after several weeks to months of treatment with the offending drug. Drugs with anti-dopaminergic action can cause symptoms that are indistinguishable from idiopathic Parkinson's disease. Typical neuroleptic antipsychotic drugs have the greatest propensity to cause drug-induced Parkinson's disease. A number of other drugs have been associated, including selective serotonin reuptake inhibitors, metoclopramide, amiodarone, reserpine, tetrabenazine, lithium, phenytoin, alpha methyldopa, valproic acid, flunarizine and cinnarizine.

How will you treat this patient?

The offending drug should be stopped; when the inducing drug is withdrawn, the Parkinsonian signs should improve, though complete resolution may require up to 6 months.

When symptoms interfere with function, it may be necessary to institute therapy with dopaminergic therapy with levodopa or a dopamine receptor agonist (pramipexole, cabergoline or ropinirole) that will offer good symptomatic benefit.

In some cases, the symptoms do not completely resolve, suggesting an underlying subclinical Parkinsonism that has been unmasked.

Key points and global issues

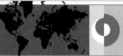 More on tremor

- The simultaneous onset of tremor in both hands is unusual for idiopathic Parkinson's disease.

See Chapter 26 of **Davidson's Principles** & **Practice** of **Medicine (21st edn)**

- The clinical picture of drug-induced Parkinson's disease differs from idiopathic Parkinson's disease in that the signs tend to be symmetrical and that tremor at rest may be less common than during posture holding.

- Lower prevalence rates of Parkinson's disease have been reported in China and West Africa.

89

Subacute confusion and amnesia

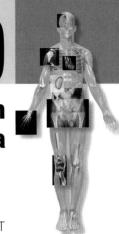

R. J. DAVENPORT

Presenting problem

A 59-year-old woman presents to the medical outpatient department. She complains of little, but her husband has noted that over the last 4 months, she has become increasingly forgetful, apathetic and has had recurrent 'turns'. He finds it difficult to describe these, but says she would typically stop talking for perhaps 15–30 s, and thereafter she would appear muddled and confused for a few minutes, before returning to normal. She is unaware of these episodes. They are occurring frequently, often several times a day. He has also been alarmed by occasional visual hallucinations, and the previous week, she told him that her parents (long since dead) had visited her, and at times she appeared muddled and argumentative. He and her family doctor thought she was depressed, although she reports no depressive symptoms on questioning.

Her past, otherwise, is unremarkable. She is taking thyroxine replacement after hypothyroidism was diagnosed 8 years previously, and 2 weeks before had been started on citalopram. She has never smoked, drinks little alcohol; her father had demented towards the end of his life, and died at the age of 82. There are no other systemic symptoms.

What would your differential diagnosis include before examining the patient?

She has presented with a subacute illness characterised by amnesia, behavioural change, visual hallucinations, and probable focal epileptic seizures, and thus the differential at this stage is wide (Box 89.1).

There is no history to suggest that this is a toxic encephalopathy due to drugs or alcohol, although this may be concealed. A primary psychiatric illness seems unlikely, given the suspicion of epilepsy. She has no other infective symptoms, and the time course is rather long for an infective encephalitis. A structural lesion(s) is possible, although the symptoms do not easily localise, and the pattern is very rapid for a degenerative disease, although dementia with Lewy bodies (DLB) can present quite abruptly. It typically causes visual hallucinations, with often quite marked diurnal variation. Parkinsonism may or may not be apparent on examination, but epilepsy would be most unusual.

The history of a subacute amnesia, epilepsy and behavioural change is very suggestive of a problem localising to the limbic system, and a limbic encephalitis (LE), either autoimmune or paraneoplastic, should be considered. The existence of Hashimoto's encephalopathy as a specific entity has been debated for many years, and is perhaps better described as a steroid responsive encephalopathy with autoimmune thyroiditis.

🔍 Examination and initial investigations

She looks well and is clinically euthyroid. There are no general medical signs. Neurologically she is intact, except for cognitive assessment; she scores 75/100 on the Addenbrooke's Cognitive Examination (ACE-R), which is clearly abnormal for her age. During the examination, she has two stereotyped episodes when she suddenly becomes vacant, with repetitive movements of her lips, after which she is briefly disorientated.

Routine blood tests are all normal, except for mild hyponatraemia (serum sodium 132 mmol/L (mEq/L)). ECG and chest X-ray are normal, as is a CT scan of the brain. Cerebrospinal fluid examination reveals normal opening pressure, normal constituents except mild elevation of protein at 0.65 g/L (0.065 g/dL). An auto-antibody screen is normal, except for strongly positive anti-thyroid peroxidase antibodies.

Have examination and initial investigations narrowed your differential diagnosis?

The absence of any persuasive localising signs is rather against a structural lesion as the explanation, and the absence of any parkinsonian signs mitigates against DLB (although does not exclude it). The witnessed 'turns' are typical for focal seizures localising to the medial temporal lobes, and the impaired ACE score would also be compatible with a limbic disorder.

Her investigations have excluded a structural explanation, as well as a metabolic cause. The positive thyroid antibodies are unsurprising given her history, but would support a diagnosis of Hashimoto's encephalopathy (assuming it exists). The hyponatraemia is potentially of significance, not as a cause for her symptoms, but because modest hyponatraemia is common in autoimmune LE.

🔍 Further investigations

An MRI of the brain demonstrates increased high signal in the medial temporal lobes bilaterally (Fig. 89.1). Paraneoplastic antibodies are negative and voltage-gated potassium channel antibodies (VGKC) are 3122 pM (normal <100 pM).

Does this narrow down your differential diagnosis?

The clinical picture and initial investigation results were suggestive of LE. Initially described in the 1950/60s, this was originally thought to be a rare paraneoplastic syndrome, associated with a poor prognosis. A number of associated antineuronal antibodies have been described, although are absent in as many as 40% of cases. In the last 10 years, however, an autoimmune form of LE has been

---

BOX 89.1

Differential diagnosis

Metabolic/toxic encephalopathy
- Drugs
- Electrolyte/glucose disturbance
- Hepatic/renal impairment
- Wernicke–Korsakoff syndrome

Psychiatric disorders
- Schizophrenia
- Depression
- Bipolar disorder

Infection
- Viral encephalitis
- Delirium associated with non-CNS infection (e.g. UTI)

Inflammation
- Hashimoto's encephalopathy
- Cerebral vasculitis
- Autoimmune limbic encephalitis

Malignancy
- Primary brain tumour
- Cerebral metastases
- Paraneoplastic syndrome (e.g. limbic encephalitis)

Degenerative
- Alzheimer's disease
- Vascular dementia
- Dementia with Lewy bodies
- Creutzfeldt–Jakob disease

described, initially in association with antibodies to voltage-gated potassium channels, but a number of other antibodies have subsequently been identified. These antibodies are thought to be pathogenic, and there appears to be a correlation between antibody titre and clinical status. The outcome is variable, but patients often respond well to immunosuppression (see below).

In this case, the clues (as always) lay in the history; LE typically presents with a subacute (usually weeks to months) onset of amnesia, seizures (focal and/or generalised), and often psychiatric symptoms such as depression, which may mislead the unwary. The low sodium is common in the autoimmune form, and provided further support for the diagnosis, and led to MR brain imaging. The temporal lobe high signal change seen is common, but not inevitably present, and the positive VGKC antibodies confirmed the diagnosis.

How will you treat this patient?

Having confirmed the diagnosis, there are two aspects to her management. First, seizure control with an anti-epileptic drug. Carbamazepine may also cause hyponatraemia and thus is best avoided. Lamotrigine is a reasonable choice, but takes several weeks to titrate to a therapeutic dose, so levetiracetam is chosen, simply because the dose can be titrated quicker, given the high frequency of seizures. However, where this drug is not available, phenytoin would be an acceptable alternative.

Immunosuppression may involve intravenous immunoglobulin (IVIG), plasma exchange, steroids or a combination of these, although the evidence is anecdotal, and there are no randomised controlled trials of therapy thus far. She was treated with IVIG and oral steroids, and had a good response. Her seizures came under control quickly, and 8 weeks later, her ACE-R had improved to 87/100, with a notable symptomatic improvement. Duration of therapy is often prolonged, with gradual tapering of the steroids.

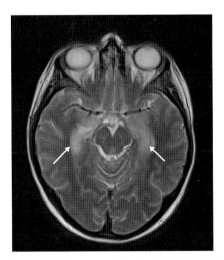

Figure 89.1 T2-weighted MR brain scan showing high signal in both medial temporal lobes (arrows).

Key points and global issues

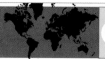

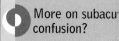

More on subacu
confusion?

See Chapter 26 of
Davidson's Principles
& **Practice** of
Medicine (21st edn)

- The global distribution of autoimmune LE is not yet well understood, and the availability of VGKC antibodies is limited (in the UK, all testing takes place in Oxford).

- In many parts of the world, phenytoin and phenobarbital remain the only anti-epileptic drugs available.

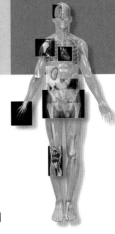

90

Functional weakness

K. R. SETHURAMAN

Presenting problem

A 20-year-old woman is brought to the Emergency Department by her parents with a main complaint of left-sided weakness of 1-h duration. She reports that when she woke up after a brief afternoon nap, she felt tightness of the throat and was breathless. When she tried to get up from the bed, she felt giddy and 'collapsed' on the floor. There was no injury due to the fall but, on trying to stand up, she realised that the left half of her body was weak and numb. She denies having any fits or twitching before or accompanying the event.

The patient has no significant past illness or known allergies and is not on any medication. On review of systems, she reports having disturbed sleep and a dull headache ('on top of my head') on and off for about 2 weeks. She had an attack of 'a rather severe headache' before falling asleep that afternoon before the onset of her symptoms. The patient has no nausea, vomiting, abdominal pain or pain in the extremities. She denies any significant head injury in the past.

The family history is notable for strokes in two of her grandparents. She is in the final year of her undergraduate studies. She is a high achiever at college, both in studies as well as in sports. She is a teetotaller. On probing further, the patient accepts having been under significant emotional stress due to her parents objecting to her wish to represent her college in a national sports event, as they felt that it would affect her scholastic achievement.

What would your differential diagnosis include before examining the patient?

It is prudent to consider organic causes and exclude them before labelling any patient as having a functional disorder. Sudden onset of motor and sensory symptoms might suggest a stroke syndrome. Stroke is less common in the young than in the elderly. In the young, the following conditions may present as a stroke: cardiac embolism, premature atherosclerosis, thrombophilia, homocystinaemia, antiphospholipid antibody syndrome, drug addiction (especially cocaine), CADASIL (cerebral autosomal dominant arteriopathy with subcortical infarcts and leucoencephalopathy), Fabry's disease, arteriovenous malformation, 'berry' aneurysm and arterial dissection. If organic disorders are excluded, dissociative disorder (conversion reaction) or factitious disorder (malingering) is more likely.

Examination

On physical examination, the patient is fully conscious, comfortable, lying supine on a stretcher and, in contrast to her parents, seems unconcerned about her symptoms. Markedly weak left extremities and slightly slurred speech are evident on an initial assessment. Vital signs reveal temperature of 37°C, blood pressure of

110/76 mmHg, heart rate of 78 beats/min, respiratory rate of 12 breaths/min and oxygen saturation of 98% on room air. Her skin appears healthy; there is no xanthelasma. She has no injury marks and her neck is supple. Heart, lung and abdominal examinations are unremarkable.

Detailed neurological examination reveals the patient to be alert and oriented to time, person and place; she exhibits left-sided hemi-neglect. The pupils are normal and react to light and accommodation. Visual field examination is equivocal and does not yield consistent findings. Extra-ocular movements are normal in range. Ocular fundi examination reveals no papilloedema. There is no facial asymmetry when the patient wrinkles her eyebrows or shows her teeth, but she is not able to puff out her left cheek. Touch and pain sensations appear to be decreased on the left side of the face. She cannot shrug her left shoulder nor use the left sternocleido-mastoid to laterally rotate her head. The swallowing and gag reflexes are intact. There is no deviation of the protruded tongue.

There is no atrophy or fasciculation of her upper or lower limbs. Although the motor power of the right arm and leg is only slightly affected (grade 4/5), the patient is unable to lift the left arm or leg (grade 2/5). The grip of the left hand is very weak (25% strength). The left half of the body has decreased touch and pain perception. On careful testing for pain, the loss of sensation extends exactly up to the midline of the torso and face. The patient is not able to perform finger-to-nose test or rapid alternating hand movements with the left extremity. Deep tendon reflexes are normal in all the four extremities. The plantar response is downward on both sides. With the patient supine, when her left hand is dropped from above her face, it deviates slightly, lands on the pillow and does not strike her face. When she is asked to lift her normal right leg off the bed against resistance, the left heel presses firmly on the bed; when this test is repeated on the affected left side, the right heel does not press on the bed. When she is coaxed to try to stand and walk a few steps, she lurches wildly in all directions and always falls in the direction (front, back of left) where the chaperone nurse is assisting her. Romberg's sign cannot be reliably tested in this setting.

Has examination narrowed down your differential diagnosis?

Yes, there are several pointers in the case history and physical findings to make a firm diagnosis in this case:

1. *In contrast to her parents, the patient seems unconcerned about the event.* Apparent lack of concern about the nature or implications of the syndrome is known as '*La belle indifference*' (the indifferent young woman).
2. *The patient had 'collapsed' on the floor without any injury due to the fall.* This is characteristic of functional disorders.
3. *The patient has no facial asymmetry and yet she is unable to puff out her left cheek*, suggesting it to be a functional weakness.
4. *The patient cannot use the left sternocleidomastoid to laterally rotate her head.* Patients with psychogenic hemiparesis often have ipsilateral weakness of the sternocleidomastoid muscle. However, this muscle, which is innervated bilaterally, is not paralysed in most cases of organic hemiparesis. This clinical sign known as 'sternocleidomastoid test' is useful to differentiate between organic and functional paralysis.
5. *When the patient is asked to lift her normal right leg off the bed against resistance, the left heel presses firmly on the bed; when this test is repeated on the affected left side, the right heel does not press on the bed.* This is known as 'The Hoover sign' of functional paralysis. In organic left-sided hemiparesis, when the patient tries to lift the affected leg, the normal heel will press on the bed and when he/she tries to lift the normal leg, the paralysed heel will remain flaccid.

6. *When the patient's left hand is dropped from above her face, it does not strike her face.* This sign is characteristic of functional paralysis.

7. *The loss of sensation extends exactly up to the midline of the patient's torso and face.* In organic lesions, the sensory loss stops short of midline as sensory innervation is bilateral close to the midline.

8. This patient is a 20-year-old woman with *emotional stress due to her parents objecting to her wish to represent her college in a national sports event.* Due to the stress, she has had *disturbed sleep and a tension-type headache.* Dissociative disorders are predominantly seen in younger women. The symptoms of a conversion are often triggered by psychosocial stressors. Her experience of having observed a stroke in two of her grandparents may have contributed to the presenting features in her case.

The firm diagnosis in this case is: Dissociative reaction – with functional left-sided motor and sensory deficits.

How will you treat this patient?

The clinical findings in this patient are typical of functional neurological deficits. It is better to avoid unnecessary referrals and investigations in such cases. Further tests could reinforce illness behaviour and disability.

Management of dissociative reactions can be quite challenging. Demonstrate by words and non-verbal clues that you believe that this patient's problems are genuine, even if there is no organic basis for them. Explain that almost half of the patients reporting to primary care do not have an organic basis for their symptoms. Educate her on the mind–body connection and how stress and unresolved conflict can provoke somatic symptoms, like paralysis. Try to establish a collaborative therapeutic partnership to manage the hemiparesis. This includes nursing care, physiotherapy and rehabilitative care until she is fully functional again. The patient, being a collegian familiar with the internet, can be guided to appropriate weblinks to learn more about somatoform disorders. Encourage her to be optimistic with the knowledge that full recovery is just a matter of time. Inform her that she needs specialist professional assessment and advice from a psychiatrist. Educate the parents of the patient not to be over protective, as it may reinforce illness behaviour and delay recovery. In this particular case, the unresolved conflict of wanting to excel in sports without losing out on scholastic performance may have triggered the dissociation. Resolving the conflict may hasten recovery and may reduce the chance of recurrence.

Key points and global issues

- Somatoform disorders are a global problem and form a significant portion of the burden of illness.

- About 40% of presenting problems in primary-care practice are likely to be medically unexplainable. Therefore, a primary healthcare provider has to acquire the competence and skills to manage these cases.

- Patients with recurrent somatoform disorders may be referred for cognitive behaviour therapy (CBT). However, be cautious in traditional communities where referral to a psychiatric service has stigma attached to it.

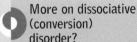

More on dissociative (conversion) disorder?

See Chapter 10 of
Davidson's Principles
& **Practice** of
Medicine (21st edn)

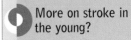

More on stroke in the young?

See Chapter 26 of
Davidson's Principles
& **Practice** of
Medicine (21st edn)

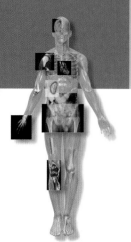

91

Anaphylaxis

S. E. MARSHALL

 Presenting problem

A 28-year-old woman is referred for assessment of possible anaphylaxis. Her first episode occurred 2 months previously, when she developed swelling of her lips associated with a generalised itchy rash 20 min after eating Chinese-style chicken, vegetables and rice. Her symptoms settled with oral antihistamines and she did not seek medical advice. Six weeks later, she developed sudden onset of flushing, lip swelling, lightheadedness and profound fear, while sitting in a café. She collapsed on to the floor and vomited profusely, but did not experience loss of consciousness. Paramedics were called and noted that her blood pressure was 80/50 mmHg. She was taken to the Accident and Emergency Department, where she received intramuscular adrenaline (epinephrine) and intravenous chlorpheniramine and hydrocortisone. She made a good recovery and was discharged after an overnight stay. On this occasion, her reaction was associated with eating a hummus (chickpea) spread.

She has mild summer hay fever, but no previous history of food allergy, asthma or eczema, and is not on any medication.

What would your differential diagnosis include before examining the patient?

Her history of sudden onset of urticaria, angioedema, breathlessness and hypotension is very suggestive of an anaphylactic reaction. This is most likely to be associated with a specific food allergy, but other causes of anaphylaxis, including medications, insect stings, latex and exercise, should be considered as possible triggers. Systemic diseases that may present with symptoms similar to anaphylaxis include phaeochromocytoma, carcinoid syndrome and mastocytosis.

 Examination

Physical examination is unremarkable.

Has examination narrowed down your differential diagnosis?

Physical examination is frequently normal in patients with a history of anaphylaxis and so may not narrow down the differential diagnosis.

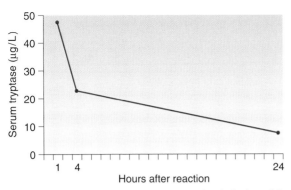

Figure 91.1 Change in serum tryptase concentrations in the hours following the anaphylactic episode. Normal range 0–14 µg/L.

Investigations

At the time of her acute admission to hospital, blood was taken for serum tryptase. This showed a very elevated tryptase immediately after the event, falling to within the normal range over 24 h (Fig. 91.1). Routine haematology, biochemistry and liver function tests are normal.

Skin prick tests to sesame and chickpeas are performed in the clinic; she develops a positive wheal and flare response to sesame.

Does this narrow down your differential diagnosis?

The sharp rise in serum tryptase at the time of clinical symptoms is pathognomonic of acute mast cell degranulation. However, this does not identify the mechanism (immunoglobulin E (IgE)-mediated or non-IgE-mediated) or the trigger. The finding of a positive skin prick test to sesame in conjunction with a consistent clinical history is very suggestive of specific allergy to sesame.

How will you treat this patient?

Exposure to sesame should be rigorously avoided. Sesame is often used for flavouring and decorative purposes in foods, and thus careful reading of package labelling is required. Sesame is also used in cosmetics, and sesame oil may occasionally be present in pharmaceuticals.

This patient should also be educated in the recognition and management of an allergic reaction in the event of inadvertent exposure. She should be prescribed oral antihistamines to be taken for mild symptoms (e.g. lip swelling). Given her history of anaphylaxis, she should also be prescribed self-injectable adrenaline (e.g. EpiPen or Anapen 1 : 1000, 0.3 mL×2 syringes), to be administered intramuscularly if she develops severe symptoms (breathlessness, syncope). Patients and their families should be shown how to use self-injectable adrenaline, and should be provided with written guidelines as to its use. She should also be advised to wear a Medic-Alert bracelet, highlighting her allergy.

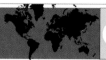

Key points and global issues

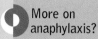

More on anaphylaxis?

See Chapter 4 of
Davidson's Principles
& **Practice** of
Medicine (21st edn)

- Between 1990 and 2005, admissions for anaphylaxis increased by 600% in the UK.

- The prevalence of allergic diseases has reached epidemic proportions in Western countries. In addition, recent studies have shown that the prevalence of allergic disorders in children is rising rapidly in recently industrialised regions, including the Indian subcontinent and Latin America. Urban centres in developing countries may have few resources to implement management programmes for these diseases in the face of multiple other demands.

- The accuracy of food labelling varies in different countries and among different manufacturers. In addition, allergen advisory statements, such as 'may contain …' or 'free from …', have no standard definitions. Thus, food labelling is often a source of confusion and limits food choices for individuals with allergic diseases.

92

The changing mole

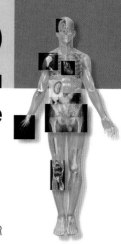

J. A. A. HUNTER

Presenting problem

A 16-year-old white girl is referred urgently by her GP to the dermatology clinic. She says that a black mole on her right calf appeared 3 months ago. It is enlarging, becoming more prominent and began to itch about 2 weeks ago. It bled, just once and a tiny amount, a week ago. On closer questioning, she thinks that there might have been a small flat brown mark near the same spot previously, but is not certain. Her general health is good and she does not take any regular medication. Although dark-haired, she has a fair skin and says that she usually burns with even short sun exposure and tans poorly (skin type II). Nevertheless, she does sunbathe and holidays in the sun every year. She has never used a sunbed. Nobody in her family has ever had a skin tumour.

What would your differential diagnosis include before examining the patient?

Her GP is obviously concerned or she would not have been referred urgently to the clinic. The sudden appearance of a black lesion on a white female's leg, together with itch and bleeding, is indeed a major *change* and should sound a loud alarm bell. First and foremost, malignant melanoma must be excluded; this diagnosis would fit in with her history of sunbathing. However, if she is lucky, this might be due to a benign pigmented lesion such as a melanocytic naevus; but why has it enlarged so much recently? A Spitz naevus (previously called juvenile melanoma) is another benign lesion; although it usually presents as a pink or red nodule, it is a possibility in this case. Dermatofibromas are common at this site and occur in this age group, but they are usually skin-coloured or just lightly pigmented. Seborrhoeic warts are most common on the trunk in older age groups, but are occasionally seen on the leg in the young. Pigmented basal cell carcinomas are almost never seen at this site in this age group. Acquired haemangiomas, including the misnamed pyogenic granuloma, are sometimes very dark and, if thrombosed, black; they should be borne in mind. A rare pigmented adnexal (from a sweat gland or hair follicle) tumour would also be at the end of the differential diagnosis list of most smart dermatologists.

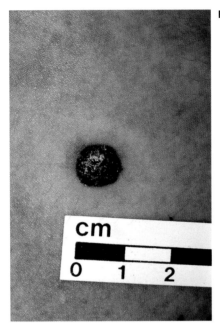

Figure 92.1 A nodule on the right calf.

Examination

The girl looks anxious but otherwise well. There is a dark brown-black nodule, measuring 1 cm in diameter, on the right calf (Fig. 92.1). On the surface of the nodule, there is a tiny area of crusting. There are no hairs. The nodule is symmetrical, the border sharply demarcated, the colour uniform and the elevation regular. There is a narrow (1–2 mm) rim of erythema around most of the nodule. She has a sprinkling (about 20–30 in all) of unexceptional-looking melanocytic naevi on her trunk and legs. There is no significant local or distal lymphadenopathy. The liver is not palpable.

Initial investigation

Examination of the lesion with a hand-held dermatoscope indicates that it is of melanocytic origin and that there are many features suggestive of malignant melanoma; the appearance rules out a heavily pigmented seborrhoeic wart and a haemangioma. Dermatoscopy is a relatively recent diagnostic aid, additional to clinical examination. Very useful in expert hands, it in no way replaces careful observation with the help of a hand lens.

Has examination narrowed down your differential diagnosis?

It seems all but certain that this is a malignant melanoma. Multiple benign melanocytic naevi (as this girl has) are a risk factor, as well as her skin type. The examination, confirmed by the dermatoscopic appearance, has ruled out most of the alternatives mentioned above, with the exception of a Spitz naevus. But, as already mentioned, these naevi are usually pink or red and seldom heavily pigmented.

The useful ABCDE (*A*symmetry, irregular *B*order, irregular *C*olour, *D*iameter >5 mm, irregular *E*levation) rule, relating to examination of the tumour, was not helpful here – a reminder that no rules are sacrosanct and that common sense must always prevail. In this case, the warning light was the history of sudden and undoubted *change* in a pigmented skin lesion.

Histological confirmation is required and the lesion should be excised straight away, under local anaesthetic, with a 5 mm margin of normal skin around (including deep to) the tumour.

Further investigations

The pathology report concludes, 'This is a nodular malignant melanoma, with incipient ulceration. Tumour thickness (Breslow): 2.5 mm'. A standard chest X-ray is reported as normal.

Does this narrow down your differential diagnosis?

Yes. The diagnosis of an intermediate-thickness, nodular malignant melanoma is confirmed.

How will you treat this patient?

Wider excision of the area is indicated. For tumours of this thickness, the margin of excision around the excision biopsy site should be 2–3 cm; more radical surgery (4–6 cm excision margins) would provide no greater benefit, in terms of local recurrence or survival. Some surgeons in specialist centres will examine a sentinel node (the first and often nearest local node in the lymphatic drainage of the tumour) at the time of wider excision, if the tumour already removed was thicker than 1.0 mm. If metastatic tumour is found in the sentinel node, then block dissection of the regional nodes (the ilio-femoral group in this case) should be performed.

If there are no facilities for sentinel node biopsy and if the local nodes are not clinically enlarged, then no further treatment is required. Prophylactic lymph node dissection is no longer advised in this group but, should clinically enlarged local nodes be noted at follow-up, then the entire lymph node basin should be removed.

The patient should be followed-up regularly to detect metastases (loco-regional and distant) and new primary melanomas (risk about 2%). Many advise lifetime follow-up but, in busy hospitals, a common regimen for a patient with an invasive melanoma is at 3-month intervals for the first 3 years and then, if all is well, 6-monthly for a total follow-up time of 5 years. At these appointments, advice about avoiding excessive sun exposure and using appropriate sunblocks should be continually reinforced and the patient taught to self-examine for loco-regional metastases and new primaries. The medical assessment should also include a whole-body examination to check for second primary melanomas. Further investigations at follow-up clinics are not routine unless there are specific clinical indications.

This patient has a clinical stage 1 malignant melanoma (primary lesion only with no nodal or distant metastases). The thickness of the tumour, measured microscopically by Breslow's method, gives a very good estimate of the prognosis. This girl has around an 80% chance of being alive and tumour-free in 5 years' time (Box 92.1). At present, there is no compelling evidence that any adjunctive chemotherapy will improve her prognosis.

BOX 92.1

Prognostic indicators in malignant melanoma

Indicator	Significance
Depth of primary tumour (Breslow)	
<0.75 mm	5-year survival 95%
0.76–1.5 mm	5-year survival 85%
1.51–3.5 mm	5-year survival 75%
>3.5 mm	5-year survival 50%
Sex	Females do better than males
Age	Prognosis worsens after 50 years of age, especially in males
Site	Prognosis is poorer for tumours on trunk, upper arms, neck and scalp
Ulceration	Signifies a poor prognosis
Sentinel node	Prognosis worsens with tumour-positive sentinel node
Clinical stage	Prognosis worsens with advancing stage

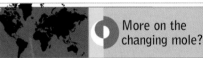

Key points and global issues

More on the changing mole?

See Chapter 27 of
Davidson's Principles & **Practice** of
Medicine (21st edn)

- Episodic exposure of fair-skinned individuals (especially those with multiple melanocytic naevi) to intense sunlight is thought to be the main cause of the steadily increasing incidence of melanoma worldwide.

- There is a higher incidence of malignant melanoma in white people living near the equator than in temperate zones.

- The highest incidence, more than 40 per 100 000 per year, is seen in white people living in Australia and New Zealand.

- The tumour is rare before puberty and in black people, Asians and Orientals; when it does occur in these races, it is most often on the palms, soles or mucous membranes.

- Sentinel node biopsy is a staging procedure and, at present, there is no evidence for better outcome in those in whom sentinel node biopsy is performed than in those whom it is not.

93

Pruritus

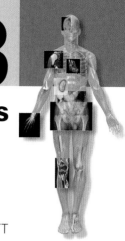

D. KEMMETT

Presenting problem

A 70-year-old man is seen in the outpatient department with a 10-year history of generalised itch. He lives alone and has a poor diet. He has been treated over the years with a large number of topical preparations, including topical corticosteroids. Other treatments have included several courses of antihistamines and antibiotics. Apart from itch, he feels otherwise well. His past medical history includes hypertension for the past 5 years, for which he takes atenolol and bendroflumethiazide. He smokes 20 cigarettes a day and admits to drinking over 30 units of alcohol per week. He has not suffered from any other skin problems and there is no relevant family history. There are no pets in the house and he denies contact with other animals.

What would your differential diagnosis include before examining the patient?

Itch can occur as a result of inflammatory processes in primary cutaneous disease or from systemic disease. Therefore, a detailed history is essential to diagnose the cause of itching. The time course, extent (generalised vs localised), severity, aggravating and alleviating factors, bathing history, past medical and drug history are the most important questions. A history of previous skin problems should always be asked. Other possible questions include involvement of other family members, contact with animals, travel history, sexual history and history of intravenous drug abuse.

Eczema, lichen planus and dermatitis herpetiformis are primary cutaneous diseases that invariably cause itch. Contrary to wide-held belief, psoriasis is often itchy. Incessant itching, worst at night-time, dominates the picture (excoriations, eczematised patches and urticated papules) caused by the human scabies mite. Infestations with lice and animal mites, as well as insect bites, must always be excluded in a patient scratching himself to bits. Our patient gives no previous history of skin problems and he denies that any close contacts are similarly afflicted, as would be likely with scabies.

A systemic cause must be excluded. Itch is a common symptom in primary biliary cirrhosis and obstructive jaundice. The itch of polycythaemia often begins some minutes after bathing. Itch is also a common symptom of chronic renal failure, particularly in patients treated with dialysis. Lymphoma is always important to consider, as pruritus may be present for many months before other signs of the disease. Only very occasionally does diabetes mellitus present with generalised pruritus. Drug eruptions are often itchy but we can exclude this cause here as our patient was symptomatic years before he started treatment for hypertension. Psychological factors, such as anxiety, depression and psychoses, can bring about and frequently worsen pruritus, whatever its cause. Some patients may be unshakably convinced that they are infested with parasites and no rational argument can convince them that they are not.

The chronicity of the symptom in our patient makes any serious underlying systemic disease unlikely. However, a diagnosis is rarely possible from the history alone; so examination should help.

Examination

Examination reveals a man, with an unkempt appearance, who looks unhappy and older than his years. Observation of his skin reveals that it is dry and that there is a symmetrical rash composed of multiple excoriated nodules on the arms (Fig. 93.1), thighs, abdomen and back. There is sparing of the mid-back (where the patient cannot reach to scratch), the so-called 'butterfly sign' (Fig. 93.2). Some of the lesions are crusted. The patient also has superficial white scars on the forearm and anterior chest, the legacy of picking. The nails are shiny, presumably due to rubbing. The oral mucosa is normal. There are no signs of the primary skin disorders mentioned above. No burrows/scabies mites or lice can be seen after a careful search. There is no significant lymphadenopathy and the liver and spleen are impalpable. Physical examination is otherwise unremarkable.

Has examination narrowed down your differential diagnosis?

The signs in our patient are exclusively secondary skin lesions of excoriation (due to picking), lichenification (due to rubbing) and scarring. Examination failed to reveal any primary skin lesions characteristic of eczema, lichen planus or psoriasis. Furthermore, a negative search for burrows and mites (scabies) and groups of small blisters (dermatitis herpetiformis) has all but ruled out these conditions. The examination suggests that the diagnosis is unlikely to be due to a specific skin disease.

Does this narrow down your differential diagnosis?

Since a primary skin disorder cannot be identified, further investigations are required to exclude a systemic cause. The laboratory work-up should include standard urine analysis, a full blood count with differential white cell count, ESR

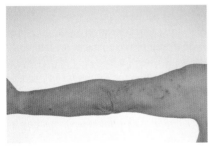

Figure 93.1 Multiple excoriated nodules are seen on the arm.

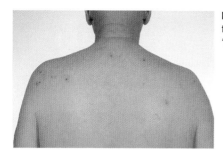

Figure 93.2 The central back is clear because the patient cannot reach to scratch (the 'butterfly sign').

and tests of renal, liver and thyroid function. A random blood glucose should be measured. In addition, a chest X-ray should be considered. As the primary lesions of dermatitis herpetiformis may be masked by the patient response of scratching and rubbing of the skin, a skin biopsy plus immunofluorescence studies might be undertaken.

Further investigations

The routine blood tests and chest X-ray are normal. Skin biopsy shows a hyperkeratotic epidermis with acanthosis (thickening). The rete ridges are elongated and irregular with a dense dermal infiltrate consisting of neutrophils, eosinophils, histiocytes and monocytes. Immunofluroescence studies are negative.

Has the diagnosis been clinched?

A primary skin disease and any serious underlying internal cause have all but been excluded. It is likely that this elderly man's skin has become itchy because it is too dry. Generalised pruritus is not uncommon in this setting and the problem may be compounded by irritation, due to over-enthusiastic scratching and the excessive use of antiseptics and soaps. It would now be worthwhile treating him under supervision, to assess if the vicious itch–scratch cycle can be broken. If the symptoms and signs remain unabated, then further follow-up and investigations (e.g. MRI or CT imaging) will be necessary.

How will you treat this patient?

The patient should attend an outpatient treatment centre for potent topical steroids and occlusive bandaging. A short course of oral prednisolone may sometimes help in the initial stages. Intra-lesional injections of corticosteroid may also help in stubborn areas. Systemic antibiotics may be necessary if the lesions become secondarily infected and antihistamines may give some partial relief of itch. The patient should be encouraged to use emollients and to avoid over exposure to soaps.

Frequent follow-up may be necessary, as the condition is often chronic with frequent relapses. In refractory cases, ultraviolet light (UVB therapy) may sometimes improve the condition. In some patients, control of pruritus may be achieved with the use of antidepressants or anti-psychotic agents.

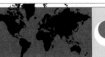
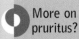
More on
pruritus?

See Chapter 27 of
Davidson's Principles
& **Practice** of
Medicine (21st edn)

- Parasitic infestation, especially due to scabies and lice, is a common cause of pruritus in the tropics and subtropics, especially in poor rural areas.

- No examination of a patient with generalised pruritus of unknown origin is complete without a thorough search for burrows (scabies) and lice (in the clothing too).

- Generalised pruritus may occur months before other manifestations of a lymphoma.

- Itch is *pruritus*, not *pruritis*.

94

Widespread scaly rash

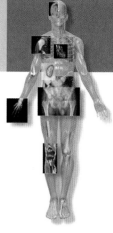

J. D. BOS

Presenting problem

A 28-year-old woman presents with a 2-week history of a widespread rash. It erupted over a few days, starting on the face and then spreading to most of the body. She complains of a deep and severe burning sensation that prevents her from sleeping. Itch is a less troubling feature. During the night, she walks around her apartment, taking cold showers and trying ointments and creams, including lotions containing menthol, without effect. She is otherwise healthy but has been treated for moderate acne with topical and systemic agents, including topical benzoyl peroxide, occasional use of topical erythromycin lotion and systemic antibiotics. There is no history of atopy. She is a hairdresser and beautician, and has never had hand eczema. Her skin is not easily irritated and she denies any allergies to cosmetics. She knows that she is allergic to nickel and avoids wearing jewellery that contains nickel.

What would your differential diagnosis include before examining the patient?

We have a patient with an eruptive and widespread red, scaly rash. Box 94.1 lists the most common causes of this presentation. Examination should help to narrow down the differential diagnosis.

Examination

On full examination of the skin, a widespread, symmetrical and somewhat violet, erythematous rash is apparent (Fig. 94.1). The eruption involves the face, trunk and extremities. There is an obvious photosensitive distribution of the rash with relative sparing of the skin unexposed to sun. The rash comprises confluent plaques which are oedematous and indurated in places. There are scattered papules between the plaques and a few tiny vesicles, some of which are haemorrhagic. There is a little scaling and no excoriations. The buccal mucosa and the nails appear normal.

> **BOX 94.1**
>
> **Sudden widespread red, scaly rashes**
>
> - Eczema
> - Psoriasis
> - Pityriasis rosea
> - Lichen planus
> - Drug eruption
> - Fungal infection

Has examination narrowed down your differential diagnosis?

Yes. We can now exclude most of the conditions in Box 94.1, but we have also to explain the photosensitive distribution. Psoriasis and eczema seem non-starters. Other than her known nickel sensitivity, the patient has no history of

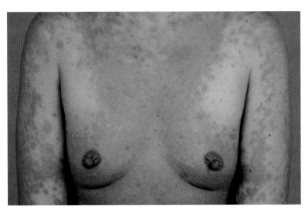

Figure 94.1 A widespread erythematous rash.

either condition in the past. The appearance of the rash, with minimal scaling, absent scalp involvement and nail changes, rules out psoriasis. Burning rather than itch, together with a paucity of vesicles and absence of weeping or crusting, does not point to a diagnosis of eczema.

There is a violet hue to the rash and acute lichen planus should be considered. This seems unlikely, however, because there is no involvement of the buccal mucosa and the classic flat shiny papules (showing Wickham's striae and the Köbner effect) are not seen. It is not pityriasis rosea. There was no 'herald plaque' preceding the generalised eruption and the typical small, oval, pink plaques with collarette scaling are not evident. The rash is too symmetrical for a fungal infection and there are no signs of peripheral scaling, vesicles or pustules at an advancing edge of the large plaques. A drug eruption is the only other common cause left in Box 94.1 and this must be a distinct possibility.

The photosensitive distribution would fit in with a reaction to a photosensitising drug, although there are some dermatoses that are initiated or exacerbated by exposure to ultraviolet radiation. These include lupus erythematosus and even photosensitive variants of psoriasis and atopic eczema. The patient is too well generally to have systemic lupus erythematosus (SLE) and there are no other systemic features of this condition, such as joint, kidney or haematological disorders. But some further investigations would exclude the possibility of this and of subacute cutaneous lupus erythematosus. The rash is not scaly enough, and is too widespread and too acute for chronic discoid erythematosus.

A phototoxic drug eruption now seems to be the most obvious diagnosis. Further enquiry about the precise use of systemic antibiotics reveals that the patient had taken oral minocycline for her acne for 2 weeks preceding the onset of skin problems.

Investigations

Urine examination reveals no proteinuria. A full blood count and erythrocyte sedimentation rate (ESR) are normal. The antinuclear antibody (ANA) test is negative and no antibodies to Ro (SSA) and La (SSB) antigens are detected.

Systemic drugs inducing photosensitivity

Phototoxic

- Amiodarone
- Retinoids
- Non-steroidal anti-inflammatory drugs (NSAIDs)
- Diuretics (chlorothiazides)
- Phenothiazines

Photoallergic

- Thiazides
- Enalapril
- NSAIDs
- Hydroxychloroquine
- Phenothiazines

Has the diagnosis been clinched?

All forms of lupus erythematosus are excluded and a confident diagnosis of minocycline-induced phototoxic rash can be made.

Photosensitivity-induced drug eruptions come in two forms. Certain compounds, when given systemically, may induce subsequent photoallergic reactions. Others are known to be phototoxic, without immunological mechanisms (Box 94.2).

How will you treat this patient?

Oral minocycline should be stopped immediately and prohibited for the rest of her life. The rash may be treated symptomatically with topical glucocorticoids of moderate strength, applied once daily in the evening. Avoidance of sun exposure is advised and a broad (ultraviolet UVA and UVB) sunscreen also prescribed. Acne therapy could be adjusted by advising the use of an androgen-inhibiting oral contraceptive (e.g. Dianette) in combination with a topical vitamin A derivative, applied once daily in the morning.

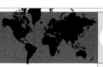

Key points and global issues

More on widespread scaly rashes and drug eruptions?

See Chapter 27 of
Davidson's Principles & **Practice** of
Medicine (21st edn)

- The incidence of drug eruptions may vary, depending on regional patterns of drug use.

- Photosensitive drug reactions are more common in the tropics and subtropics than in temperate climates.

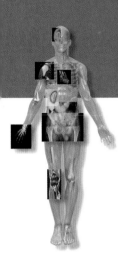

95

Palpable purpura

O. M. SCHOFIELD

Presenting problem

A 65-year-old woman who has a long history of psoriasis and psoriatic arthritis presents with a 4-day history of a rash on her lower limbs, lethargy and fever. The rash is quite different to her psoriasis. Rather than being red and scaly, it is purplish and in some areas, almost black. She says that these lesions started off as small papules, some of which blistered. The affected area has extended and now there are large purplish lesions which are beginning to 'break down'. Besides psoriasis, this woman has a history of hypertension and type 2 diabetes mellitus. She has had bilateral knee replacements in the past. Her current medication includes diclofenac, aspirin, omeprazole, metformin, lisinopril, amlodipine and tramadol. She is being treated with weekly oral methotrexate for her psoriasis, and she has been treated with myocrisin and etanercept unsuccessfully for her psoriatic arthritis in the past.

What would your differential diagnosis include before examining the patient?

The differential diagnosis of a purple-coloured skin eruption would include purpura and vasculitis. Purpura does not blanch on pressure and can be traumatic in origin, related to a low platelet count or abnormal clotting, or secondary to a Gram-negative coccal septicaemia. Clinically, vasculitis is characterised by palpable purpura and can be due to a wide variety of causes: in particular, a drug eruption, infections, connective tissue disease or an underlying malignancy (Box 95.1).

> **BOX 95.1**
>
> **Causes of vasculitis**
>
> - Drugs
> - Infection
> - Connective tissue disease
> - Malignancy
> - Idiopathic (Henoch–Schönlein purpura)

Examination

The woman is pale, apyrexial and in some pain from her rash. She has significant signs of chronic arthritis with ulnar deviation of her fingers and reduced grip strength. She has reduced range of movement of several large joints but no evidence of active synovitis of any joints. General examination shows no features to cause concern: in particular, no breast lumps or lymphadenopathy. She has evidence of ongoing chronic plaque psoriasis on her back, extensor surfaces and scalp. She has nail changes of pitting and onycholysis consistent with this condition. On her legs, she has an eruption that consists of individual scattered lesions, which are palpable and purpuric, ranging from a few millimetres to 5 cm in size.

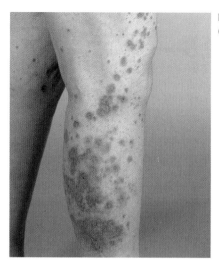

Figure 95.1 The rash of cutaneous vasculitis (palpable purpura).

Some of the lesions have vesicles within them and larger areas are beginning to show necrosis of the superficial portion of skin (the epidermis) (Fig. 95.1).

Has examination narrowed down your differential diagnosis?

This woman has a florid vasculitis evident in the skin of her legs. Her medication has not changed recently and so it is unlikely that a drug is causative. Further investigations are needed to determine the cause of the patient's vasculitis.

Further investigations

Initially and most importantly, urinalysis is performed to look for haematuria, which might indicate renal involvement. A full 'vasculitis screen' is performed, including a full blood count, erythrocyte sedimentation rate (ESR) and C-reactive protein (CRP), urea and electrolytes, liver function tests, serum immunoglobulins, antinuclear factor and anti-double-stranded DNA antibody, rheumatoid factor, antineutrophil cytoplasmic antibodies (ANCA), viral and hepatitis serology, cryoglobulins, a throat swab and chest X-ray. The results of her investigations are shown in Box 95.2. A skin biopsy is taken from one of the lesions on her leg and confirms the diagnosis of a small-vessel vasculitis with leucocytoclasis. A section of the biopsy is sent for immunofluorescence examination and shows deposition of immunoglobulin (Ig) A, IgM and C3 within small vessels.

Does this narrow down your differential diagnosis?

The histology confirms the diagnosis of vasculitis. This is a leucocytoclastic vasculitis, with the presence of large numbers of neutrophils. Taken together with the direct immunofluorescence results and elevated serum IgA, this is typical of the idiopathic form of vasculitis, Henoch–Schönlein purpura. This condition can be seen at all ages and has no clear precipitating cause. It can occur as one attack or become more chronic with repeated attacks. As with all causes of vasculitis, it can affect several organs.

How will you treat this patient?

In view of the severity of this patient's rash and the localised areas of ulceration, she is treated with oral prednisolone starting at a dose of 40 mg daily. The effect of prednisolone on her diabetes makes it likely that she will need insulin temporarily. Topically, she has a very potent topical corticosteroid (clobetasol propionate 0.05%) applied 12-hourly to the lesions on her legs and a topical antibacterial cream (silver sulfadiazine 1% cream) under a Jelonet dressing applied to any ulcerated areas. For her psoriasis she just has simple emollients applied. As the rash improves, her treatment with oral steroids is slowly reduced. In the case of severe recurrent attacks, treatment with an alternative form of immunosuppressant, such as azathioprine, should be considered. The systemic steroids are phased out over several months to avoid a significant flare-up of her psoriasis.

BOX 95.2

Further investigations

Urinalysis	Negative for blood and protein
Haemoglobin	102 g/L (10.2 g/dL)
ESR	99 mm/h
CRP	154 mg/L
ANF	1:40
Anti-dsDNA	Negative
ANCA	Negative
RF	Negative
Cryoglobulins	Negative
Serum immunoglobulins	IgG normal, IgM normal, IgA elevated
Hepatitis serology	Negative
Viral serology	Negative
Chest X-ray	Mild cardiomegaly, lung fields clear

Key points and global issues

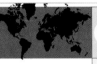 More on vasculitic rash?

See Chapter 27 of
**Davidson's Principles
& Practice** of
Medicine (21st edn)

- About half of all cases of leucocytoclastic vasculitis are idiopathic.

- The most common cause of vasculitis globally is likely to be post-infectious; appropriate screening investigations are required for local concerns and risks.

- Around 1% of cases are due to underlying malignancy which, if suspected, should be investigated by appropriate directed tests.

- Besides the skin, the most commonly affected organs are joints, gastrointestinal tract and kidneys.

- Renal involvement is the most serious complication of vasculitis; involvement of the kidneys should be carefully monitored and investigated early if suspected.

- Although leucocytoclastic vasculitis is more common in a younger age group, there is a significant incidence in older people. In the elderly, there is a significant risk of gastrointestinal involvement in Henoch–Schönlein purpura.

96

Dermatomyositis

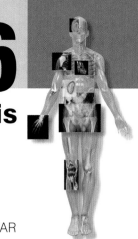

T. AZHAR

Presenting problem

A 47-year-old woman presents with a history of progressive lethargy associated with an erythematous rash, involving the face and hands. The rash developed about 8 months ago and was associated with painless swelling of the finger joints. She has since become progressively lethargic, with generalised muscle weakness over the last few months. There is no history of photosensitivity or oral ulcers. There is a history of diffuse thinning of hair with loss of appetite and weight.

What would your differential diagnosis include before examining the patient?

Some form of connective tissue disorder seems very likely, particularly systemic lupus erythematosus (SLE). The facial rash, joint swelling and hair thinning are common features of SLE. The age of onset is a little older than usual, since SLE commonly presents in the 2nd or 3rd decade.

Examination and initial investigations

On examination, the patient is found to be pale, cachectic and afebrile. There is no jaundice or clubbing. Cervical and axillary lymph nodes are not palpable. In the inguinal region, some shotty nodes are palpable. Macular erythematous lesions are noted over the malar region with sparing of the upper eyelid and the nasolabial folds, and there is just a hint of infraorbital oedema. There are streaks of erythema overlying the extensor tendons on the backs of the hands and dusky erythema of the proximal nail folds. Tortuous capillaries in the proximal nail folds and flat-topped papules on the digits are especially striking (Fig. 96.1, from another patient). The scalp shows diffuse non-scarring alopecia. There are no oral ulcers. Neck examination reveals a 1 cm non-tender, solitary right thyroid nodule. There are no palpable breast lumps. There is hepatomegaly of 5 cm below the right subcostal margin, which is firm in consistency with a nodular surface. The spleen is not palpable and there are no other masses palpable in the abdomen. Respiratory and cardiovascular examination is unremarkable. Blood pressure is 130/80 mmHg and pulse is 80/min. Results of initial investigations are provided in Box 96.1.

Initial investigations

Haemoglobin	93 g/L (9.3 g/dL)
WCC	7.3×10^9/L (10^3/mm³)
Platelets	340×10^9/L (10^3/mm³)
ESR	52 mm/1st hour
Blood smear	Normochromic, normocytic anaemia with anisopoikilocytosis; no target cells, sickling, nucleated red blood cells or Howell–Jolly bodies
Blood urea, sodium, potassium, serum creatinine	All normal
Bilirubin	4.3 μmol/L (0.26 mg/dL)
Albumin	32 g/L (3.2 g/dL)
ALT	26 U/L
AST	96 U/L
Alkaline phosphatase	181 U/L
CRP	6.7 mg/L (normal <6)
Creatine kinase	96 U/L (normal 24–195)
Rheumatoid factor, antinuclear antibody, HBsAg, Anti-HCV antibody, HIV antibody	All negative

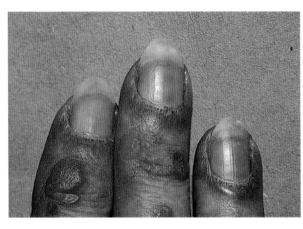

Figure 96.1 The erythema, dilated and tortuous nail capillaries in the proximal nail folds, and the flat-topped (Gottron's) papules on the digits are important diagnostic features of dermatomyositis.

Have examination and initial investigations narrowed down your differential diagnosis?

Considering the muscle weakness and skin signs, dermatomyositis with an underlying malignancy is top of the list. The enlarged firm nodular liver is compatible with a multicentric primary hepatocellular carcinoma or secondaries from elsewhere. SLE can cause hepatomegaly but not nodularity. The right thyroid nodule needs to be investigated. Small differentiated thyroid malignancies (follicular and papillary) do not normally metastasise early and tend to constitute a locoregional disease in the early stages. This may not be true of tumours with an anaplastic histology where haematogenous dissemination can occur early. The patient is a little young to develop an anaplastic carcinoma of the thyroid.

Initial investigations show a mild normocytic normochromic anaemia, associated with a moderately elevated erythrocyte sedimentation rate (ESR), but these

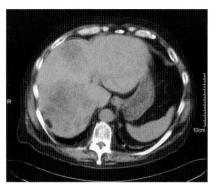

Figure 96.2 CT showing multiple lesions in the liver compatible with metastatic deposits.

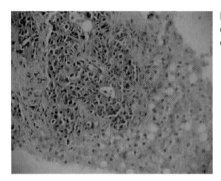

Figure 96.3 Histopathological examination of one of the masses in the liver shows malignant cells arranged in a glandular formation.

are non-specific findings. The creatine kinase level is not raised; this is unusual in dermatomyositis but can occasionally happen when the brunt of the reaction involves skin rather than muscles. Underlying malignancy is now high on the differential diagnosis list and the obviously enlarged nodular liver needs to be investigated.

Further investigations

Computed tomography (CT) of the abdomen reveals multiple heterogeneous lesions scattered in both lobes of the liver and ranging from 1 to 5 cm in diameter. The main portal vein is intact. There is partial compression of the inferior vena cava. The spleen, pancreas, kidneys and uterus are normal. There is no para-aortic lymphadenopathy. The bowels are normal and no ascites is detectable.

An ultrasound-guided liver biopsy is carried out. Histopathological examination of the biopsy specimen reveals malignant cells arranged in sheets with some glandular formation (Figs 96.2, 96.3). The stain for mucin is positive.

Imaging studies of potential primary sites are undertaken. An ultrasound scan of the thyroid shows that the nodular lesion is primarily cystic; an ultrasound-guided fine-needle aspiration reveals no cytological features of malignancy. An ultrasound of the breast is normal. Transvaginal ultrasound shows normal uterus and ovaries and no adnexal masses. Upper gastrointestinal endoscopy shows mild pan-gastritis, with no ulcers or masses. A colonoscopy and a barium enema are entirely normal. A CT of the neck and thorax is entirely normal, except for the previously documented right thyroid nodule. Results of serum tumour markers are provided in Box 96.2.

BOX 96.2	
Serum tumour markers	
α-Fetoprotein	9.15 µg/L (ng/mL) (normal <15)
CA125	13 kU/L (U/mL) (normal <35)
CEA	5176 µg/L ng/mL) (normal <5)

Does this narrow down your differential diagnosis?

Yes. The presenting symptoms of a facial/hand rash and joint swelling associated with muscle weakness can be attributed to a paraneoplastic dermatomyositis syndrome.

Dermatomyositis appearing after the age of 40 should always make a physician suspicious of underlying malignancy. Different series report different risks but the increased risk in this patient is not less than three-fold. The biopsy findings are suggestive of an underlying mucin-secreting adenocarcinoma. Primary liver tumours (hepatocellular carcinoma) are not mucin-secreting. These must be metastatic deposits from another primary site such as the lung, the breast or the gut. Further imaging and endoscopic investigations did not reveal any obvious primary site. The very high levels of carcinoembryonic antigen (CEA) are compatible with a tumour arising from the gut, although breast and lung tumours can also lead to high CEA levels.

How will you treat this patient?

A two-pronged approach should be taken. First of all, systemic corticosteroid treatment should help the woman's myositis and make her feel generally much better and less lethargic. Occasionally, if progress is slow, prednisolone needs to be supplemented with an immunosuppressive agent.

Second, consideration needs to be given to the treatment of the metastatic adenocarcinoma of unknown origin. This is a difficult situation and the evidence base for management is poor. Clearly, there is a distinction between patients with an unknown primary who have been insufficiently investigated and those in whom exhaustive investigation has been unhelpful. In most instances, this represents the end stage of the natural history of the malignancy. If an individual has a good performance status, then chemotherapy can be considered. The choice of regimen may be determined by the pattern of disease. Thus, for example, isolated peritoneal disease in a woman should generally be managed as ovarian cancer; isolated axillary lymph nodes in a woman should be managed as breast cancer; and isolated malignant pleural effusion should be managed as primary lung cancer (although mesothelioma needs to be excluded).

In this case, the elevated CEA is consistent with, but by no means diagnostic of, a gastrointestinal primary. The main aim of management is palliation, along with the provision of both physical and emotional support for the woman and her family. This being so, a few cycles of 5-fluorouracil (5-FU), or its orally-administered precursor capecitabine, could be recommended and with this, a significant clinical response may be seen. The treatment itself is generally well tolerated. Some oncologists favour a more aggressive regimen of either oxaliplatin and 5-FU or cisplatin and gemcitabine, but this is clearly associated with a higher side-effect profile.

Key points and global issues

More on dermato-myositis?

See Chapters 11 and 25 of **Davidson's Principles** & **Practice** of **Medicine (21st edn)**

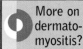

- Adenocarcinoma of unknown primary is not infrequent in oncology practice.

- Common presenting sites are the head and neck region, and the regional nodes; rarely, the skin may be involved.

- In the majority of cases, the primary is never established, even at postmortem.

- Careful pathological analysis is a vital part of the investigation of these patients. Immunocytochemical profiling (including CK7, CK20, TTF1 and CEA) is available in many centres and may help to indicate a likely site of origin.

- No fewer than 30% of adults with dermatomyositis have an underlying malignancy. Hunt for this in the middle-aged and elderly, but not in juvenile cases.

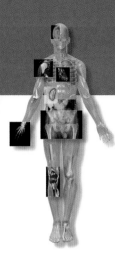

97

A non-healing leg ulcer

M. J. TIDMAN

Presenting problem

A 73-year-old man presents with an uncomfortable enlarging ulcer over his left calf of 6 weeks' duration. He is known to have type 2 diabetes mellitus, controlled with dietary measures, and after complaining to his GP of being tired, he has recently been found to have anaemia (Box 97.1).

What would your differential diagnosis include before examining the patient?

The most common cause of leg ulceration in the UK is venous hypertension, but varicose/venous ulcers typically occur over the malleolar regions. An arterial (ischaemic) ulcer is a possibility, for which this man's diabetes would be a risk factor, as it is for neuropathic ulcers. However, these are usually painless and situated over pressure points. Necrobiosis lipoidica, a cutaneous manifestation of diabetes that usually involves the shins, may ulcerate. Cutaneous malignancy, particularly basal cell and squamous cell carcinomas, should always be considered in chronic leg ulceration, especially if there is background actinic damage. Remember that, very occasionally, chronic venous ulcers may undergo malignant change to a squamous cell carcinoma ('Marjolin ulcer').

BOX 97.1	
Initial investigations	
Haemoglobin	96 g/L (9.6 g/dL)
MCV	101 fL
WCC	3.7×10^9/L (10^3/mm³)
Platelets	86×10^9/L (10^3/mm³)

Leg ulcers may be the result of an underlying vasculitis, either confined to the skin or as part of a systemic condition such as rheumatoid arthritis. Hypertension is said to predispose to painful leg ulceration (Martorell's ulcer), typically situated more proximally than a venous ulcer. Infections of bacterial (including mycobacterial), fungal, parasitic or treponemal aetiology have also to be considered, especially in tropical regions. Pyoderma gangrenosum, a necrotising inflammatory disorder, may also be confined to the legs. Haemoglobinopathies, such as sickle-cell disease and spherocytosis, and genetic predisposition, such as prolidase deficiency, would probably have been diagnosed earlier in life, and thrombophilic disorders, such as antiphospholipid syndrome and platelet aggregability, may need to be excluded. Certain drugs, such as hydroxyurea and methotrexate, may cause leg ulcers. Finally, leg ulcers may

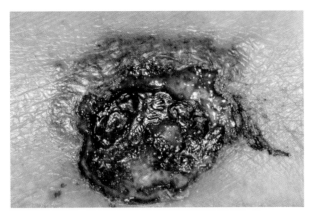

Figure 97.1 Typical clinical presentation of pyoderma gangrenosum, showing an ulcer with an undermined inflamed margin.

be self-inflicted (dermatitis artefacta), but this is usually a diagnosis made by excluding other causes.

Examination

The ulcer measures several centimetres in diameter. The margin is duskily erythematous and somewhat undermined, and the base is covered with a purulent slough (Fig. 97.1). The absence of bolstering of the ulcer edge is reassuring that this is not a malignant ulcer, and there are no signs of venous hypertension (such as pinpoint purpura, pigmentation, atrophie blanche and venular dilatation) or arterial insufficiency (pallor, mottled skin, poor capillary filling and dystrophic nails). The patient's pedal pulses are easily palpable and there are no objective signs of peripheral sensory loss. The absence of palpable purpura elsewhere on his legs militates against a vasculitic aetiology.

Has examination narrowed down your differential diagnosis?

The appearance of the margin suggests that this ulcer is pyoderma gangrenosum. This condition is diagnosed principally on its clinical features; the histology is not specific, although characterised by a neutrophil-abundant inflammatory process. Although the clinical signs may be typical of pyoderma gangrenosum, a biopsy from the ulcer edge is always advisable for definite exclusion of infection, malignancy and vasculitis.

An important aspect of pyoderma gangrenosum is that, in up to 80% of cases, it is associated with an underlying disease, most commonly inflammatory bowel disease, rheumatoid arthritis, plasma cell dyscrasias (monoclonal gammopathy and myeloma) and myeloproliferative disorders (leukaemia and myelofibrosis). When associated with haematological malignancy, pyoderma gangrenosum may present as a haemorrhagic blister.

Further investigations

Histological examination of a skin biopsy from the lesion shows the features of an abscess with haemorrhage, tissue necrosis and vascular thrombosis. Bacterial and fungal culture of a sample of skin reveals no organisms.

The full blood count, as well as showing mild anaemia, also demonstrates low white cell and platelet counts, i.e. a pancytopenia. Vitamin B$_{12}$ and folate levels are within the normal range and a subsequent bone marrow examination shows features consistent with myelofibrosis.

Does this narrow down your differential diagnosis?

The association of a chronic ulcer, characterised by a bluish, undermined margin and a neutrophil-rich histology, and a myeloproliferative disorder, makes the diagnosis of pyoderma gangrenosum very likely. A note of caution, however, is that the absence of an objective diagnostic test means that pyoderma gangrenosum is, perhaps, too freely diagnosed. This clinical scenario is an example of how changes in the skin can, quite frequently, act as a window for the diagnosis of internal disorders.

How will you treat this patient?

The management of pyoderma gangrenosum depends on the extent and degree of inflammation. If there is an underlying medical problem, this will require appropriate treatment. In this particular case of a single lesion, the combination of the daily application of a topical antiseptic, such as potassium permanganate (1 : 10 000 dilution), with the 12-hourly application of a very potent topical corticosteroid, such as clobetasol propionate, under polythene occlusion, is a reasonable initial therapeutic option. However, if this is not quickly effective in settling the inflammation, a tapering course of prednisolone is indicated. Other systemic therapeutic options include minocycline and ciclosporin. Surgical excision is contraindicated, as this may precipitate aggressive recurrence because of the phenomenon of pathergy (hyper-reactivity of the skin) that characterises pyoderma gangrenosum.

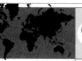

Key points and global issues

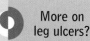

More on leg ulcers?

See Chapter 27 of
Davidson's Principles
& **Practice** of
Medicine (21st edn)

- Yaws, leishmaniasis, leprosy, syphilis, tuberculosis and atypical mycobacterial infections can all cause indolent leg ulcers; although rare in Western Europe, they should be considered in other ethnicities.

- A Buruli ulcer is caused by *Mycobacterium ulcerans* and occurs in rural African areas. It is the third most common mycobacterial infection worldwide after tuberculosis and leprosy. Surgery is the treatment of choice.

- Cutaneous amoebiasis, blastomycosis, cryptococcosis and tropical ulcer may mimic pyoderma gangrenosum.

98

Blistering disorder

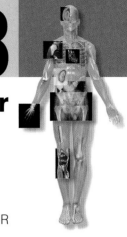

J. A. A. HUNTER

Presenting problem

A 70-year-old white man presents at a skin clinic with numerous, discrete, large, tense blisters on his trunk. These developed over 10 days, appearing within red and irritable patches. The patient does not feel ill. His general health has been good in the past and he is not taking any form of medication.

What would your differential diagnosis include before examining the patient?

Not many conditions need to be considered with such a concise history. The inherited forms of epidermolysis bullosa would have presented early in life. Lack of pain, the large size of the blisters and lack of systemic symptoms rule out widespread herpes simplex and herpes zoster (also excluded, as unilateral blisters are not described). Dermatitis herpetiformis would have declared itself earlier in life; characteristically, its lesions are itchy and vesicular (a few millimetres in diameter) rather than bullous and appear mostly on the elbows, shoulders and buttocks. Toxic epidermal necrolysis is a non-starter; although this may appear initially as widespread blistering, the blisters soon coalesce and the blister roofs peel off, leaving large, painful, moist denuded areas like a scald. It cannot be a bullous drug eruption because the patient is not taking any drugs. Bullous pemphigoid must be at the top of the list of possibilities, but pemphigus, bullous erythema multiforme, acquired epidermolysis bullosa, cicatricial pemphigoid and even bullous impetigo need to be excluded. Examination should help here.

Examination

The patient is apyrexial and remarkably unperturbed by the extensive blisters. The eruption is bullous (blisters >0.5 cm in diameter) rather than vesicular (blisters <0.5 cm in diameter) and predominantly involves the trunk (especially flexures) and limbs (Fig. 98.1). The bullae are tense and filled with clear fluid; many have an erythematous rim and there are discrete urticarial-like plaques with small blisters developing within them. There are scattered erosions at the site of some previous blisters. Shearing stress on normal-looking skin between the blisters does not produce an erosion (negative Nikolsky sign).

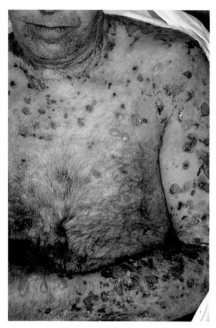

Figure 98.1 Bullous pemphigoid.

There are no blisters in the mouth. Physical examination is otherwise unremarkable.

Has examination narrowed down your differential diagnosis?

The appearance of many skin diseases is diagnostic, providing the whole skin is examined carefully and under optimal conditions. The history and clinical findings here are so typical of bullous pemphigoid that subsequent investigations will only be necessary for confirmation. Patients with pemphigus vulgaris invariably feel ill, the mouth is usually involved, the blisters are flaccid, numerous erosions are seen and the Nikolsky sign may be positive. There are no purple, target-like lesions with an acral distribution to suspect bullous erythema multiforme, and in this condition, the mucous membranes of the mouth, conjunctivae and genitalia are frequently involved. The blisters of porphyria cutanea tarda are induced by minor trauma, occur only on exposed skin and leave milia in their wake. Acquired epidermolysis bullosa can be excluded because there is no history of blisters developing as a result of trauma, and there are no milia at the site of previous blisters. In this condition, the blisters appear on normal skin rather than within urticarial-like plaques. Cicatricial pemphigoid differs from bullous pemphigoid in that its blisters occur mainly on mucous membranes such as the conjunctivae, mouth and genital tract. As the name suggests, these lesions heal with scarring. Bullous impetigo is more common in children but may be seen in the elderly, especially those immunosuppressed. The bullae are flaccid, often contain pus and are frequently grouped or located in body folds.

Has the diagnosis been clinched?

The clinical picture is all but diagnostic, but histology of a small fresh blister with immunofluorescence will confirm it.

Further investigations

Histology reveals a subepidermal blister filled with eosinophils. Direct immunofluorescence shows a linear band of immunoglobulin (Ig) G and C3 along the basement membrane zone.

Circulating IgG antibodies, reacting with the basement membrane zone of skin, are found in 70% of patients. The test is simple and (stored) serum from the patient, acquired before starting treatment, may easily be sent to a laboratory offering this service. Tzanck smears remain popular in some countries. A blister roof is removed and cells taken from the base of the blister with a surgical blade. These cells are smeared on to a glass slide, fixed with methanol and then stained with Giemsa, toluidine blue or Wright's stain. Distinctive cells are seen in pemphigus (acantholytic cells) and herpes simplex/zoster infections (multinucleate giant cells). A fresh blister swab would reveal no bacterial growth in bullous pemphigoid (compare *Staphylococcus aureus* in bullous impetigo). Immunofluorescent studies on salt-split human skin, to detect more precisely the site of the target antigen, and immunoblotting studies, to determine the molecular weight of the target antigen, are essentially research techniques.

How will you treat this patient?

Systemic corticosteroids (provided there are no contraindications) should be given straight away, without waiting for the results of confirmatory diagnostic tests. In the acute phase, prednisolone at a dosage of 40–60 mg/day should control the eruption, but other immunosuppressive agents may also be required. The patient should be followed-up regularly, with urine and blood screening standard for a patient taking a prolonged course of corticosteroids. The dosage is gradually reduced as soon as fresh blisters stop appearing and, within a month or two, the patient should end up on a low-maintenance regimen (e.g. prednisolone 5–10 mg on alternate days) of systemic corticosteroids, until stopped. Bullous pemphigoid is usually self-limiting and treatment can often be stopped after 1–2 years.

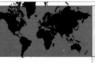

Key points and global issues

More on blistering diseases?

See Chapter 27 of **Davidson's Principles** & **Practice** of **Medicine (21st edn)**

- Bullous pemphigoid is relatively common in the West but uncommon in the East. Pemphigus vulgaris is more common than bullous pemphigoid in India and Pakistan.

- Dermatitis herpetiformis appears to be less common in Asia and the USA, compared with Europe.

- In a case as typical as this, it could be argued that further investigations in a developing country would be an expensive luxury that would simply confirm a very sound clinical diagnosis. However, in developed countries, confirmation would be required with a biopsy of a small recent blister and immunofluorescent investigations.

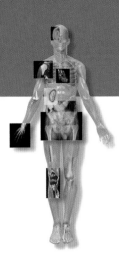

99

Multiple hypopigmented lesions

B. KUMAR

Presenting problem

A 14-year-old Indian boy presents with multiple hypopigmented lesions over the trunk and extremities. Three years ago, he noticed a hypopigmented dry patch over his right forearm. Since then he has noted an increase in the size of this lesion and has developed similar patches over his trunk and limbs. He had not bothered to seek medical attention because the lesions were almost asymptomatic. Over the last 6 months he has developed numbness and weakness of the right hand, which is now interfering with his daily activities. The use of some indigenous medication produced no improvement. There has been no significant medical or dermatological illness in the past and he has no systemic complaints.

What would your differential diagnosis include before examining the patient?

Hypopigmented lesions are a common finding in practice. There are several conditions which can produce them. A careful history regarding the evolution of the lesions and a thorough systematic examination greatly help to limit the differential diagnoses. In this boy, the absence of systemic features, at present or in the past, makes malignant, metabolic and endocrine causes of hypopigmentation most unlikely. Most of the stable lesions are likely to be congenital and progressive lesions are usually inflammatory or immunological.

Causes of hypopigmented patches include pityriasis alba, pityriasis versicolor, post-inflammatory hypopigmentation and leprosy (Box 99.1). Pityriasis alba is especially common in children. A few hypopigmented, minimally scaly patches with ill-defined margins usually appear on the face, but may also involve the trunk and limbs. They take weeks to months to subside. Pityriasis versicolor is a common superficial fungal infection of the skin caused by *Malassezia furfur*. These lesions are seen in young adults with dark skin as multiple small hypopigmented macules with powdery scales, and are generally distributed over the chest and upper back. In those

BOX 99.1
Causes of hypopigmented lesions
Common
• Pityriasis alba
• Pityriasis versicolor
• Post-inflammatory hypopigmentation
• Vitiligo
• Leprosy
Rare
• Sarcoidosis
• Idiopathic guttate hypomelanosis
• Progressive macular hypopigmentation
• Tuberous sclerosis
• Naevus anaemicus
• Naevus depigmentosus
• Hypomelanosis of Ito
• Mycosis fungoides
• Lichen sclerosus

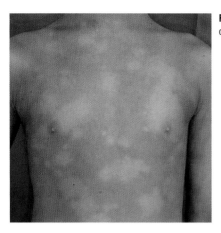

Figure 99.1 Multiple hypopigmented patches over the trunk.

99

with white skin, the initial lesions appear as fawn areas standing out against the light background. The lesions are often asymptomatic but may occasionally be itchy. In the tropics, the patches of hypopigmentation may be large with raised margins, covering large parts of the body. Post-inflammatory hypopigmentation is another common cause of such a presentation. It may follow a variety of inflammatory dermatoses, including psoriasis, pityriasis rosea, adverse cutaneous drug reactions, trauma and contact dermatitis. Vitiligo, also known as leuco-derma, is characterised by milky white or depigmented lesions, sometimes with a hyperpigmented border. However, evolving lesions may sometimes be hypo-pigmented. The sharply defined lesions of the generalised type of vitiligo are especially common on the backs of the hands, the wrists, the fronts of knees and the neck and around body orifices.

Leprosy is undoubtedly the most important cause of hypopigmented lesions and often, for months or even years, this is the only manifestation of the disease before a neurological deficit develops. For those practising in a non-endemic country who are not familiar with this disease, the diagnosis may be missed and subsequent neurological symptoms may be attributed to some other disease. An insidious onset and slow progression of these often asymptomatic or anaesthetic hypopigmented lesions in a patient living in an endemic country, or in an immi-grant from such a part of the world, should raise a high index of suspicion. Further clinical examination of the lesions and peripheral nerves will help to confirm the diagnosis.

Some rarer causes of hypopigmented skin lesions are also listed in Box 99.1.

Examination

The patient is apparently healthy and remarkably unperturbed by the skin lesions, more than 30, distributed over his body. The hypopigmented and slightly indurated lesions are of varying sizes, measuring up to 10 cm (Fig. 99.1). The lesions have sparse hair and, within them, there is partial loss of sensation, including temperature. The boy's right ulnar nerve (above the elbow) is thickened and non-tender, with associated sensory impairment and weak-ness of small muscles of the hand on the ulnar side (ulnar claw hand). His greater auricular nerves, radial cutaneous nerves and left lateral popliteal nerve are also thickened.

Has examination narrowed down your differential diagnosis?

Often in dermatology, there is not always an easy spot diagnosis (as the morphology of many dermatoses is so similar), and astute observation, with correlation of the findings, helps the physician to arrive at the final diagnosis. But the combination of typical skin and neurological signs in this case positively proclaim a diagnosis of leprosy! The diagnosis and classification of leprosy are based on the clinical features and skin smears when facilities are available. The clinical diagnosis of leprosy is based on patients having one or more of the three cardinal signs (Box 99.2).

BOX 99.2

Cardinal signs of leprosy

- Hypopigmented or erythematous skin lesion(s) with definite loss or impairment of sensation
- Involvement of the peripheral nerves, as demonstrated by definite thickening with sensory impairment
- Slit skin smear positive for acid-fast bacilli

Further investigations

A slit skin smear (SSS) was performed and was positive for acid-fast bacilli with a bacteriological index (BI) of 2+ and a morphological index (MI) of 1%. A skin biopsy revealed perivascular, peri-appendageal and perineural lymphocytic infiltrates, granulomas in the dermis and foam cells filled with lepra bacilli. These findings are consistent with a diagnosis of borderline lepromatous (BL) leprosy.

How will you treat this patient?

The treatment of leprosy is based on the type of disease. Patients with paucibacillary leprosy (≤ 5 skin lesions or negative SSS) are treated with the World Health Organization (WHO) recommended multidrug therapy (MDT) paucibacillary (PB) regimen. Patients with multibacillary (MB) leprosy (>5 skin lesions or positive SSS or involvement of two or more nerves) are treated with the WHO MDT multibacillary (MB) regimen. This young man has multibacillary disease and should be treated with the WHO-MDT-MB regimen (Box 99.3). A course of systemic corticosteroids (prednisolone) for 4–6 months will be required for the recent neurological deficit involving the right hand. Physiotherapy, counselling for compliance with the treatment, advice for care of hands and feet, and examination of close household contacts are important components of total treatment.

BOX 99.3

MDT-MB regimen for multibacillary leprosy (12 months) in a child of 10–14 years

Dapsone

- 50 mg given daily

Rifampicin

- 450 mg given once a month under supervision

Clofazimine

- 50 mg given daily *and*
- 150 mg given once a month under supervision

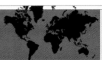

Key points and global issues

 More on leprosy?

- Leprosy is caused by *Mycobacterium leprae*. It is a chronic granulomatous disease with a long incubation period, and primarily affects skin and peripheral nerves.

See Chapter 13 of
Davidson's Principles
& **Practice** of
Medicine (21st edn)

- Leprosy is the most common cause of peripheral nerve thickening and associated neuropathy.

- Leprosy still remains a public health problem in some highly populated countries of the world. Pockets of high endemicity exist in some areas of Angola, Brazil, the Central African Republic, the Democratic Republic of the Congo, India, Madagascar, Mozambique, Nepal and the United Republic of Tanzania.

- The number of leprosy cases reported to WHO shows that there were 244 796 registered prevalent cases at the beginning of 2010; 211 903 cases were registered in 2009, mainly in the African and South-East Asia regions.

- Slit skin smears are useful for confirming the diagnosis and monitoring response to treatment.

- MDT, recommended by the WHO in 1982, has rapidly become the standard treatment of leprosy. It consists of three drugs: dapsone, rifampicin and clofazimine. PB patients are treated with an MDT-PB (rifampicin + dapsone) regimen for 6 months, and MB patients are treated with an MDT-MB (rifampicin + dapsone + clofazimine) regimen for 12 months.

- In countries where this disease is uncommon, a high index of suspicion is required to diagnose, treat early and prevent the transmission of infection and development of deformities. Biopsy of the lesion is mostly confirmatory.

- With increased migration, leprosy will occur globally until the disease is eradicated.

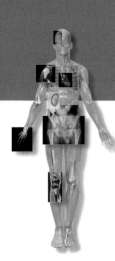

100

Bilateral swollen, red legs

M. J. TIDMAN

Presenting problem

A 64-year-old man with long-standing skin thickening, redness and swelling of both legs, and a history of recurrent bilateral 'cellulitis', necessitating multiple courses of antibiotics, is referred by his GP. An episode of leg ulceration resulted in hospital assessment the previous year. Coincident medical conditions include morbid obesity and osteoarthritis of the knees, causing him to be virtually housebound. He also has type 2 diabetes mellitus, ischaemic heart disease and a sex chromosome mosaicism (46XY/47XXY).

What would your differential diagnosis include before examining the patient?

Venous hypertension is the most common cause of leg ulceration in the UK. Chronic elevation of venous blood pressure predisposes to pedal oedema and dermatitis ('venous', 'varicose', 'stasis' or 'gravitational' eczema) within the gaiter regions (the lower third of the legs), as well as atrophie blanche and punctate purpura. It may also ultimately cause *lipodermatosclerosis*, a panniculitis consisting of inflammatory change (which may be mistaken for cellulitis) and sclerosis within the subcutaneous fat, eventually resulting in firm, bound-down skin giving an 'inverted champagne bottle' appearance to the legs.

Bilateral (in contrast to unilateral) cellulitis of the legs, while not impossible, is highly unusual in clinical practice, although not if judged by the frequency with which this putative diagnosis is suggested (the bacteria that cause cellulitis are not noted for their sense of symmetry).

Chronic lymphoedema of the legs may cause the skin to become erythematous, thickened and deeply folded, often with a 'cobblestone' texture and secondary epidermal changes such as warty hyperkeratosis, superficial erosions and retained scale.

Simple excess of adipose tissue (*lipoedema*) can sometimes masquerade as lymphoedema, and the distinguishing clue is that in lipoedematous legs, the feet are relatively normal, whereas in lymphoedematous legs, the feet are almost always swollen.

Of interest in this particular case is that some patients with Klinefelter's syndrome have an increased thrombotic tendency with subsequent development of post-thrombotic changes and venous ulcers.

Examination

He is apyrexial. He has tense, thickened, erythematous skin circumferentially involving the legs almost to knee level, with marked pitting oedema

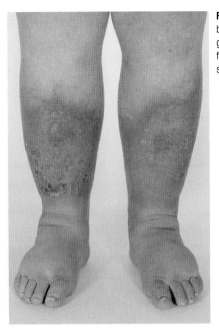

Figure 100.1 Anterior view of legs showing bilateral, swollen, erythematous, deeply-grooved skin, also involving the dorsa of the feet and toes: impetiginisation and adherent scale are evident on the shins.

(Fig. 100.1). There are areas of impetiginisation (golden crusts indicative of *Staphylococcus aureus* infection), particularly on the right, and a significant degree of adherent scale. Both feet are swollen, and a number of his toe webs are macerated. His pedal pulses are impalpable. There is no inguinal lymphadenopathy and no lymphangitis. There are no clinical signs of cardiac failure. His BMI is 58 kg/m^2, and he has great difficulty undertaking even minimal physical activity because of pain in his knees.

Has examination narrowed down your differential diagnosis?

The cutaneous changes are those of chronic lymphoedema, the result of inadequate lymphatic drainage. There are often a number of factors contributing to chronic lymphoedema, and in this particular case general immobility, and consequent absence of an effective muscle pump, is likely to be important. There may have been an underlying tendency to venous hypertension, although the clinical features suggest that this is not the primary problem. The presence of ischaemic heart disease raises the possibility of cardiac or renal elements, and hypoalbuminaemia should be excluded. A primary deficiency of lymphatic drainage should be considered, as should an obstructive cause in the pelvis or abdomen. The absence of foreign travel in this case effectively excludes parasitic (filariasis) or infective (deep mycosis) aetiology. Occasionally, the classical form of Kaposi's sarcoma may present as lymphoedema and, exceptionally, pretibial myxoedema may mimic chronic lymphoedema.

Initial investigations

His inflammatory markers (ESR and CRP), differential white cell count and routine renal and hepatic biochemistry are unremarkable, and his chest X-ray and pelvic ultrasound are normal. A swab from the skin on his right leg grows *Staphylococcus aureus*. Doppler measurement of his pedal blood pressures confirms satisfactory arterial perfusion.

Does this narrow down your differential diagnosis?

Staphylococcus aureus is a common coloniser in this setting. Examination and the investigations exclude cellulitis. Obstruction in the pelvis has been excluded as a cause of the lymphoedema, which is most likely due to his immobility and obesity.

How will you treat this patient?

Undoubtedly, in this particular instance, measures to improve mobility and reduce weight are the aspects of management most likely to be helpful in the long term. Unfortunately, chronic lymphoedema secondary to mechanical factors such as poor mobility tends to be resistant to diuretic therapy. Drawing an analogy between waterlogged skin and a wet sponge helps to illustrate that squeezing the skin dry by means of compression bandaging or customised graduated compression hosiery, supplemented by elevation of the legs when possible (ankles above pelvis), is much more likely than diuretics to be of benefit. However, establishing that there is no danger of compromising the arterial supply to the feet (Doppler blood pressure measurement) must precede such measures.

Waterlogged skin is prone to infection (particularly cellulitis) and possible ulceration. Regular immersion of lymphoedematous skin in an antiseptic, such as potassium permanganate (1 : 10 000) solution or a benzalkonium chloride-containing emollient, is more likely to cleanse the skin of potentially invasive bacteria than systemically administered antibiotics. However, bacteria may gain entry into the skin through macerated or fissured toe webs, and scrupulous attention to toe-web hygiene will close this portal for infection.

Removal of the adherent scale by gentle but firm rubbing with arachis oil or olive oil may also help to reduce the risk of bacterial infection, and the regular application of an emollient will help to maintain the integrity and suppleness of the epidermis.

Key points and global issues

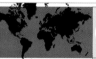

More on swollen, red legs?

See Chapter 27 of
Davidson's Principles
& **Practice** of
Medicine (21st edn)

- Worldwide, the commonest causes of lymphoedema are conditions endemic to the tropics, particularly filariasis, although the aetiology of lymphoedema in the tropics is often obscure.

- Bilateral swollen red legs are usually *not* due to cellulitis, especially in the absence of pyrexia, regional lymphadenopathy, lymphangitis and a neutrophilia, although episodes of superimposed cellulitis will exacerbate chronic lymphoedema.

- Chronic lymphoedema may be due to more than one factor, and careful clinical examination and investigation are necessary to elucidate the underlying cause.

- Consideration of compression therapy for chronic lymphoedema necessitates the demonstration of adequate arterial perfusion.

Appendix

S. W. WALKER

Biochemical and haematological values

A.1

Urea and electrolytes in venous serum

Analyte	Reference range	
	SI units	**Non-SI units**
Sodium	135–145 mmol/L	135–145 mEq/L
Potassium	3.6–5.0 mmol/L	3.6–5.0 mEq/L
Chloride	95–107 mmol/L	95–107 mEq/L
Urea	2.5–6.6 mmol/L	15–40 mg/dL
Creatinine	60–120 μmol/L	0.68–1.36 mg/dL

A.2

Arterial blood analysis

Analyte	Reference range	
	SI units	**Non-SI units**
Bicarbonate	21–29 mmol/L	21–29 mEq/L
Hydrogen ion	37–45 nmol/L	pH 7.35–7.43
$PaCO_2$	4.5–6.0 kPa	34–45 mmHg
PaO_2	12–15 kPa	90–113 mmHg
Oxygen saturation	>97%	

A.3

Hormones in venous blood

Hormone	Reference range	
	SI units	Non-SI units
Adrenocorticotropic hormone (ACTH) (plasma)	1.5–11.2 pmol/L (0700–1000 h)	7–51 pg/dL
Aldosterone		
Supine (at least 30 min)	30–440 pmol/L	1.08–15.9 ng/dL
Erect	110–860 pmol/L	3.97–31.0 ng/dL
Cortisol	Dynamic tests are required	
Follicle-stimulating hormone (FSH)		
Male	1.0–10.0 U/L	1.0–10.0 mU/dL
Female	3.0–10 U/L (early follicular; days 1–5)	3.0–10 mU/dL
	>30 U/L (postmenopausal)	>30 mU/dL
Gastrin (plasma, fasting)	<120 ng/L	<120 pg/dL
Growth hormone (GH)	A single GH measurement is of limited value. Suppression/ stimulation tests are essential	
Insulin	Highly variable and interpretable only in relation to plasma glucose and body habitus	
Luteinising hormone (LH)		
Male	1.0–9.0 U/L	–
Female	2.5–9.0 U/L (early follicular, luteal)	–
	>20 U/L (postmenopausal)	–
17β-Oestradiol		
Male	<160 pmol/L	<43 pg/dL
Female	75–140 pmol/L (early follicular)	20–39 pg/dL
	<150 pmol/L (postmenopausal)	<41 pg/dL
Parathyroid hormone (PTH)	1.1–6.8 pmol/L	10–65 pg/dL
Progesterone (female)	Only of use in assessing fertility in normally menstruating women. Collect at days 18–24 of 28-day cycle, or 7–10 days before next expected menses. Repeat in 3 cycles if needed, to allow for variation between cycles	
Prolactin (PRL)	60–500 mU/L	–
Renin activity		
Supine (at least 30 m)	0.5–2.6 ng/dL/h	–
Erect	1.0–4.2 ng/dL/h	–
Testosterone		
Male	10–30 nmol/L	2.88–8.64 ng/dL
Female	0.4–3.0 nmol/L	0.12–0.87 ng/dL
Thyroid-stimulating hormone (TSH)	0.2–4.5 mU/L	–
Thyroxine (free) (free T$_4$) (Male, non-pregnant female)	9–21 pmol/L	700–1634 pg/dL
Triiodothyronine (T$_3$) (Total)	0.9–2.4 nmol/L	59–156 ng/dL

Notes

1. A number of hormones are unstable and collection details are critical to obtaining a meaningful result. Refer to local laboratory handbook.

2. Values in the table are only a guideline; hormone levels can often only be meaningfully understood in relation to factors such as sex (e.g. testosterone), age (e.g. FSH in women), time of day (e.g. cortisol) or regulatory factors (e.g. insulin and glucose, PTH and [Ca^{2+}]).

3. Reference ranges may be critically method-dependent.

A.4

Other common analytes in venous blood in adults

Analyte	Reference range	
	SI units	Non-SI units
α_1-Antitrypsin	1.1–2.1 g/L	110–210 mg/dL
Alanine amino-transferase (ALT)	10–50 U/L	–
Albumin	35–50 g/L	3.5–5.0 g/dL
Alkaline phosphatase	40–125 U/L	–
Amylase	<100 U/L	–
Aspartate amino-transferase (AST)	10–45 U/L	–
Bilirubin (total)	3–16 µmol/L	0.18–0.94 mg/dL
Calcium (total)	2.1–2.6 mmol/L	8.4–10.4 mg/dL
Carboxy-haemoglobin	0.1–3.0% total Hb	–
Caeruloplasmin	0.2–0.6 g/L	20–60 mg/dL
Cholesterol (total)	Ideal level varies according to cardiovascular risk (see cardiovascular risk chart, p. 359) so reference ranges can be misleading. The following values were described by the European Atherosclerosis Society: Mild increase 5.2–6.5 mmol/L 200–250 mg/dL Moderate increase 250–300 mg/dL 6.5–7.8 mmol/L Severe increase >7.8 mmol/L >300 mg/dL	
HDL-cholesterol	Ideal level varies according to cardiovascular risk so reference ranges can be misleading. According to the National Cholesterol Education Programme Adult Treatment Panel III (ATPIII), a low HDL-cholesterol is: <1.0 mmol/L <40 mg/dL	
Copper	10–22 µmol/L	64–140 µg/dL
C-reactive protein	<5 mg/L Highly sensitive CRP assays also exist which measure lower values and may be useful in estimating cardiovascular risk	
Creatine kinase (total)		
Male	55–170 U/L	–
Female	30–135 U/L	–
Creatine kinase MB isoenzyme	<6% of total CK	–
γ-Glutamyl transferase (GGT)		
Male	5–55 U/L	–
Female	5–35 U/L	–
Glucose (fasting)	3.6–5.8 mmol/L	65–104 mg/dL
Glycated haemoglobin (HbA$_{1c}$)	5.0–6.5% 20–42 mmol/mol Hb	–
Immunoglobulin A	0.8–4.5 g/L	80–450 mg/dL
Immunoglobulin G	6.0–15.0 g/L	600–1500 mg/dL
Immunoglobulin M	0.35–2.90 g/L	35–290 mg/dL
Lactate	0.6–2.4 mmol/L	5.40–21.6 mg/dL

Continued

A.4

Other common analytes in venous blood in adults—cont'd

Analyte	Reference range	
	SI units	Non-SI units
Lactate dehydrogenase (total)	208–460 U/L	–
Lead	<0.5 μmol/L	<10.4 μg/dL
Magnesium	0.7–1.0 mmol/L	1.4–2.0 mEq/L
Osmolality	280–296 mmol/kg	–
Osmolarity	280–296 mosm/L	–
Phosphate (fasting)	0.8–1.4 mmol/L	2.48–4.34 mg/dL
Protein (total)	60–80 g/L	6–8 g/dL
Triglycerides (fasting)	0.6–1.7 mmol/L	53–150 mg/dL
Troponins	Values consistent with 'myocyte necrosis' or myocardial infarction are crucially dependent upon which troponin is measured (I or T) and on the method employed	
Urate		
Male	0.12–0.42 mmol/L	2.0–7.0 mg/dL
Female	0.12–0.36 mmol/L	2.0–6.0 mg/dL
Vitamin D		
25(OH)D	25–170 nmol/L	10–68 ng/dL
1,25(OH)2D	20–120 pmol/L	7.7–46 pg/dL
Zinc	11–22 μmol/L	72–144 μg/dL

A.5

Haematological values

Analyte	Reference range	
	SI units	Non-SI units
Bleeding time (Ivy)	<8 min	–
Blood volume		
Male	75±10 mL/kg	–
Female	70±10 mL/kg	–
Coagulation screen		
Prothrombin time	10.5–13.5 s	–
Activated partial thromboplastin time	26–36 s	–
D-dimer		
Routine (for DVT assessment)	Threshold 500 ng/dL	–
DIC	<200 ng/dL	–
Erythrocyte sedimentation rate	Higher values in older patients are not necessarily abnormal	
Adult male	0–10 mm/h	–
Adult female	3–15 mm/h	–

A.5

Haematological values—cont'd

Analyte	Reference range	
	SI units	Non-SI units
Ferritin		
Male	20–300 µg/L	–
Pre-menopausal female	14–150 µg/L	–
Fibrinogen	1.5–4.0 g/L	0.15–0.4 g/dL
Folate		
Serum	5.0–20 µg/L	–
Red cell	257–800 µg/L	–
Haemoglobin		
Male	130–180 g/L	13–18 g/dL
Female	115–165 g/L	11.5–16.5 g/dL
Haptoglobin	0.4–2.4 g/L	0.04–0.24 g/dL
Iron		
Male	14–32 µmol/L	78–178 µg/dL
Female	10–28 µmol/L	56–156 µg/dL
Leucocytes (adults)	$4.0–11.0 \times 10^9$/L	$4.0–11.0 \times 10^3$/mm^3
Differential white cell count		
Neutrophil granulocytes	$2.0–7.5 \times 10^9$/L	$2.0–7.5 \times 10^3$/mm^3
Lymphocytes	$1.5–4.0 \times 10^9$/L	$1.5–4.0 \times 10^3$/mm^3
Monocytes	$0.2–0.8 \times 10^9$/L	$0.2–0.8 \times 10^3$/mm^3
Eosinophil granulocytes	$0.04–0.4 \times 10^9$/L	$0.04–0.4 \times 10^3$/mm^3
Basophil granulocytes	$0.01–0.1 \times 10^9$/L	$0.01–0.1 \times 10^3$/mm^3
Mean corpuscular haemoglobin (MCH)	27–32 pg	–
Mean corpuscular volume (MCV)	78–98 fL	–
Packed cell volume (PCV) or haematocrit		
Male	0.40–0.54	–
Female	0.37–0.47	–
Platelets	$150–350 \times 10^9$/L	$150–350 \times 10^3$/mm^3
Red cell count		
Male	$4.5–6.5 \times 10^{12}$/L	$4.5–6.5 \times 10^6$/mm^3
Female	$3.8–5.8 \times 10^{12}$/L	$3.8–5.8 \times 10^6$/mm^3
Red cell lifespan		
Mean	120 days	–
Half-life (51Cr)	25–35 days	–
Reticulocytes (adults)	$25–85 \times 10^9$/L	$25–85 \times 10^3$/mm^3
Transferrin	2.0–4.0 g/L	0.2–0.4 g/dL
Transferrin saturation		
Male	25–56%	–
Female	14–51%	–
Vitamin B_{12}	251–900 ng/L	–

A.6

Cerebrospinal fluid analysis

Analyte	Reference range	
	SI units	Non-SI units
Cells	$<5 \times 10^6$ cells/L (all mononuclear)	<5 cells/mm^3
Glucose	2.3–4.5 mmol/L	41–81 mg/dL
IgG index[a]	<0.65	–
Total protein	0.14–0.45 g/L	0.014–0.045 g/dL

[a]A crude index of increase in IgG attributable to intrathecal synthesis.

Cardiovascular risk prediction charts

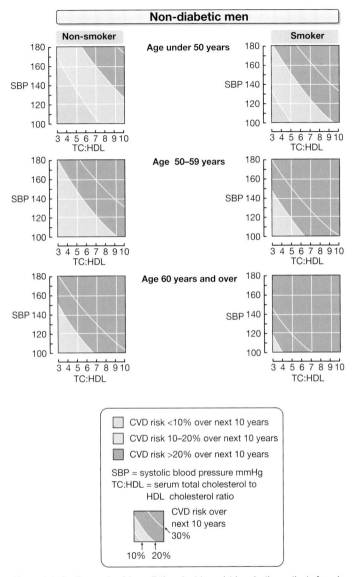

Figure A.1 Cardiovascular risk prediction chart to assist in selecting patients for primary prevention therapy. *Continued on p. 360*

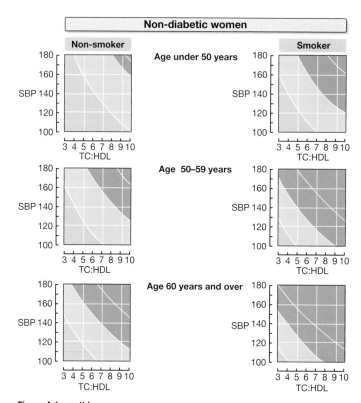

Figure A.1, cont'd

- To estimate an individual's absolute 10-year risk of developing cardiovascular disease (CVD), choose the panel for the gender, smoking status and age. Within this, define the level of risk from the point where the coordinates for SBP and ratio of the total to high-density lipoprotein (HDL)-cholesterol cross. If no HDL-cholesterol result is available, assume it is 1.0 mmol/L and use the lipid scale as total serum cholesterol.
- Highest-risk individuals (red areas) are those whose 10-year CVD risk exceeds 20%, which is approximately equivalent to a 10-year coronary heart disease risk of >15%.
- The chart also assists in identification of individuals with a moderately high 10-year CVD risk – in the range of 10–20% (orange area) and those in whom it is lower than 10% (green area).
- Smoking status should reflect lifetime exposure to tobacco.

Index

Note: Entries in cases have been referenced to the page numbers of each case and not the specific page on which the indexed term appears. References have been given to the more possible or likely differential diagnoses in addition to the correct diagnoses. Numbers in bold indicate the title of each case which is usually (but not always) the major presenting symptom of a case.

fungal infections
hepatosplenomegaly, 248–251
skin, 346–349
fungus ball (aspergilloma), 104–106

galactorrhoea, 157–159
gallstones, 207–209
gastroenteritis, *Salmonella*, 37–40
gastrointestinal tract
dissemination malignancy from, 61–64
magnesium loss relating to, 133–135
potassium loss relating to, 126–128
generalised tonic–clonic disorder, 298–300
geniospasm, hereditary, 308–310
genital herpes, 1–3
genital ulceration, 1–3
giant cell (temporal) arteritis, 283–285, 287–289
Giardia lamblia, 195–198
gingival bleeding, and rash on lower limbs,
256–259
Gitelman's syndrome, 133–135
glatiramer acetate delaying multiple sclerosis
onset after optic neuritis, 301–303
glomerulonephritis
chronic, 147–150
post-streptococcal, 136–138
glomerulosclerosis, focal and segmental, 139–142
glucocorticoid therapy *see* steroid therapy
glucose (blood)
high, newly discovered, 177–180
low, spontaneous low, 174–176
gluten-sensitive enteropathy (coeliac disease),
195–198
goitres, 151–156
gonadotrophin deficiency, 157–159
gonorrhoea, 4–6
gout, 271–273
granuloma, pyogenic, 321–324
granulomatous disorders, hypercalcaemia,
160–162
Graves' disease, 151–153
gum bleeding and rash on lower limbs, 256–259

haemangiomas (skin), acquired, 321–324
haematemesis, 192–194
haematological causes of hepatosplenomegaly,
239–241
haematuria, 136–138
haemophilias, 252–255
haemoptysis
anorexia and weight loss with, 104–106
pleuritic chest pain and, 139–142
haemorrhage *see* bleeding
haemorrhagic fevers, viral, 25–28, 256–259
hair follicle tumour, pigmented, 321–324
Hashimoto's encephalopathy, 311–313
head injury, coma, 293–296

headache
chronic, 287–289
fronto-parietal, with insomnia and
generalised itch, 239–241
orgasmic, 283–285
heart
arrhythmias, 79–82
infective endocarditis complications, 86–89
heart block, 2nd degree, 79–82
heart disease
coronary, 68–74
rheumatic, 90–93
syncope due to, 274–276
valvular, 72–74, 90–93
heart failure
congestive, 72–74
in myocardial infarction, 68–71
helminths and tropical pulmonary eosinophilia,
41–44
HELP syndrome, 207–209
hemiparesis, psychogenic, 315–317
Henoch–Schönlein purpura, 332–334
heparin
deep venous thrombosis, 267–270
pulmonary embolism, 101–103, 280–282
hepatic veins
central occlusion, 214–217
thrombosis, 214–217
hepatitis, acute, 210–213
viral, 25–28, 192–194, 207–213
HAV, 210–213
HCV, 192–194
HEV, 207–209
hepatocellular cancer, 192–194
hepatosplenomegaly, 13–17, 192–194, 239–241,
248–251
hepatotoxicity of antituberculous drugs, 112–115
hereditary geniospasm, 308–310
hereditary motor and sensory demyelinating
neuropathy type 1, 287–289
herpes simplex
blistering, 343–345
genital infection, 1–3
proctitis, 7–9
herpes zoster, 343–345
hip
osteoporosis, 277–279
pain after fall in elderly, 225–228
histoplasmosis, hepatosplenomegaly, 248–251
HIV infection (and AIDS)
adrenal insufficiency, 170–173
fever, 13–17
kala-azar, 245–247
malnutrition, 221–224
testing with risk of, 4–9
tuberculosis and, 13–17, 72–74
see also antiretroviral drugs